DC Dutta's

Clinics in
GYNECOLOGY

Cover Image

FIG: Unruptured tubal ectopic pregnancy, salpingectomy was done. The specimen is cut open to show the embryo of 7 weeks gestation (see discussion Chapter 46)

DC Dutta's
Clinics in GYNECOLOGY

DC Dutta MBBS DGO MO (Cal)
Professor and Head, Department of Obstetrics and Gynecology
Nilratan Sircar Medical College and Hospital, Kolkata, India

Edited by

Hiralal Konar (Hons; Gold Medalist)
MBBS (Cal) MD (PGI) DNB (India)
MNAMS FACS (USA) FRCOG (London)
Professor and Head, Department of Obstetrics and Gynecology, KPC Medical College and Hospital, Kolkata, India
FOGSI Representative to Asia Oceania Federation of Obstetricians and Gynecologists (AOFOG)
Member, Oncology Committee of AOFOG
Chairman, Indian College of Obstetricians and Gynecologists (2013)
Formerly
Professor and Head, Department of Obstetrics and Gynecology
Agartala Govt. Medical College and GB Pant Hospital, Tripura, India
Professor, Department of Obstetrics and Gynecology
Calcutta National Medical College and Hospital, Kolkata

Professor and Head, Department of Obstetrics and Gynecology
Midnapore Medical College and Hospital, West Bengal University of Health Sciences, Kolkata

Rotation Registrar in Obstetrics, Gynecology and Oncology
Northern and Yorkshire Region, Newcastle-upon-Tyne, UK
Examiner
National: MBBS, DGO, MD and PhD of different Universities and
National Board of Examination, New Delhi
International: Royal College of Obstetricians and Gynaecologists (MRCOG), London
Royal College of Physicians of Ireland (MRCPI)
Recipient, "Pride of FOGSI" award – 2019, for exemplary efforts toward upliftment of Women's Health in India

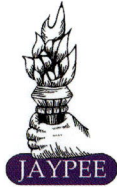

JAYPEE BROTHERS MEDICAL PUBLISHERS
The Health Sciences Publisher
New Delhi | London

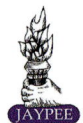
Jaypee Brothers Medical Publishers (P) Ltd

Headquarters
Jaypee Brothers Medical Publishers (P) Ltd
4838/24, Ansari Road, Daryaganj
New Delhi 110 002, India
Phone: +91-11-43574357
Fax: +91-11-43574314
Email: jaypee@jaypeebrothers.com

Corporate Office
Jaypee Brothers Medical Publishers (P) Ltd
4838/24, Ansari Road, Daryaganj
New Delhi 110 002, India
Phone: +91-11-43574357
Fax: +91-11-43574314
Email: jaypee@jaypeebrothers.com

Overseas Office
J.P. Medical Ltd
83 Victoria Street, London
SW1H 0HW (UK)
Phone: +44 20 3170 8910
Fax: +44 (0)20 3008 6180
Email: info@jpmedpub.com

Website: www.jaypeebrothers.com
Website: www.jaypeedigital.com

© Copyright reserved by Mrs Madhusri Konar

The views and opinions expressed in this book are solely those of the original contributor(s)/author(s) and do not necessarily represent those of editor(s) of the book.

All rights reserved. No part of this publication may be reproduced, stored or transmitted in any form or by any means, electronic, mechanical, photocopying, recording or otherwise, without the prior permission in writing of the publishers.

All brand names and product names used in this book are trade names, service marks, trademarks or registered trademarks of their respective owners. the publisher is not associated with any product or vendor mentioned in this book.

Medical knowledge and practice change constantly. This book is designed to provide accurate, authoritative information about the subject matter in question. However, readers are advised to check the most current information available on procedures included and check information from the manufacturer of each product to be administered, to verify the recommended dose, formula, method and duration of administration, adverse effects and contraindications. It is the responsibility of the practitioner to take all appropriate safety precautions. Neither the publisher nor the author(s)/editor(s) assume any liability for any injury and/or damage to persons or property arising from or related to use of material in this book.

Medical knowledge and practice change constantly. This book is designed to provide accurate, authoritative information about the subject matter in question. However, readers are advised to check the most current information available on procedures included and check information from the manufacturer of each product to be administered, to verify the recommended dose, formula, method and duration of administration, adverse effects and contraindications. It is the responsibility of the practitioner to take all appropriate safety precautions. Neither the publisher nor the author(s)/editor(s) assume any liability for any injury and/or damage to persons or property arising from or related to use of material in this book.

This book is sold on the understanding that the publisher is not engaged in providing professional medical services. If such advice or services are required, the services of a competent medical professional should be sought.

Every effort has been made where necessary to contact holders of copyright to obtain permission to reproduce copyright material. If any have been inadvertently overlooked, the publisher will be pleased to make the necessary arrangements at the first opportunity.

Inquiries for bulk sales may be solicited at: jaypee@jaypeebrothers.com

DC Dutta's Clinics in Gynecology

First Edition: 2022, Reprint: **2024**

ISBN: 978-93-5465-139-7

Printed at: Samrat Offset Pvt. Ltd.

Dedicated

to

those who strive relentlessly
to develop quality care
for
women's health

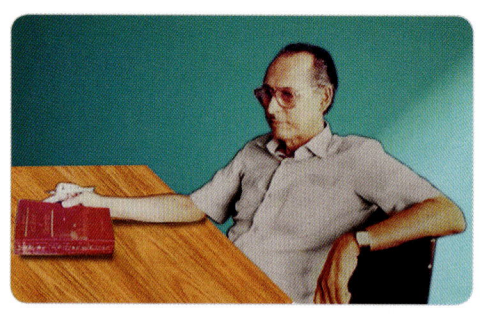

Professor DC Dutta

Professor DC Dutta was an Obstetrician, Gynecologist, a teacher par excellence and above all a noble human being. He came out with his first book entitled, **Textbook of Obstetrics** in 1983, while he was the Professor in Obstetrics and Gynecology at Sir Nil Ratan Sircar Medical College and Hospital, Kolkata, India. He was the first author in Obstetrics and Gynecology to remove the complexity of management with a most simple approach of the text information and the management flowchart, based on science and available resources. *Textbook of Obstetrics* soon became very popular nationally and internationally for which he received many accolades. DCD, as he was known to all his colleagues and students, was the doyen in Obstetrics and Gynecology in his era. His '**Textbook of Gynecology**' was published in 1989 from the same institute and department while he was the Professor and Head. This book also fetched more name and fame.

His deep interest in emergency obstetric care, is reflected by his several publications in the national journals. Presently, the best publication award, under the Federation of Obstetric and Gynecological Societies of India (FOGSI), every year, goes by his name. He is well-known for his fast surgical skill. He retired from the same institution in 1993, after a long and distinguished career. He died on 29th December 1995. His charming personality and the profound knowledge, made him very popular to the generations of students, professionals, practitioners and the patients. His legacy continues. He is remembered with great affection and professional respect by all, who knew him.

PREFACE

Dutta's Clinics in Gynecology is an up-to-date comprehensive review for the postgraduates. The current edition has been made more widened and prepared with recent advances in gynecology extensively.

Approach for this book is entirely different from a standard textbook. Any attempt to cover the entire subject of gynecology is presently impossible for anyone in the discipline. Technology driven advances from embryo biopsy to robotics for gynecology oncology, have given us a huge new insight. The topics are selected depending on the necessity to learn and practice with the available resources.

This book has been designed for all categories of medical students and the residents that they are striving to keep themselves abreast with the progress of science and technology for improved patient care. Practicing gynecologists will equally be benefitted to update themselves for the quality care. This book focuses on all the practical aspects of clinical diagnosis and management. The book covers several hundreds of problems in Gynecology, in a concise mode of discussion within a well-deigned structured framework.

As the concept of precision medicine is the trend, attempts have been made to provide a comprehensive summary of each subject under the subspecialty. My sincere attempt was to provide a global view for the standard of teaching, training and evaluation. A framework for the international standard of postgraduate examinations have been provided. This book is enriched with a good number of illustrations, numerous charts, tables, boxes, photographs of rare variety. *Suggested Reading* has been added for additional information to know the other management options.

Clinics in Gynecology provides a scholarly and updated answer for any question related to the subject as discussed in the different sections of subspecialty. While writing the book, I have tried my best to analyze critically the events, researches, trials and the literatures that appeared most clinically relevant. At the end, the author has expressed his experience and judgment as regard the care of an individual patient.

Hiralal Konar

ACKNOWLEDGMENTS

I am deeply indebted to my esteemed colleagues, residents and students, Department of Obstetrics and Gynecology of all the medical institutions of the country and abroad for their generous support while writing this book. I thank all the readers who have contacted me with suggestions and seeking explanations through e-mails. Their inputs have been invaluable and much appreciated. I wish I could mention their names individually.

I thank Professor Gautam Joarder, Principal, Professor Ashok Mondal, Chief Medical Director and Adviser to the Principal and Dr Saurav Ghosh, Medical Director, KPC Medical College and Hospital, Kolkata, India for the support.

I sincerely thank World Health Organization Regional Office of South-East Asia (WHO-SEARO) for supporting me to include the important chapter "Safe Abortion Service and WHO Guidelines" in the book. I also sincerely acknowledge the valuable inputs and contributions of Dr Neena Raina, Senior Advisor, Maternal, Child and Adolescent Health and Aging and Dr Meera Thapa Upadhyay, Technical Officer, Reproductive Health, WHO-SEARO and technical experts from Sexual and Reproductive Health (SRH)/Prevention of Unsafe Abortion (PUA) unit at WHO, Geneva.

I sincerely acknowledge the help specially Shri Jitendar P Vij (Group Chairman), Mr Ankit Vij (Managing Director), Mr MS Mani (Group President) and Dr Madhu Choudhary (Publishing Head–Education) of M/s Jaypee Brothers Medical Publishers (P) Ltd, New Delhi for all round support as and when needed. I thank, Md Jakir Hossain MSc, BEd, ADCA, Consultant Software for the technological support while composing the draft.

I am grateful to Dr Arindam Halder, Associate Professor, Dinajpur Medical College and Hospital, Dr (Mrs) Picklu Choudhury, Professor and Head, Department of Obstetrics and Gynecology, Rampurhat Medical College and Hospital, Dr Pallab Mistri, Associate Professor, Medical College, Kolkata, Prof Malabika Misra, JIMSH, Kolkata, Dr Chandrachur Konar, Assistant Professor SDUMC, Dr Roshni R, Senior Resident MVJ Medical College and Dr Lisley Konar, Resident, SDUMC for their tireless efforts to review the manuscripts.

I am ever grateful to Mrs Madhusri Konar for her sincere secretarial job and the all round support for this project.

At the end, I am grateful to all who have taught me most—all the patients and my beloved students.

I always welcome the views of the students, and the teachers through on line access to:
        e-mail: *h.kondr@gmail.com* and websites: *hirlalkonar.com* and *dcdutta.com*

CONTENTS

Section 1: Gynecology (OSCE)

1. **Objective Structured Clinical Examination (OSCE) in Gynecology** 3
   - A. **General Gynecology**
     - Case 1: Polycystic ovarian syndrome (PCOS)   3
     - Case 2: Endometriosis—A   5
     - Case 3: Endometriosis—B   7
     - Case 4: Pelvic pain   8
     - Case 5: Hydatidiform mole   9
     - Case 6: Cervical fibroid   10
     - Case 7: Menopause and hormonereplacement therapy (HRT)   11
   - B. **Adolescent Gynecology**
     - Case 8: Primary amenorrhea   12
   - C. **Menstrual Abnormalities**
     - Case 9: Secondary amenorrhea   14
     - Case 10: Hematocolpos (cryptomenorrhea)   14
   - D. **Infertility**
     - Case 11: Infertility—A   16
     - Case 12: Infertility—B   17
   - E. **Oncology**
     - Case 13: Hysterectomy and oophorectomy   19
     - Case 14: Postmenopausal bleeding   19
     - Case 15: Carcinoma cervix—A   21
     - Case 16: Carcinoma cervix—B   24
     - Case 17: Carcinoma cervix—C   25
     - Case 18: Carcinoma endometrium   26
     - Case 19: Carcinoma of the ovary   27
     - Case 20: Inherited cancers and the management   29

2. **Self-Assessment in Gynecology** 31

Section 2: Gynecology Discussion

3. **Recurrent Pregnancy Loss** 57
4. **Heavy Menstrual Bleeding** 62
5. **Congenital HIV Infection and AIDS** 66
6. **Urinary Incontinence** 68
7. **Fibroid Uterus: Management Issues** 70
8. **Polycystic Ovarian Syndrome** 73
9. **Hyperandrogenemia** 78
10. **Association of Subfertility with Endometriosis** 80
11. **Management of Pain in Endometriosis** 83

12. Adenomyosis Uterus 87
13. High Intensity Focused Ultrasound in the Management of Leiomyomas and Adenomyosis 89
14. Menopause and the Management Issues 91
15. Abnormal Uterine Bleeding 94
16. Abnormal Uterine Bleeding: Investigations and Management Issues 96
17. Management of Adnexal Mass in Peri- and Post-menopausal Women 100
18. Use of Selective Progesterone Receptor Modulators in Gynecology 104

Section 3: Infertility and Assisted Reproductive Technology (ART)

19. Current Concept in Physiology of Ovulation 109
20. Infertility Evaluation and Management 113
21. Female Infertility 115
22. Male Infertility 123
23. Assisted Reproductive Technology (ART) 126
24. Reproductive Outcome in Women with Advanced Maternal Age 133
25. Anti-Mullerian Hormone in Reproductive Biology 135
26. Fertility Management Strategies for Low Responder 137
27. Surrogacy 140

Section 4: Contraception

28. Advances in Contraception including Contraceptive Measures Following Treatment of GTD 145
29. Long-acting Reversible Contraceptives 150
30. Male and Female Sterilization 152
31. Safe Abortion Service and WHO Guidelines 157

Section 5: Gynecological Oncology

32. Carcinoma of the Endometrium (Early Stage Disease) 167
33. Surgical Management of Endometrial Carcinoma 170
34. Role of Pelvic and Para-aortic Lymph Node Dissection in the Surgical Management of
    Endometrial Cancer 172
35. Ovarian Tumor with Low Malignant Potential 174
36. Gestational Trophoblastic Disease 177
37. Human Chorionic Gonadotropin and the Management of Gestational Trophoblastic Disease 181
38. Fertility Preservation in Women 183
39. Fertility Preserving Options for Women with Ovarian Cancer 185
40. Fertility Preserving Options for Women with Cervical Cancer 187
41. Fertility Preserving Options for Women with Endometrial Cancer 189
42. Chemotherapy in Gynecological Cancers 190
43. Radiotherapy in Gynecological Cancers 194
44. Sentinel Lymph Node Mapping in Gynecologic Cancers 197

Section 6: Operative Gynecology

45. Abdominal Incisions 201
46. Tubal Ectopic Pregnancy 204
47. Cervical Insufficiency (Incompetence) 206
48. Surgical Management of Heavy Menstrual Bleeding 209
49. Surgical Site Infection 214
50. Endoscopy in Gynecology (Laparoscopic Surgery) 218
51. Prevention of Urinary Tract Injuries in Gynecological Laparoscopic Surgery 220
52. Management of Urinary Tract Injuries Following Laparoscopic Surgery 222
53. Place of Prophylactic Salpingectomy or Salpingo-oophorectomy in Current Gynecologic Practice ... 225
54. Surgical Management of Polycystic Ovarian Disease 227
55. Bariatric Surgery in Gynecology and Obstetrics 229
56. Robotic Surgery in Gynecology 232
57. Interventional Radiology in Obstetrics and Gynecology 235

Section 7: Maternal Sepsis

58. Maternal Sepsis: Prevention, Recognition and Management 241
59. Guidelines for use of Antimicrobials/Antibiotics in Gynecology 245

Section 8: Practice of SBA and EMQs

60. Model Questions and Answers for Practice of SBA 249
61. Model Questions and Answers for Practice of EMQs 258

Section 9: History in Obstetrics and Gynecology

62. Histoy in Obstetrics and Gynecology 265

Index *269*

ABBREVIATIONS

AACE:	American Association of Clinical Endocrinology	**CDMR:**	Cesarean Delivery on Maternal Request
AC:	Abdominal Circumference	**CECT:**	Contrast-enhanced Computed Tomography
ACA:	Anticardiolipin Antibodies	**CEE:**	Conjugated Equine Estrogens
ACE:	Angiotensin Converting Enzyme	**CEMACH:**	Confidential Enquiry into Maternal and Child Health
ACHOIS:	Australian Carbohydrate Intolerance Study		
ACOG:	American College of Obstetricians and Gynecologists	**cff-DNA:**	Cell-free Fetal DNA
		CFTR:	Cystic Fibrosis Transmembrane Regulator
ACS:	Acute Chest Syndrome	**CFU:**	Colony-forming Unit
ACTH:	Adrenocorticotropic Hormone	**CGH:**	Comparative Genomic Hybridization
ADA:	American Diabetes Association	**CIN:**	Cervical Intraepithelial Neoplasia
AEDF:	Absent End-diastolic Flow	**CIS:**	Carcinoma in situ
AEDs:	Antiepileptic Drugs	**CMV:**	Cytomegalovirus
AFASS:	Affordable, Feasible, Accessible, Sustainable and Safe	**CNS:**	Central Nervous System
		CO:	Combined Obesity
AFC:	Antral Follicle Count	**COCs:**	Combine Oral Contraceptives
AFE:	Amniotic Fluid Embolism	**COS:**	Controlled Ovarian Stimulation
AFP:	Alpha-fetoprotein	**COX:**	Cycloxygenase
AFS:	American Fertility Society	**CPD:**	Cephalopelvic Disproportion
AI:	Aromatase Inhibitors	**CPP:**	Chronic Pelvic Pain
AIDS:	Acquired Immune Deficiency Syndrome	**CPR:**	Cardiopulmonary Resuscitation
ALT:	Alanine Transaminase	**CPR:**	Cumulative Pregnancy Rate
AMH:	Anti-Müllerian Hormone	**CPT:**	Complete Perineal Tear
APA:	Antiphospholipid Antibody	**CREST:**	Calcinosis, Raynaud Phenomenon, Esophageal Dysmotility, Sclerodactyly, and Telangiectasia
APAS:	Antiphospholipid Antibody Syndrome		
API:	Association of Physicians of India	**CRH:**	Corticotropin-releasing Hormone
APS:	Antiphospholipid Syndrome	**CRS:**	Congenital Rubella Syndrome
ARDS:	Acute Respiratory Distress Syndrome	**CS:**	Cesarean Section
ARM:	Artificial Rupture of the Membranes	**CSF:**	Cerebrospinal Fluid
ART:	Assisted Reproductive Technology	**CSP:**	Cesarean Scar Pregnancy
ASB:	Asymptomatic Bacteriuria	**CT:**	Computed Tomography
ASRM:	American Society for Reproductive Medicine	**CTG:**	Cardiotocography
AST:	Aspartate Transaminase	**CTPA:**	Computed Tomographic Pulmonary Angiography
ASTEC:	A Study in the Treatment of Endometrial Cancer		
ATA:	American Thyroid Association	**CVD:**	Cardiovascular Disease
AUB:	Abnormal Uterine Bleeding	**CVS:**	Chorionic Villus Sampling
BBT:	Basal Body Temperature	**CZ:**	Carbimazole
BC:	Blood culture	**D and C:**	Dilatation and Curettage
BMD:	Bone Mineral Density	**DF:**	Dominant Follicle
BMI:	Body Mass Index	**DHEA:**	Dehydroepiandrosterone
BP:	Blood Pressure	**DHEAS:**	Dehydroepiandosterone Sulphate
BRCA:	BReast CAncer gene	**DIC:**	Disseminated Intravascular Coagulation
BSO:	Bilateral Salpingo-oophorectomy	**DMPA:**	Depot Medroxyprogesterone Acetate
BTB:	Breakthrough Bleeding	**DPG:**	Diphosphoglycerate
CAH:	Congenital Adrenal Hyperplasia	**DTIC:**	Distal Tubal Intraepithelial Carcinoma
C and S:	Culture and Sensitivity	**DVT:**	Deep Vein Thrombosis
CBAVD:	Congenital Bilateral Absence of Vas Deferens	**E2:**	Estradiol
CBC:	Complete Blood Count	**EC:**	Endometrial Curettage
CC:	Clomiphene Citrate	**ECG:**	Electrocardiogram
CCCT:	Clomiphene Citrate Challenge Test	**EGF:**	Epidermal Growth Factor
CCU:	Clean Catch Urine	**EOCs:**	Epithelial Ovarian Cancers
CDC:	Centers for Disease Control and Prevention	**EPAU:**	Early Pregnancy Assessment Unit

ESBL:	Extended-spectrum beta-lactamase	ICSI:	Intracytoplasmic Sperm Injection
ESHRE:	European Society of Human Reproduction and Embryology	ICU:	Intensive Care Unit
		IDDM:	Insulin-dependent Diabetes Mellitus
FBC:	Full Blood Count	IFA:	Immunofluorescence Assay
FDP:	Fibrinogen Degradation Products	IGF:	Insulin-like Growth Factor
FET:	Frozen Embryo Transfer	IOTA:	International Ovarian Tumor Analysis
FFP:	Fresh Frozen Plasma	IPV:	Inactivated Polio Vaccine
FIGO:	International Federation of Gynaecology and Obstetrics	ISMINIM:	International Society for Minimally Invasive and Noninvasive Medicine
FISH:	Fluorescence in situ Hybridization	ITP:	Idiopathic Thrombocytopenic Purpura
FL:	Femur Length	ITS:	Indian Thyroid Society
FOGSI:	Federation of Obstetricians and Gynecologists of India	ITU:	Intensive Therapy Unit
		IUCD:	Intrauterine Contraceptive Device
FSH:	Follicle Stimulating Hormone	IUD:	Intrauterine Device
FVS:	Fetal Varicella Syndrome	IUI:	Intrauterine Insemination
G-6PD:	Glucose-6-phosphate dehydrogenase	IVC:	Inferior Vena Cava
GAS:	Group A Streptococcus (Streptococcus pyogenes)	IVF-ET:	In vitro Fertilization and Embryo Transfer
GBS:	Group B Streptococci	IVH:	Intraventricular Hemorrhage
GBS:	Group B Streptococcus (Streptococcus agalactiae)	IVIG:	Intravenous Immunoglobulin
GC:	Gonococcus (Neisseria gonorrhoeae)	LAC:	Lupus Anticoagulant
GDM:	Gestational Diabetes Mellitus	LARC:	Long-acting reversible contraceptives
GIFT:	Gamete Intrafallopian Transfer	LARVT:	Laparoscopic Assisted Radical Vaginal Trachelectomy
GIT:	Gastrointestinal Tract		
GnRH:	Gonadotropin Releasing Hormone	LAVH:	Laparoscopic Assisted Vaginal Hysterectomy
GO:	Generalized Obesity	LBC:	Liquid-based Cytology
GSI:	Genuine Stress Incontinence	LDH:	Lactate Dehydrogenase
GTD:	Gestational Trophoblastic Disease	LDL:	Low Density Lipoprotein
GTN:	Gestational Trophoblastic Neoplasia	LE:	Leucocyte Esterase
HAART:	Highly Active Antiretroviral Therapy	LFT:	Liver Function Test
HAIR-AN:	Hyperandrogenism, Insulin Resistance and Acanthosis Nigricans	LGSOC:	Low-grade Serous Ovarian Cancer
		LH:	Luteinizing Hormone
HAPO:	Hyperglycemia and Adverse Pregnancy Outcome	LLETZ:	Large Loop Excision of the Transformation Zone
HAV:	Hepatitis A Virus	LMP:	Last Menstrual Period
HbF:	Fetal Hemoglobin	LMWH:	Low Molecular Weight Heparin
HBV:	Hepatitis B Virus	LNG-IUD:	Levonorgestrel-intrauterine Device
HC:	Head Circumference	LNG-IUS:	Levonorgestrel-intrauterine System
hCG:	Human Chorionic Gonadotropin	LOD:	Laparoscopic Ovarian Drilling
HCV:	Hepatitis C Virus	LOS:	Laparoscopic Ovarian Surgery
HDFN:	Hemolytic Disease of the Fetus and Newborn	LPD:	Luteal Phase Defect
HDL:	High Density Lipoprotein	LSCS:	Lower Segment Cesarean Section
HDR:	High Dose Radiation	LUF:	Luteinized Unruptured Follicle
HDU:	High Dependency Unit	LVS:	Low Vaginal Swab
HFEA:	Human Fertilization and Embryology Authority	LVSI:	Lymphovascular Space Involvement
hGH:	Human Growth Hormone	MAHA:	Microangiopathic Hemolytic Anemia
HGSOC:	High-grade Serous Ovarian Cancer	MAP:	Mean Arterial Pressure
HIFU:	High Intensity Focused Ultrasound	MC:	Monochorionic
HIV:	Human Immunodeficiency Virus	MCA:	Middle Cerebral Artery
HLA:	Human Leukocyte Antigen	MCA-PSV:	Middle Cerebral Artery Peak Systolic Velocity
HMB:	Heavy Menstrual Bleeding	MCDA:	Monochorionic Diamniotic
HMG:	Human Menopausal Gonadotropin	MCTP:	Monochorionic Twin Pregnancy
HPL:	Human Placental Lactogen	MDTA:	Multidisciplinary Team Approach
HPV:	Human Papilloma Virus	MEA:	Microwave Endometrial Ablation
HRT:	Hormone Replacement Therapy	MESA:	Microsurgical Epididymal Sperm Aspiration
HVS:	High Vaginal Swab	MFR:	Monthly Fecundity Rate
HWY:	Hundred Woman Years (Pregnancy)	MgSO4:	Magnesium Sulfate
IAI:	Intra-amniotic infection (Chorioamnionitis)	MHV:	Mechanical Heart Valves
IAP:	Intrapartum Antibiotic Prophylaxis	MMK:	Marshall-Marchetti-Krantz
ICD:	International Statistical Classification of Disease	MMR:	Maternal Mortality Rate

MNM:	Maternal Near Miss	**PUL:**	Pregnancy of Unknown Location
MOM:	Multiple of the Median	**PVD:**	Peripheral Vascular Disease
MPGS:	Massively Parallel Genomic Sequencing	**RALH:**	Robotic Assisted Laparoscopic Hysterectomy
MRg FUS:	MR-guided Focused Ultrasound	**RCOG:**	Royal College of Obstetrics and Gynecology
MRI:	Magnetic Resonance Imaging	**RCTs:**	Randomized Controlled Trials
MRSA:	Meticillin-resistant *Staphylococcus aureus*	**RMI:**	Risk of Malignancy Index
MSAFP:	Maternal Serum Alpha-fetoprotein	**ROMA:**	Risk of Ovarian Malignancy Algorithm
MSU:	Midstream urine	**RPL:**	Recurrent Pregnancy Loss
MTCT:	Mother-to-child Transmission	**RVT:**	Radical Vaginal Trachelectomy
MTHFR:	Methylenetetrahydrofolate Reductase	**SAMM:**	Severe Acute Maternal Morbidity
MTP:	Medical Termination of Pregnancy	**SCCA:**	Squamus Cell Carcinoma Antigen
MTX:	Methotrexate	**SCJ:**	Squamocolumnar Junction
MVA:	Manual Vacuum Aspiration	**SGA:**	Small for Gestational Age
N:	Nitrites	**SHBG:**	Sex Hormone Binding Globulin
NICE:	National Institute for Health and Clinical Excellence	**SIL:**	Squamous Intraepithelial Lesion
NICHD:	National Institute of Child Health and Human Development	**SIS:**	Saline Infusion Sonography
		SLE:	Systemic Lupus Erythematosus
NIPT:	Noninvasive Prenatal Testing	**SOFA:**	Sequential Organ Failure Assessment
NSAIDs:	Nonsteroidal Antiinflammatory Drugs	**SSI:**	Surgical Site Infection
NTD:	Neural Tube Defects	**STIC:**	Serous Tubal Intraepithelial Carcinoma
OAB:	Overactive Bladder	**STIs:**	Sexually Transmitted Infections
OAT:	Oligoasthenoteratozoospermia	**SUI:**	Stress Urinary Incontinence
OGTT:	Oral Glucose Tolerance Test	**SUZI:**	Subzonal Insemination
OHSS:	Ovarian Hyperstimulation Syndrome	**TAH:**	Total Abdominal Hysterectomy
OP:	Occiput Posterior	**TBEA:**	Thermal Balloon Endometrial Ablation
OSCE:	Objective Structured Clinical Examination	**TCRE:**	Transcervical Resection of Endometrium
OTA:	Oligoasthenoteratozoospermia	**TEC:**	Thromboembolic Complications
P-PROM:	Pre-term Premature Rupture of Membranes	**TESE:**	Testicular Sperm Aspiration
PAPP-A:	Pregnancy Associated Plasma Protein-A	**TIC:**	Tubal Intraepithelial Carcinoma
PCOS:	Polycystic Ovarian Syndrome	**TLH:**	Total Laparoscopic Hysterectomy
PCR:	Polymerase Chain Reaction	**TNFs:**	Tumor Necrosis Factors
PDA:	Patent Ductus Arteriosus	**TOT:**	Transobturator Tape
PE:	Pulmonary Embolism	**TPO:**	Thyroid Peroxidase
PESA:	Percutaneous Epididymal Sperm Aspiration	**TPOAbs:**	Thyroid Anti-TPO Antibodies
PET:	Positron Emission Tomography	**TRAP:**	Twin Reverse Arterial Perfusion
PGD:	Prenatal Genetic Diagnosis	**TRH:**	Thyrotropin Releasing Hormone
PID:	Pelvic Inflammatory Disease	**TSHRAbs:**	Thyrotropin Receptor Autoantibodies
PMB:	Postmenopausal Bleeding	**TV:**	Trichomonas Vaginalis
PMS:	Premenstrual Syndrome	**TVS:**	Transvaginal Sonography
PO:	Post Operative	**TVT:**	Tension-free Vaginal Tape
POC:	Product of Conception	**TZ:**	Transformation Zone
POD:	Pouch of Douglas	**UAE:**	Uterine Artery Embolization
POF:	Premature Ovarian Failure	**UE3:**	Unconjugated Estriol
POP:	Pelvic Organ Prolapse	**UFH:**	Unfractionated Heparin
POP:	Progestin only Pill	**UI:**	Urinary Incontinence
PORTEC:	Postoperative Radiation Therapy in Endometrial Cancer	**USG:**	Ultrasonography
		UTI:	Urinary Tract Infection
PPA:	Primary Peritoneal Adenocarcinoma	**VaIN:**	Vaginal Intraepithelial Neoplasia
PPIUCD:	Postpartum Intrauterine Contraceptive Devices	**VAMA:**	Very Advanced Maternal Age
PR:	Pulse Rate	**VCB:**	Vaginal Cuff Brachytherapy
PRBCs:	Packed Red Blood Cells	**VEGF:**	Vascular Endothelial Growth Factor
PSOC:	Papillary Serous Ovarian Cancer	**VIA:**	Visual Inspection using Acetic Acid
PSP1:	Pregnancy Specific Protein 1	**VKA:**	Vitamin K Antagonist
PSTT:	Placental Site Trophoblastic Tumor	**VTE:**	Venous Thromboembolism
PT:	Prothrombin Time	**VVF:**	Vesicovaginal Fistula
PTD:	Postpartum Thyroid Dysfunction	**WHO:**	World Health Organization
PTT:	Partial Thromboplastin Time	**WLTC:**	Women with Life-threatening Condition

Section 1: Gynecology (OSCE)

Section Outline

Ch. 1. Objective Structured Clinical Examination (OSCE) in Gynecology

A. General Gynecology
- Case 1: Polycystic Ovarian Syndrome (PCOS)
- Case 2: Endometriosis—A
- Case 3: Endometriosis—B
- Case 4: Pelvic Pain
- Case 5: Hydatidiform Mole
- Case 6: Cervical Fibroid
- Case 7: Menopause and Hormone Replacement Therapy (HRT)

B. Adolescent Gynecology
- Case 8: Primary Amenorrhea

C. Menstrual Abnormalities
- Case 9: Secondary Amenorrhea
- Case 10: Hematocolpos (Cryptomenorrhea)

D. Infertility
- Case 11: Infertility—A
- Case 12: Infertility—B

E. Oncology
- Case 13: Hysterectomy and Oophorectomy
- Case 14: Postmenopausal Bleeding
- Case 15: Carcinoma Cervix—A
- Case 16: Carcinoma Cervix—B
- Case 17: Carcinoma Cervix—C
- Case 18: Carcinoma Endometrium
- Case 19: Carcinoma of the Ovary
- Case 20: Inherited Cancers and the Management

Ch. 2. Self-assessment in Gynecology

Chapter 1: Objective Structured Clinical Examination (OSCE) in Gynecology

A. GENERAL GYNECOLOGY

CASE 1: POLYCYSTIC OVARIAN SYNDROME (PCOS)

Case Summary

Mrs UC, 30-year-old receptionist, married for 3 years, was seen with the problem of oligomenorrhea-amenorrhea and infertility. She also complained of excess body hair (Fig. 1.1).

Her height was 5'1" and she weighed 80 kg. Her hormone assay done on D-2 of the cycle revealed FSH 5.0 IU/L, LH 13.01 IU/L. Testosterone 3.8 nmol/L prolactin 60 ng/mL; TSH 3.8 mU/L.

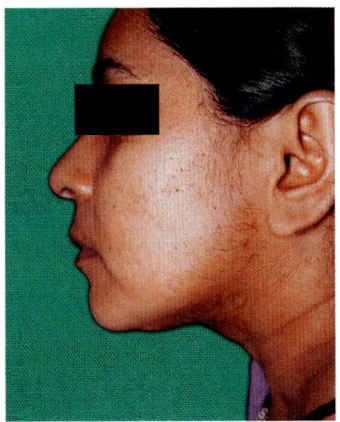

Fig. 1.1: Excess growth of facial (upper lip, cheek, chin and male-pattern beard) hair.

Q.1 What is the likely diagnosis?
Ans. Polycystic ovarian syndrome

Q.2 What is the current diagnostic criteria for PCOS?
Ans. According to ASRM/ESHRE, 2018 diagnosis of PCOS is based upon the presence of any two of the following three criteria:
1. Oligo and/or anovulation
2. Hyperandrogenism (clinical and/or biochemical)
3. Polycystic ovaries.
Other causes of hyperandrogenic conditions (adrenal) are to be excluded.

Q.3 What are the symptoms of PCOS?
Ans.
- Obesity
- Infertility
- Menstrual abnormality: Oligomenorrhea, amenorrhea, abnormal uterine bleeding (AUB)
- Hirsutism
- Characteristic skin changes (acanthosis nigricans)
- Acne
- HAIR-AN syndrome (*See* Dutta's Textbook of Gynecology, 8th Edition, p. 385).

Q.4 What are the characteristic changes in the ovary of a woman with PCOS?
Ans. Ovaries are enlarged in volume. The capsule is thickened. On cut section multiple (≥ 2) follicular cysts measuring about 2–9 mm in diameter are seen peripherally (Fig. 1.2). There is stromal hyperthecosis. Transvaginal sonography (TVS) can demonstrate the enlarged ovarian volume with peripherally arranged cysts.

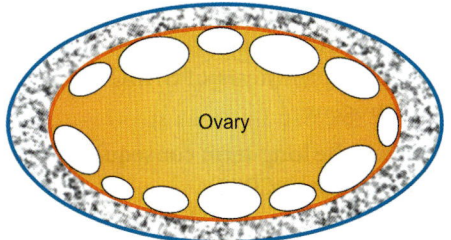

Fig. 1.2: Polycystic ovary.

Q.5 What other investigations would be appropriate for her?
Ans.
- Ultrasound scan (TVS) (Figs. 1.3A and B)
- To detect polycystic ovarian changes
- Investigations for other factors for infertility, e.g., tubal patency test and husband's semen analysis.

Q.6 What is the basic underlying pathology in this condition of PCOS?
Ans. Hyperandrogenic state and chronic anovulation.

Q.7 What are the biochemical abnormalities seen in a case of PCOS?
Ans.
- Hyperandrogenemia [(↑) testosterone, DHEA, androstenedione)]
- Hyperinsulinemia (insulin resistance)
- Hypersecretion of luteinizing hormone (LH)

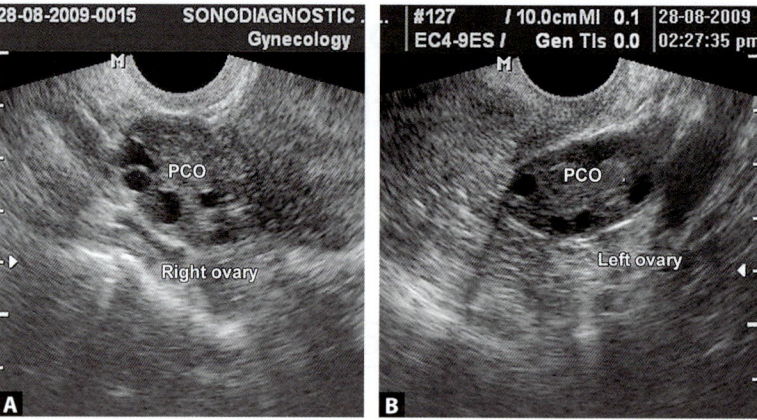

Figs. 1.3A and B: (A) Ultrasonography of the pelvis showing polycystic ovary (right); (B) Ultrasonography of the same patient showing polycystic ovary (left).
Courtesy: Dr (Mrs) S Ghosh, Professor BN Chakravorty, IRM, Kolkata, India.

- Hyperprolactinemia
- (↑) Serum estrogen
- (↓) Sex hormone-binding globulin (SHBG)
- (↑) Lipids.

Q.8 How can obesity and hyperinsulinemia cause hyperandrogenism?

Ans.
- **Obesity** → increased insulin resistance and raised insulin level stimulate → ovary (theca cells) → androgens (↑) : **Obesity** → (↓) SHBG → (↑) androgens (free).
- **Hyperinsulinemia** → ovarian theca cells → (↑) androgens: *increased insulin* → (↓) hepatic synthesis of SHBG → more (↑) free androgens.

Q.9 What are the long-term consequences in a woman suffering from PCOS?

Ans.
- Risk of developing diabetes mellitus due to insulin resistance.
- Risk of endometrial carcinoma due to unopposed action of estrogen.
- Risk of developing hypertension and cardiovascular disease due to abnormal lipid profile (dyslipidemia).

Q.10 What is the aim of management of PCOS?

Ans. Aim of treatment is to individualize the patient for her presenting symptoms like infertility, obesity or menstrual abnormality. In obese patients, weight reduction is essential.

Q.11 How do you treat hyperandrogenemia?

Ans.
- Weight reduction
  - Combined oral contraceptive pills
  - GnRH agonists
  - Cyproterone acetate
  - Spironolactone
  - Flutamide.

Q.12 What medical management will improve her fertility status?

Ans. Weight reduction and induction of ovulation. Adjuvant drugs may be needed (e.g., metformin, bromocriptine) depending upon the associated abnormalities.

Q.13 If the woman is desirous of pregnancy how can you help her?

Ans. Ovulation of induction is to be done as she suffers from chronic anovulation. However, other factors (male factor, tubal patency tests) should be normal.

Q.14 What drug is commonly used for induction of ovulation?

Ans.
- Clomiphene citrate
  - However, clomiphene citrate is to be combined with other drugs when other biochemical abnormalities are associated.
    - Clomiphene citrate + metformin → where there is obesity and hyperinsulinemia.
    - Clomiphene citrate + bromocriptine → where there is associated hyperprolactinemia.

Q.15 What is the place of insulin sensitizers in the management of women with PCOS desiring for conception?

Ans. Women with PCOS with body mass index more than 25 are often found insulin resistant. Along with weight reduction, treatment with metformin (insulin sensitizer) is found to reduce hyperinsulinemia and hyperandrogenemia. Pioglitazone and rosiglitazone are also being used in cases, resistant to metformin. Metformin is given in a dose 500 mg thrice daily.

Q.16 What are the different surgical methods?

Ans. Laparoscopic ovarian drilling (LOD) or laser (CO_2) vaporization of the cysts is usually done. LOD reduces systemic and intraovarian androgen levels. The woman ovulates spontaneously following LOD (*See* Ch 54).

CASE 2: ENDOMETRIOSIS—A

Case Summary

Mrs PL, 24-year-old lady, married for 1 year, complaining of pelvic pain and deep dyspareunia. She was advised diagnostic laparoscopy which revealed the pathology (Fig. 1.4). She does not wish to become pregnant at present.

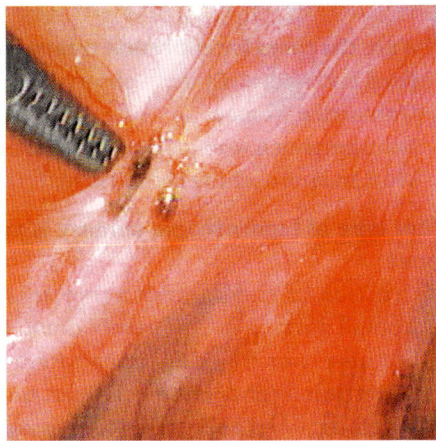

Fig. 1.4: Pelvic endometriosis.

Q.17 What is the likely diagnosis?
Ans. Pelvic endometriosis.

Q.18 What is endometriosis?
Ans. It is the presence of functioning endometrium (both glands and stroma) in sites other than the uterine mucosa.

Q.19 What are the common sites of endometriosis?
Ans.
- Ovary
- Uterosacral ligaments
- Rectovaginal septum
- Pouch of Douglas (POD)
- Sigmoid colon
- Abdominal scar.

Q.20 What are the other symptoms?
Ans. Abnormal menstruation like menorrhagia, dysmenorrhea (secondary), dyspareunia, pain during defecation, rectal bleeding. She may be asymptomatic.

Q.21 What is the naked eye appearance of pelvic endometriotic lesions?
Ans. Lesions may appear as:
- Small black dots (powder burns)
- Red flame shaped areas
- White patches
- Peritoneal windows
- Subovarian adhesions
- Puckering of peritoneum
- Ovaries may be involved—chocolate cysts
- White peritoneal areas.

Q.22 What are the important symptoms of pelvic endometriosis?
Ans.
- Some patients remain asymptomatic (25%)
- Dysmenorrhea (50%)
- Abnormal menstruation—menorrhagia, polymenorrhea
- Infertility (40–60%)
- Dyspareunia
- Pelvic pain
- Abdominal pain
- Bladder symptoms (dysuria)
- Bowel symptoms (rectal bleeding)
- Pain during defecation.

Q.23 How the diagnosis of pelvic endometriosis is confirmed?
Ans. It is commonly done by diagnostic laparoscopy.

Q.24 What is the place of serum CA-125 in the diagnosis of pelvic endometriosis?
Ans. Measurement of serum CA-125 levels is not a diagnostic tool because of its low sensitivity (< 50%). It may be used to predict the recurrence of endometriosis after therapy.

Q.25 What are the causes of infertility in a woman with pelvic endometriosis?
Ans. The possible cause of infertility are:
- **Ovarian dysfunction:** Anovulation, defective folliculogenesis or luteal phase defect.
- **Tubal dysfunction:** Pelvic adhesions, causing distorsion of normal tube ovary relationship.
- **Others:** Abnormal peritoneal fluid, implantation failure, miscarriage.

Q.26 What are the endocrine abnormalities associated with endometriosis?
Ans.
- Corpus luteum insufficiency
- Raised prolactin level
- Luteolysis due to increased PGF2α.

Q.27 What associated condition such a patient may present with?
Ans. Infertility.

Q.28 What are the complications of endometriosis?
Ans.
- Leakage or rupture of chocolate cyst
- Infection of chocolate cyst
- Infertility
- Obstructive features (ureteral obstruction).

Q.29 What are the different modalities of therapy for pelvic endometriosis?
Ans.
- Expectant
- Medical NSAIDs: Hormonal
- Surgery
- Conservative

- Combined surgical and medical
- Definitive
- Assisted reproduction (*See* Ch 23).

Q.30 What are the factors that determine the type of treatment to a particular woman?
Ans. To an individual woman the determining factors are:
- Age of the woman
- Size and extent of lesion
- Severity of symptoms
- Desire for a child
- Stage of the disease [American Fertility Society (AFS) scoring system—*See* Dutta's Textbook of Gynecology, 8th Edition, p. 257]
- Results of previous therapy.

Q.31 What are the different hormones that can be used for the treatment of pelvic endometriosis?
Ans.
- Combined oral contraceptives (COCs)
- Progestogens
  - Oral:
    - Medroxyprogesterone acetate
    - Dydrogesterone
    - Dienogest
  - Parenteral (IM): Medroxyprogesterone
  - Intrauterine contraceptive device (IUCD): Levonorgestrel intrauterine system (LNG-IUS)
- Danazol
- Gestrinone
- GnRH analogs.

Q.32 What are the important side effects of danazol and GnRH analogs?
Ans.
- ***Danazol:*** It causes symptoms due to pseudomenopause and it is less tolerated.
- ***GnRH analogs:*** It works by creating medical oophorectomy compared to danazol, GnRH analogs are well-tolerated.

Q.33 What are the indications of surgery for pelvic endometriosis?
Ans.
- Symptomatic endometriosis which is not responsive to hormone therapy.
- Severe endometriosis—to correct the distortion of pelvic anatomy or for improvement of symptoms.
- Chocolate cyst ≥ 4 cm needs ovarian cystectomy and adhesiolysis.

Q.34 What are the different types of surgery that can be done?
Ans. Either by laparotomy or laparoscopy.

Q.35 What is meant by conservative surgery?
Ans. Preservation of the reproductive organs and restoration of their anatomy for enhancement of fertility (function).

Q.36 What is meant by expectant treatment?
Ans. Expectant treatment means doing nothing actively. The woman is kept under observation.

Q.37 What is the place of expectant treatment?
Ans. Role of any treatment for minimal to mild endometriosis is controversial. Cumulative pregnancy rate is similar following expectant treatment and that after conservative surgery.

Q.38 Who are the cases for expectant treatment?
Ans. Minimal endometriosis when observed in
- Unmarried women
- Young married woman who is desirous of a baby
- Women approaching menopause.

Q.39 What type of laparoscopic surgery is commonly done?
Ans. Destruction of endometriotic implants over the peritoneal surface is commonly done. It is done by diathermy or by laser vaporization. Ovarian endometrioma (chocolate cyst) can be resected laparoscopically. Laparoscopic uterosacral nerve ablation (LUNA) is done when pain is very severe.
Division of adhesions (adhesiolysis) can also be done by laparoscopy.

Q.40 What are the treatment options for this woman?
Ans. **Combined oral contraceptive pill** for a period of 6–9 months would be most appropriate for her. Continuous therapy without the usual 7 days break would make her amenorrheic. This will help regression of the endometriotic deposits. This will also improve her symptoms. At the same time contraception is also provided.
Other options depending on the severity of endometriosis would be:
- ***Medical therapy:*** Continuous progestogen, dienogest or GnRH analogs.
- ***Surgical therapy:*** Laparoscopic laser or electrodiathermy to ablate the endometriotic implants.

Q.41 What would be the appropriate management when she desires to conceive?
Ans. Pregnancy itself provides remission to the problem. For this case, following the initial treatment, expectant management would be appropriate for next 6 months. About 60–70% women will become pregnant within a year provided there is no other factor for infertility.

Q.42 What is the optimum treatment for scar endometriosis?
Ans. Treatment is done by excision. Hormone therapy is ineffective.

Q.43 What is adenomyosis?

Ans. Adenomyosis is a condition when there is ingrowth of endometrium (both the glands and stroma) directly within the myometrium (*See* Ch 12).

Q.44 How does a woman with adenomyosis present?

Ans. Usually the woman is parous, with age above 40 years.
Common symptoms are:
- Menorrhagia
- Dysmenorrhea.

Q.45 How can you differentiate a fibroid uterus from an adenomyosis?

Ans. *See* Ch 12.

Q.46 What should be the treatment of adenomyosis in a parous and elderly woman?

Ans.
- Treatment of adenomyosis (Figs. 1.5A and B) is predominantly surgical.
- Medical management (hormones) is often ineffective.
- Conservative surgery includes partial resection of adenomyomata.
- Total hysterectomy with or without bilateral salpingo-oophorectomy is the optimum treatment for a woman who is parous and aged.
- Currently, LNG-IUD is being used and found to be effective in improving the symptoms of menorrhagia and pelvic pain.

CASE 3: ENDOMETRIOSIS—B

Case Summary

Mrs BK, 24-year-old, married lady has been examined in the outpatient clinic for her pelvic pain which gets worse during menstruation.

Q.47 What more relevant questions you will ask her to make the provisional diagnosis?

Ans. Regarding the pain, e.g., character of pain, duration, exact relationship with the period, deep dyspareunia and fertility status.

Q.48 What clinical signs will help you to make the differential diagnosis?

Ans. Pelvic tenderness, nodularity in the pouch of Douglas, fixed retroversion of the uterus, adnexal mass, tenderness and bulky uterus. The differential diagnosis includes pelvic endometriosis, adenomyosis, chronic pelvic inflammatory disease.

Q.49 To confirm the diagnosis what single investigation would be most valuable?

Ans.
- Diagnostic laparoscopy by double puncture procedure.
- Laparoscopy revealed the diagnosis (Fig. 1.6).

Q.50 Is this pathology going to affect her future fertility?

Ans. There is an association of pelvic endometriosis and infertility. Amongst the infertile patients, 15%

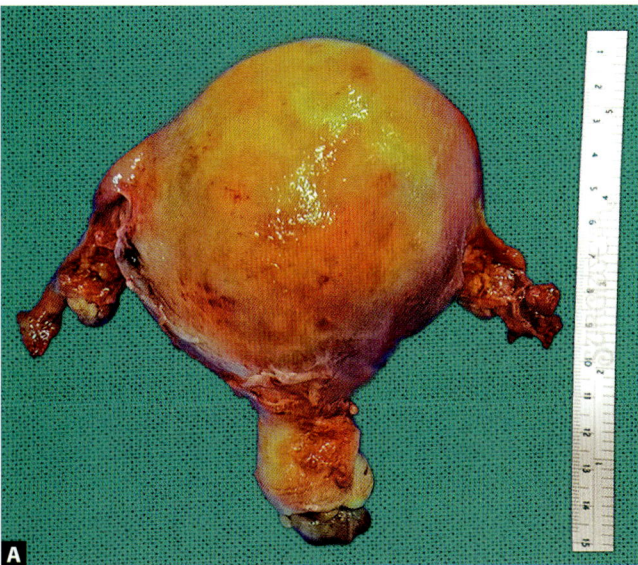
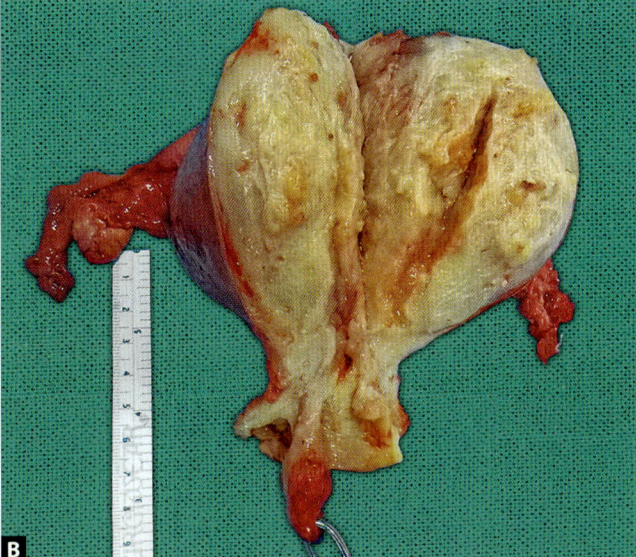

Figs. 1.5A and B: (A) Postoperative specimen of a uterus with tubes and ovaries. Mrs SE, a 46-year-old, parous lady, was admitted for menorrhagia and intractable dysmenorrhea. She did not respond to any medical therapy. She was investigated. She underwent hysterectomy and bilateral salpingo-oophorectomy. The uterus is seen uniformly enlarged; (B) The specimen of the same patient is cut opened to show myohyperplasia with hemorrhagic spots within the myometrium.

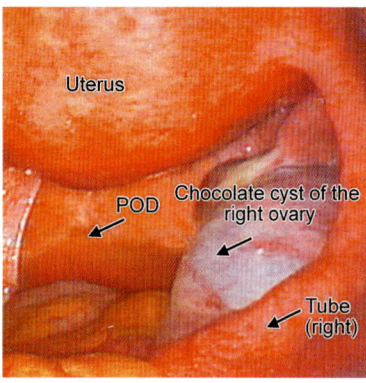

Fig. 1.6: Chocolate cyst of the right ovary (arrows).

suffer from endometriosis. Whereas patients with endometriosis suffer from infertility in 40–60% cases. The possible explanations are—anovulation, luteal phase defect, luteinized unruptured follicle syndrome, pelvic adhesions, dyspareunia, increased macrophage activity, altered prostaglandin balance and altered immune response.

Q.51 Should a patient with mild endometriosis be treated?
Ans. There is no advantage of any therapy over expectant management in cases with minimal or mild endometriosis. The association of infertility and endometriosis is not absolute unless there is tubal obstruction or extensive pelvic adhesions.

Q.52 What would be the appropriate treatment for this patient?
Ans. The content of chocolate cysts can be drained and the cavity is to be lavaged with normal saline. The lining of the cyst wall is then separated from the ovarian tissue. This may be done either by laparoscopy or by laparotomy. The principle of surgery is similar to ovarian cystectomy. Bleeding points are electrocoagulated by bipolar diathermy. In a small size chocolate cyst, the contents are aspirated and the cavity is irrigated repeatedly. This may be done under TVS guidance or laparoscopically under anesthesia.

Q.53 What is the overall result of laparoscopic cystectomy for endometrioma?
Ans. It is effective in relieving pain in about 74% of cases of mild to moderate disease. Pregnancy rate is about 60% in cases with moderate disease. However, improved pregnancy rate is observed within the first 6 months of conservative surgery.

CASE 4: PELVIC PAIN

Case Summary
Mrs CM, 36-year-old lady, had been suffering from lower abdominal pain and severe deep dyspareunia for last 8 months.

Q.54 What are the common causes of acute pelvic pain in gynecology?
Ans.
- Acute pelvic inflammatory disease (PID)
- Ruptured chocolate cyst
- Twisted ovarian cyst
- Ruptured corpus luteum cyst
- Disturbed tubal ectopic pregnancy
- Ovarian hyperstimulation syndrome.

Q.55 What are the common causes of chronic pelvic pain?
Ans.
- Dysmenorrhea
- Premenstrual tension syndrome
- Pelvic endometriosis
- Ovarian remnant syndrome—trapped or residual ovarian syndrome
- Psychosomatic
- Pelvic vericosities
- Uterine fibroid
- Adenomyosis
- Ovarian cyst
- Pelvic inflammatory disease (PID) (chronic)
- Retroversion or prolapse of the uterus

Q.56 What are the causes of dyspareunia?
Ans. *Superficial*
- Narrow introitus
- Tough hymen
- Tender perineal scar
- Vulval infection
- Vulvar vestibulitis syndrome
- Vaginal—septum, infection, agenesis.

Deep
- Pelvic endometriosis
- Chronic PID
- Prolapsed ovary in the polycystic ovarian disease (POD).

Q.57 Mention some of the important causes of postmenopausal bleeding.
Ans.
- Senile endometritis
- Senile vaginitis
- Dysfunctional uterine bleeding
- Decubitus ulcer
- Genital malignancy:
    - Carcinoma of the cervix, endometrium, vagina, vulva, fallopian tube
    - Uterine sarcoma.
- Retained foreign body—pessary, IUCD (Fig. 1.7)
- Urethral caruncle
- Withdrawal bleeding following estrogen intake.

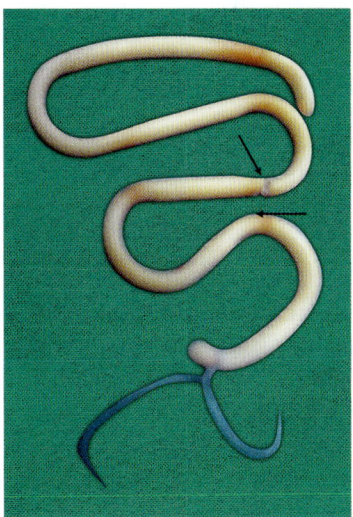

Fig. 1.7: Lippes loop. This has been removed from a 65-year-old lady hysteroscopically. She presented with postmenopausal bleeding. She had this at her age of 27 years. It was embeded within the endometrium and became brittle (arrows).

CASE 5: HYDATIDIFORM MOLE

Case Summary

Mrs AL, 24-year-old lady, was admitted in her first pregnancy at 16 weeks of amenorrhea with vaginal bleeding and passage of grape-like structures. On examination she looked pale, uterus was found 20 weeks size. There was no FHS on auscultation.

Q.58 What is the provisional diagnosis?
Ans. Hydatidiform mole.

Q.59 What investigations should be done for her?
Ans. Ultrasonography of the uterus (Fig. 1.8) and urine or serum for β-hCG. Once the diagnosis is confirmed, other investigations are complete hemogram, ABO and Rh-grouping, LFT and X-ray chest and thyroid profile.

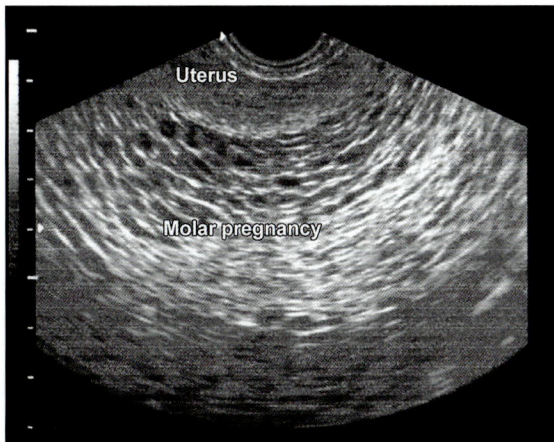

Fig. 1.8: Ultrasonography—snowstorm appearance in hydatidiform mole.
Courtesy: Dr (Mrs) S Ghosh, Professor BN Chakravorty, IRM Kolkata, India.

Q.60 What is the initial management for this problem?
Ans.
- Correction of anemia with blood transfusion
- To prevent infection
- Suction and evacuation of the uterus with or without oxytocin drip should be done. Tissue should be sent for histological examination.

Q.61 What are the common complications of this problem?
Ans.
- Hemorrhage
- Infection
- Pre-eclampsia
- Perforation of the uterus
- Respiratory distress due to pulmonary embolization of trophoblastic cells
- Coagulation failure
- Development of choriocarcinoma (2–10% cases).

Q.62 How should this patient be followed up and for how long?
Ans. Serial urinary β-hCG estimation weekly till negative. Usually, it becomes negative by 4–6 weeks time. Once negative, she is followed up at every month with serum hCG report for 6 months to 1 year.

Q.63 What precautionary measures she should be advised while on follow-up?
Ans. She should avoid pregnancy for at least 6 months to 1 year. For contraception, she can use barrier methods. Combined oral pills (low dose) may be used following normalization of β-hCG.

Q.64 What are the reasons that the patient needs to be followed up following initial treatment?
Ans.
- Detection of cases with persistent trophoblastic disease.
- Early detection of choriocarcinoma.

Q.65 What is her prospect of future pregnancy and chance of recurrence of the problem?
Ans. Prospect of future successful pregnancy is high, provided she is followed up. The risk of recurrence is less than 5%.

Q.66 What is the karyotype pattern of a complete hydatidiform mole and that of a partial mole?
Ans. In complete moles—karyotype pattern in majority is normal—46XX (90%). There is fertilization of 'an empty ovum' by a single sperm carrying 23 chromosomes. The usual 46XX chromosome pattern is the result of doubling of the paternal set of chromosomes (Fig. 1.9).

In about 10% cases, an empty ovum is fertilized by two sperm (dispermy), one carrying X and the other carrying Y chromosome. The chromosomal pattern is 46XY. All the chromosomes are derived paternally.

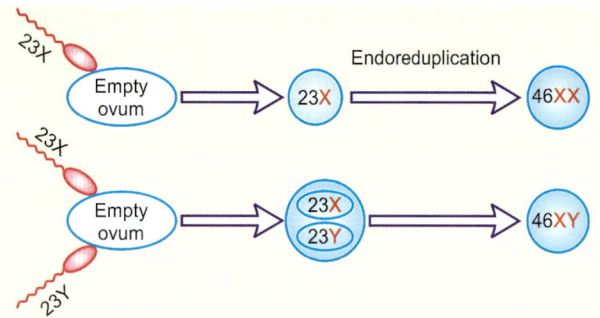

Fig. 1.9: Karyotype pattern of a complete mole—genome is entirely paternal in origin.

Partial moles (Fig. 1.10) consist of both the placenta and the fetus. Partial moles usually (90%) have triploid karyotype (Fig. 1.11). A normal ovum is fertilized by double sperm (dispermy), resulting in 69 chromosomes with sex chromosome configuration of 69XXX, 69XXY and 69XYY. The extra haploid set of chromosomes usually is derived from the father. The fetus is usually triploid, dies in the first trimester or is growth retarded with multiple malformations (syndactyly, hydrocephaly).

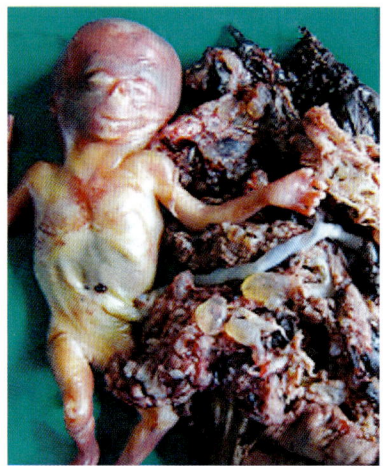

Fig. 1.10: Partial mole with a stillborn baby.
Courtesy: Dr S Mitra, Professor, Department of G and O, KPC Medical College, Kolkata.

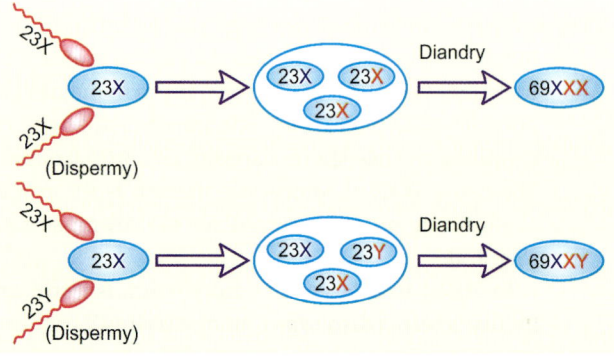

Fig. 1.11: Triploid chromosomal pattern of a partial mole. Genome is both paternal and maternal in origin.

CASE 6: CERVICAL FIBROID

Case Summary

Mrs CR, 40-year-old, had undergone surgery to remove her pathology. The specimen is seen in Figure 1.12.

Q.67 What is the diagnosis?
Ans. Posterior cervical fibroid.

Q.68 With what signs and symptoms she may have presented?
Ans. Vaginal discharge, pressure symptoms:
- **Bowel:** Constipation, incomplete evacuation.
- **Urinary:** Frequency, retention.
- Lateral pelvic wall pressure to cause leg pain or edema.

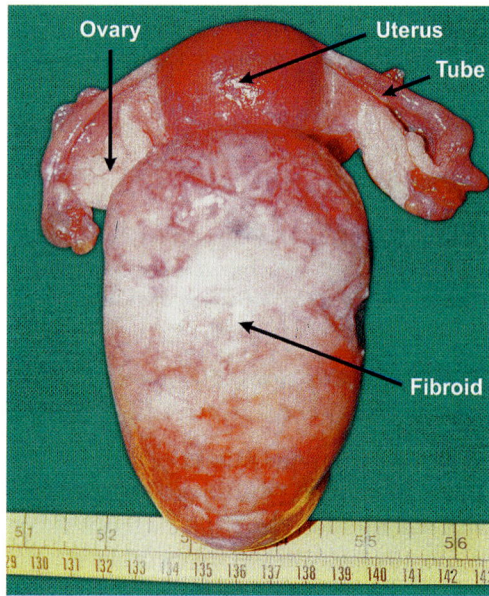

Fig. 1.12: Huge cervical fibroid.

Q.69 What surgery had been done for her?
Ans. Total abdominal hysterectomy with bilateral salpingo-oophorectomy.

Q.70 What are the dangers of this operation?
Ans. Hemorrhage, injury to bladder, rectum and the ureter.

Q.71 How the dangers could be minimized?
Ans.
- Delineation of the course as well as the proximity of the ureters to the fibroid could be done preoperatively by intravenous urography.
- Ureteric catheterization may be done preoperatively as a precautionary measure.
- Enucleation of the myoma first followed by hysterectomy.
- Preoperative GnRH analog therapy for 3 months may facilitate surgery.

CASE 7: MENOPAUSE AND HORMONE REPLACEMENT THERAPY (HRT)

Case Summary

Mrs VL, 55-year-old school teacher, was seen in the clinic for the problem of postmenopausal bleeding. She did not have any history of pelvic pain, recent weight gain or weight loss. Clinical examination did not reveal any abnormality.

Q.72 What are the common causes of postmenopausal bleeding?

Ans. Senile vaginitis, senile endometritis, cervical carcinoma, endometrial carcinoma.

Q.73 What investigations should you organize for her?

Ans. Ultrasonography to assess endometrial thickness and/or any of the biopsy methods as:
- Pipelle endometrial biopsy
- Hysteroscopy and endometrial biopsy
- Fractional curettage and endometrial biopsy.

Q.74 What abnormality will guide her to go for hysterectomy?

Ans. Significant endometrial pathology and risks of endometrial carcinoma are as follows:

Type of endometrial hyperplasia and the risk of endometrial carcinoma.

Typical
- Simple (cystic without atypia): 1%
- Complex (adenomatous without atypia): 3%.

Atypical
- Simple (cystic with atypia): 8%
- Complex (adenomatous with atypia): 29%
  The risk of malignancy with atypical hyperplasia is high. This may necessitate hysterectomy.

She is aware of menopause and osteoporosis. She wants to know the following.

Q.75 Has she got any of the risk factors for osteoporosis?

Ans. Risk factors are:
- Family history
- Early menopause
- Low body weight
- Excess caffeine intake
- Smoking
- Sedentary habit or use of some drugs (corticosteroids).

Q.76 What preventive measures can she take to prevent osteoporosis?

Ans. Exercise, adequate dietary intake of calcium, vitamin D and nonhormonal treatment (biphosphonate) or HRT.

Q.77 What HRT would be appropriate for her?

Ans. If the uterus is intact, combined estrogen and progestin cyclically. Progestin is added for last 12–14 days of each month or she can have low dose estrogen and progestin combined and continuous. Otherwise, following hysterectomy she should take estrogen only. There is reduction in the risk of osteoporosis, coronary heart disease and colon cancer.

Q.78 What other benefits can she have with HRT?

Ans.
- Improvement of vasomotor symptoms (hot flushes, night sweats)
- Prevention of atrophic changes in the skin, genital and urinary tract epithelium
- Protection against cardiovascular disease
- Reduction in the problems of anxiety, insomnia, irritability and depression.

Q.79 Is there any risk for continuing HRT?

Ans. In a well-selected case, risks are generally less compared to the benefits. In most of the studies (WHO 2003, Million Women Study 2003), there is no increased risk of breast cancer when estrogen is only used (in a hysterectomized woman). Currently low dose estrogen (conjugated equine estrogen 0.3 mg or ethinyl estradiol 1 mg) is recommended. However, the woman needs to be counseled.

But regular breast self-examination (BSE) monthly, clinical breast examination (CBE) yearly and mammography yearly (ACOG-2000) should be carried out as a part of breast screening.

There is an increased risk of deep vein thrombosis (DVT) from 10 to 30 per 10,000 users.

Q.80 What are the contraindications of HRT?

Ans. Contraindications are:
- Undiagnosed genital tract bleeding
- Estrogen-dependent cancer in the body
- Active liver disease
- History of venous thromboembolism
- Gallbladder disease.

Q.81 What are different routes through which HRT can be administered?

Ans. HRT can be administered orally, through the skin as patches, gel, subcutaneous implant or nasal spray. It can also be administered by vaginal route as creams or pessaries. Use of oral route and the first pass liver metabolism has its beneficial effects on the lipoproteins.

Q.82 How long can HRT be taken?

Ans. The optimal duration of use for HRT is currently debatable. Small dose and short-term use for a period of 3–5 years has been recommended for bone protection.

B. ADOLESCENT GYNECOLOGY

CASE 8: PRIMARY AMENORRHEA

Case Summary

A 18-year-old school girl has been seen in the gyne clinic due to failure to commence menstruation. Secondary sex characters were well-developed. On systemic examination there was no abnormality. Pelvic examination revealed as shown in Figure 1.13.

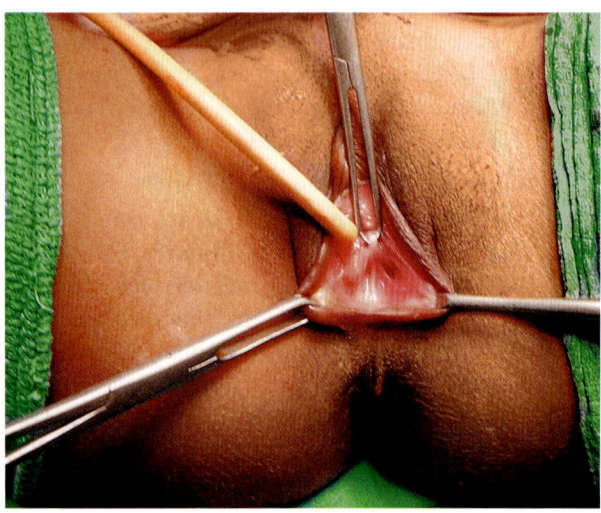

Fig. 1.13: Complete absence of vagina.

Q.83 What is most likely the diagnosis?
Ans. A case of vaginal agenesis.

Q.84 How do you define primary amenorrhea?
Ans. A young girl who has not menstruated by 16 years of age is defined as primary amenorrhea.

Q.85 When do you start investigations for primary amenorrhea?
Ans.
- No menstruation by the age of 16 years, when other secondary sex characters are normal.
- No menstruation by the age of 14 years when there is absence of growth and/or development of secondary sex characters.

Q.86 What are the factors essential for the onset and continuation of normal menstruation?
Ans.
- Normal female chromosomal pattern (46XX).
- Coordinated function of the hypothalamopituitary ovarian axis.
- Anatomical presence and patency of the outflow tract.
- Responsive endometrium.
- Active support of thyroid and adrenal gland.

Q.87 What is cryptomenorrhea?
Ans. It is a condition where the menstrual blood fails to come out from the genital tract due to an obstruction present in the passage.

Q.88 What are the common causes of cryptomenorrhea?
Ans.
- **Congenital**
  - Imperforate hymen
  - Transverse vaginal septum.
- **Acquired**
  - Cervical stenosis following amputation
  - Vaginal stricture following traumatic (instrumental delivery).

Q.89 What are the common causes of primary amenorrhea?
Ans.
- **Hypogonadotrophic hypogonadism**
  - Delayed puberty
  - Hypothalamic and pituitary dysfunction (stress, weight loss, anorexia nervosa)
  - Kallmann syndrome
  - CNS tumors—craniopharyngioma.
- **Hypergonadotrophic hypogonadism**
  - Primary ovarian failure
  - Galactosemia.
- **Abnormal chromosomal pattern**
  - Turner's syndrome (45X)
  - Various mosaic states (45X/46XX)
  - Testicular feminization (46XY).
- **Developmental defect of genital tract**
  - Müllerian agenesis (MRKH syndrome)
  - Imperforate hymen
  - Transverse vaginal septum
  - Vaginal agenesis (Fig. 1.13).
- **Thyroid and adrenal disorders**
- **Metabolic disorders (juvenile diabetes)**
- **Systemic illness (tuberculosis)**
- **Others:** Uterine synechiae, unresponsive endometrium (receptor defect).

Q.90 What are the characteristic features of Mayer-Rokitansky-Kuster-Hauser syndrome?
Ans.
- Stature—average
- Breasts—normal
- Sexual hair—normal
- External genitalia—normal
- Internal genitalia:
  - Vagina—absent
  - Uterus—absent/rudimentary
  - Ovaries—normal
  - Karyotype—normal (46XX)
  - IVP—Urinary tract abnormalities (30%)
- Primary amenorrhea.

Q.91 What are the characteristic features of Turner's syndrome?
Ans.
- Stature—short.
- Secondary sex character—poorly developed

- Webbing of the neck
- Shield chest
- Wide apart nipples
- Cubitus valgus
- Coarctation of aorta
- 'Streak' gonads
- Serum gonadotropins—high
- Karyotype: 45XO or 45XO/46XX (Fig. 1.14)
- Primary amenorrhea.

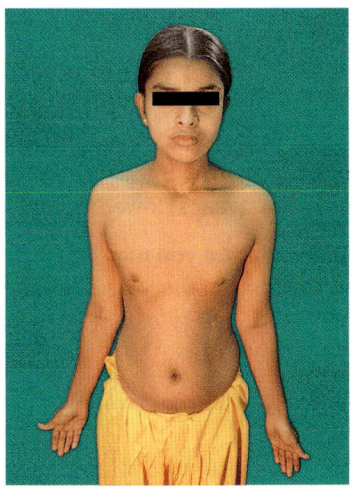

Fig. 1.14: A 19-year-old girl with features of Turner's syndrome. Karyotype: 45XO.

Q.92 What are the characteristic features of androgen insensitivity syndrome [testicular feminization syndrome (Fig. 1.15)]?

Ans.
- Stature—average
- Scanty pubic and axillary hair
- Breast development—normal
- Vagina—short and blind
- Uterus and tubes—absent
- Gonads—at labia or intra-abdominal or at inguinal region
- Gonadal biopsy—testicular tissue
- Serum testosterone—equal to normal males
- Karyotype: 46XY
- Primary amenorrhea.

Q.93 What are the characteristic features of adrenogenital syndrome? (Fig. 1.16)

Ans.
- Stature: Average
- Phenotypically: Normal female

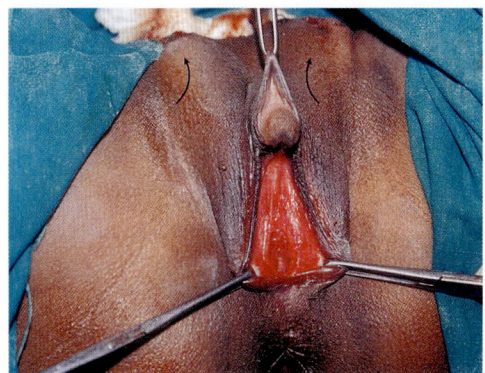

Fig. 1.15: Testicular feminization syndrome showing short and blind vagina, scanty pubic hair, clitoromegaly and labial gonads (arrows).

- Labial fusion
- Enlargement of clitoris
- Uterus: Normal
- Ovaries: Normal
- Vagina: Normal
- Karyotype: 46XX
- Serum 17-OHP: Elevated
- Urinary pregnanetriol: Elevated
- Primary amenorrhea.

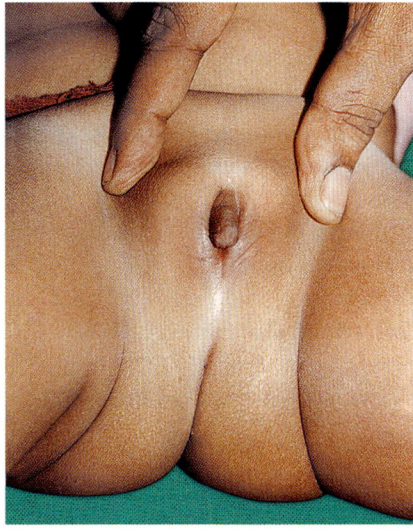

Fig. 1.16: A 14-month-old girl with adrenogenital syndrome showing labial fusion and enlarged clitoris. Congenital adrenal hyperplasia is commonly due to 21-hydroxylase deficiency.

C. MENSTRUAL ABNORMALITIES

CASE 9: SECONDARY AMENORRHEA

Case Summary

Mrs JL, 42-year-old woman, was seen in the gyne clinic with the problem of cessation of menstruation for the last 7 months. Her urine test for pregnancy was negative.

Q.94 What is her present problem?
Ans. Secondary amenorrhea.

Q.95 How do you define secondary amenorrhea?
Ans. It is the absence of menstruation for 6 months or more in a woman who has menstruated normally in the past.

Q.96 What are the common 'uterine factors' that may cause secondary amenorrhea?
Ans.
- Tubercular endometritis
- Synechiae
- Surgical removal (hysterectomy)
- Transcervical resection of endometrium (TCRE).

Q.97 What are the 'ovarian factors' that may cause secondary amenorrhea?
Ans.
- Polycystic ovarian syndrome
- Premature ovarian failure
- Surgical removal
- Radiation.

Q.98 Dysgenetic gonads are the common 'hypothalamic factors' that may cause secondary amenorrhea?
Ans.
- Stress
- Anorexia nervosa
- Strenuous exercise
- Trauma
- Infection (tuberculosis)
- Psychogenic drugs (phenothiazine)
- Tumors (craniopharyngioma, meningioma).

Q.99 What are the common causes of secondary amenorrhea?
Ans.
- Stress
- Polycystic ovary syndrome (PCOS)
- Premature ovarian failure
- Synechiae (Asherman's syndrome)
- Drugs (phenothiazine)
- Postpill amenorrhea.

Q.100 What is PCOS?
Ans. See Ch 8.

CASE 10: HEMATOCOLPOS (CRYPTOMENORRHEA)

Case Summary

Miss LN, 17-year-old young girl, presented in the outpatient clinic with cyclical lower abdominal pain. She had normal physical growth and development of secondary sexual characters. Pelvic examination revealed as shown in Figure 1.17.

Q.101 What is the diagnosis?
Ans. Imperforate hymen with hematocolpos.

Q.102 What other symptoms she might have?
Ans. Urinary retention, dysuria, lower abdominal heaviness and cyclical lower abdominal pain.

Q.103 What investigation you may do for her?
Ans. Ultrasonography of the lower abdomen to ascertain the extent of pathology, e.g., hematocolpos, hematometra, hematosalpinx.

Q.104 What would be the appropriate treatment for her?
Ans. Incision (cruciate) and drainage under general anesthesia, antibiotic coverage.

Q.105 What is the prospect of her future reproductive career?
Ans. Normal.

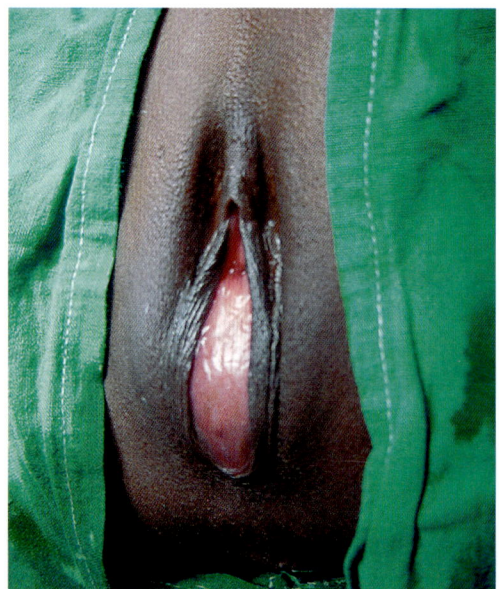

Fig. 1.17: Hematocolpos showing the hymen tense, bluish and bulged.

Q.106 What is the basic underlying abnormality of this condition?

Ans. It is due to failure of disintegration of the central cells of the Müllerian eminence that projects into the urogenital sinus. Depending upon the amount of blood so collected, it may present with hematocolpos (blood in the vagina), hematometra (blood in the uterus) or hematosalpinx (blood within the fallopian tubes).

Q.107 What is crypyomenorrhea?

Ans. There is periodic shedding of the endometrium and bleeding but the menstrual blood fails to come out from the genital tract due to obstruction in the passage.

Q.108 What are the common causes?

Ans.
- **Congenital:**
  - Imperforate hymen
  - Transverse vaginal septum
  - Vaginal atresia in the upper part
- **Acquired:**
  - Stenosis of the cervix following amputation, conization
  - Secondary vaginal atresia following difficult vaginal delivery.

D. INFERTILITY

CASE 11: INFERTILITY—A

Case Summary

A 28-year-old woman has been seen for her problem of primary infertility. Her husband's semen analysis was normal. On further investigation she was found to suffer from anovulation. Her tubes were patent.

Q.109 According to WHO, how the ovulatory disorders are classified?

Ans. *Group I:* Hypothalamic-pituitary failure (hypogonadotrophic hypogonadism).
Group II: Hypothalamic pituitary dysfunction (normogonadotrophic normogonadism).
Group III: Ovarian failure (hypergonadotropic hypogonadism).

Q.110 How the problems of anovulatory infertility is treated?

Ans. Induction of ovulation is done. Different drugs are used depending upon the response. Clomiphene citrate is the commonly used drug. It is usually prescribed 50 mg twice daily from D-3 to D-7 (5 days) of the cycle. Ovulation usually occurs 5–7 days after the last day of therapy.

Q.111 What are the indications of gonadotrophin therapy for induction of ovulation?

Ans. Women with infertility due to:
- Hypogonadotrophic hypogonadism (WHO group I)
- Women who have either failed or are resistant to clomiphene citrate (WHO group II)
- Women with unexplained infertility.

Q.112 When are GnRH analogs used for induction of ovulation?

Ans.
- Patients who are refractory to gonadotropins.
- Patients with elevated LH.
- Patients with premature ovulation due to premature LH surge.
- Patients with premature follicular luteinization.

Q.113 How do you manage the woman with WHO groups I, II or III ovulatory disorders?

Ans. *WHO group I*
- Gonadotropins: Follicle-stimulating hormone (FSH), LH.
- GnRH (pulsatile).

WHO group II
- Clomiphene citrate
- FSH
- For premature LH surges—GnRH agonist/antagonist
- For insulin resistance—insulin sensitizer
- Adrenal androgens—glucocorticoids.

WHO group III
- Cyclic hormone replacement therapy
- Gonadotropins—high dose
- Chance of spontaneous pregnancy—occasional
- Assisted reproductive technology (ART) (*See* Ch 23)
- Oocyte donation.

Q.114 What are the different types of surgery done for the management of infertility?

Ans. Surgery may be needed both for female as well as male factors for infertility.

For female
- Laparoscopic ovarian diathermy (drilling) (LOD).
- Wedge resection of ovary in cases with PCOS (not commonly done) (*See* Ch 54).
- Surgery for pituitary prolactinomas.
- Salpingo-ovariolysis—laparoscopically.
- Proximal tubal block: Cannulation and balloon tuboplasty: This is done under hysteroscopic guidance.
- Midtubal block: Recanalization procedure (reversal of tubal ligation).
- Distal tubal block:
  - Fimbrioplasty
  - Neosalpingostomy
- Tubal reconstruction (tuboplasty) following sterilization operation.

Q.115 What is assisted reproductive technology (ART)? What are the different methods of ART?

Ans. ART encompasses all procedures that involve manipulation of gametes and embryos for the treatment of infertility. For the rest (*See* Ch 23).

Q.116 What are the indications of in vitro fertilization-embryo transfer (IVF-ET)?

Ans.
- Tubal disease
- Unexplained infertility
- Endometriosis
- Male factor infertility
- Cervical hostility
- Failed ovulation induction.

Q.117 What are the indications of intrauterine insemination (IUI)?

Ans.
- Cervical stenosis
- Immunological factors for infertility (male and female)
- Oligospermia or asthenospermia
- Unexplained infertility.

Q.118 What are the principle steps of an ART cycle?
Ans.
- Down regulation using GnRH analog
- Controlled ovarian stimulation (COS)
- Monitoring of follicular growth
- Oocyte retrieval
- Fertilization *in vitro* [IVF, intracytoplasmic sperm injection (ICSI)]
- Transfer of gametes or embryos
- Luteal support with progesterone.

Q.119 How is the monitoring of follicular growth done?
Ans. It is done by:
- Sonographic (TVS) measurement of follicular diameter
- Serum estradiol level 3 or more follicles > 18 mm in diameter and serum E_2 levels: 100–150 pg/mL/follicle is optimum. Injection hCG 5000–10,000 IU is given IM. Oocytes are retrieved 36 hours after hCG administration.

Q.120 What is the procedure for embryo transfer?
Ans. Transfer is done at 4–8 cell stage (48–72 hours later) transcervically. Usually two embryos are transferred.

Q.121 What is ovarian hyperstimulation syndrome (OHSS)?
Ans. It is characterized by multiple follicular development and ovarian enlargement following hCG stimulation. It may be a serious complication.

It is clinically manifested by bilateral ovarian enlargement, abdominal pain, nausea, vomiting, ascites, hypotension, hemoconcentration, oliguria, disseminated intravascular coagulation (DIC), thrombosis and sometimes adult respiratory distress syndrome.

Q.122 How can OHSS be prevented and managed?
Ans. *See* Dutta's Textbook of Gynecology, 8th Edition, p. 444.

Q.123 How endometrial receptivity could be improved in an IVF cycle?
Ans. Exact understanding of endometrial receptivity is lacking. Importance of many adhesion molecules (integrins) have been considered. However supplemental progesterone therapy is started after oocyte retrieval in all IVF programs as a routine. This is mainly because GnRH analog use and oocyte aspiration impair the secretion of endogenous progesterone from the ovary (corpus luteum).

Q.124 How is egg retrieval done in an IVF cycle?
Ans. Ultrasound-guided needle aspiration of oocyte through the vagina is done. This is done under IV sedation. The complications may be injury to bowel, bladder or infection.

Q.125 How can a man without any sperm to ejaculate, father children?
Ans. ICSI is the optimum procedure for this man, if he can produce sperm on testicular biopsy. ICSI is also helpful to men with congenital absence of vas deferens.

Q.126 Should a woman with hydrosalpinx be considered for IVF-ET?
Ans. IVF is considered to bypass the function of the blocked tubes. But presence of hydrosalpinges causes implantation failure with reduced pregnancy rate in IVF cycles. So, it is recommended to remove the tubes (prophylactic salpingectomy) prior to IVF in these women. The tubes may be clipped laparoscopically to get the same benefits.

CASE 12: INFERTILITY—B

Case Summary

Mrs ZR, 26-year-old, $P_{0+0+1+0}$ woman with H/O one previous miscarriage, presented in the clinic with problems of inability to conceive. Hormone study revealed that she is ovulating and the report of her husband's semen analysis (done recently) was normal. She had an investigation as shown in Figure 1.18.

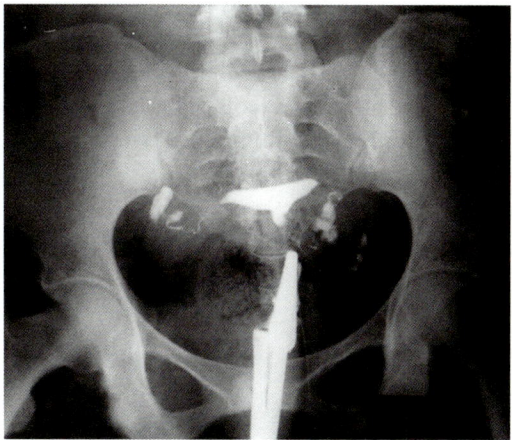

Fig. 1.18: Hysterosalpingogram showing bilateral hydrosalpinx without any spillage of dye.

Q.127 What is this investigation?
Ans. Hysterosalpingography.

Q.128 What is the pathology revealed by the procedure?
Ans. Bilateral hydrosalpinx without any spillage of dye.

Q.129 What is the basic pathology for this abnormality?
Ans. In majority, it is the sequelae of ascending infection from the lower genital tract. *Chlamydia trachomatis* (85%), *N. gonorrhoeae* and other pyogenic infections (*E. coli*) are responsible. Mixed infections (aerobic and anaerobic) are more common. Infection and inflammation cause destruction of tubal epithelium and pus formation known as ***pyosalpinx***. There is

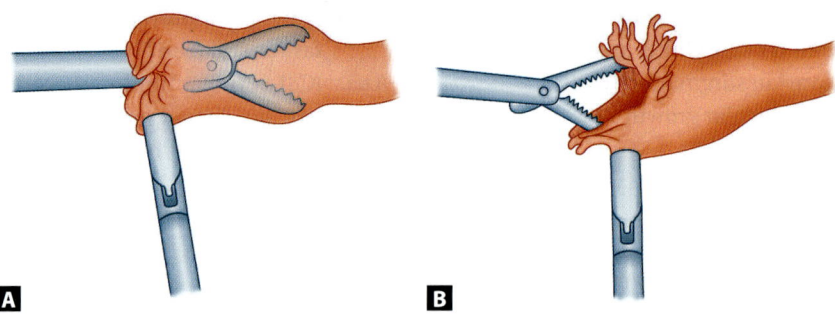

Figs. 1.19A and B: (A) Laparoscopic fimbrioplasty by introducing the closed forceps within the closed ostium; (B) The phimotic ostium is opened up and the fimbrial folds are released by opening up the forceps blades.

peritubal adhesion formation and agglutination of the fimbriae. Gradually when the inflammation subsides, the pus settles down and the tube is filled with a clear fluid called **hydrosalpinx**. The tube is dilated, retort-shaped with closed abdominal ostium.

Q.130 Is there any other method of evaluation?
Ans. Diagnostic laparoscopy and chromopertubation under general anesthesia. It may reveal tubal edema, hyperemia, dilated tubes (hydrosalpinx), fimbrial adhesion and/or peritubal adhesions.

Q.131 What are the treatment options that may resolve her problem of infertility?
Ans. Tubal reconstructive surgery (tuboplasty) may be attempted. This may be in the form of releasing the peritubal adhesions (adhesiolysis) and/or opening up the fimbrial end (fimbrioplasty or salpingostomy).

As the tubal epithelium is often destroyed, the results of such operations are not always successful. Pregnancy rate following laparoscopic fimbrioplasty is 30–35%. Ectopic pregnancy rate is 5–10% (Figs. 1.19A and B).

Q.132 What other options are left to her?
Ans. Assisted reproduction—IVF-ET.

Q.133 What are the different methods of assisted reproductive technology that you know?
Ans.

> **IVF-ET:** *In vitro* fertilization and embryo transfer
> **GIFT:** Gamete intrafallopian transfer
> **ICSI:** Intracytoplasmic sperm injection
> **TESE:** Testicular sperm extraction
> **MESA:** Microsurgical epididymal sperm aspiration
> **PESA:** Percutaneous epididymal sperm aspiration

E. ONCOLOGY

CASE 13: HYSTERECTOMY AND OOPHORECTOMY

Case Summary

Mrs CJ, 46-year-old, parous, woman had been admitted for hysterectomy due to the problem of multiple fibroid uterus. She had been adequately counseled for this operation. She is further interested to know about the current status of prophylactic-oophorectomy during hysterectomy. You have to discuss with her in this regard.

Q.134 What are the risks of bilateral oophorectomy during hysterectomy?

Ans. Risks are mainly due to loss of endocrine function of the ovaries. Loss of estradiol function is significant. Moreover, ovarian stroma secretes androgen precursors which are converted to estrogen in adipose tissue (peripheral endocrine organs). Major health hazards following oophorectomy are osteoporosis, fracture and cardiovascular risk. Additional morbidities are due to atrophy of the genital and urinary organs (dyspareunia, dysuria), vasomotor instability (hot flushes) and psychological disturbances (irritability, insomnia, mood swing).

Q.135 What are the benefits of doing bilateral oophorectomy during hysterectomy?

Ans. Bilateral oophorectomy protects the woman against the risks of developing ovarian cancer (100%) and peritoneal cancer (95%). It reduces residual ovarian syndrome (3–5%) and risks of relaparotomy (5–10%) for any benign or malignant ovarian lesions. It also reduces the risk of breast cancer by 50%. It eliminates the problems of chronic pelvic pain and dyspareunia.

Q.136 What is the risk of age (46 years in this case) in developing ovarian cancer?

Ans. Yes, this age has its own independent risk. The current information about the age and the risk of ovarian cancer as follows:

> Age < 40 years = infrequent; age 40–45 years = 15–16/100,000; age 60–70 years = 57/100,000 and the median age for ovarian cancer is 63 years.

Q.137 What are the benefits and risks of hysterectomy alone in relation to ovarian cancer and menopause problems?

Ans. The current information in this regard is, a woman who had undergone hysterectomy alone had a long-term reduced risk of epithelial ovarian cancer. However, hysterectomy is associated with earlier onset of menopause (3.7–4.4 years) even if the ovaries are preserved.

Q.138 What is familial ovarian cancer and how common it is?

Ans. Mutations of certain genes (*BRCA1* and *BRCA2*) are associated with higher risk of ovarian and breast cancers. However, of all the epithelial ovarian cancers 1 out of 10 is hereditary. Familial ovarian cancer has an earlier onset of disease.

Q.139 Is there any current guidelines for prophylaxis of oophorectomy during hysterectomy?

Ans. Nothing is specifically recommended till date. It should be based on individual woman's risk and the family history. However, prophylactic oophorectomy during hysterectomy is performed at a median age of 48 years or 5 years before the index case with the family history of ovarian cancer whichever is earlier. Once oophorectomy is done, management of surgical menopause with nonhormonal or hormonal method should be considered.

All these needs informed consent of the individual concerned.

CASE 14: POSTMENOPAUSAL BLEEDING

Case Summary

Mrs AB, 58-year-old woman presented with postmenopausal bleeding (PMB). She was thoroughly investigated and diagnosed to have endometrial carcinoma. Her clinical staging (FIGO) was stage IB, G2. You are asked to discuss the pros and cons of different risk factors, investigations and the stage of endometrial carcinoma.

Q.140 What are the common causes of PMB?

Ans. In the developing countries including India genital malignancy particularly carcinoma cervix is the most common cause of PMB. Other causes are:
- Atrophic endometritis
- Endometrial hyperplasia
- Endometrial polyps
- Dysfunctional uterine bleeding (DUB)
- Decubitus ulcer
- Retained (forgotten) pessary or IUCD (Fig. 1.20)
- Endometrial carcinoma.

Q.141 Who are the high-risk women to develop endometrial carcinoma?

Ans.
- Unopposed estrogen stimulation
- Delayed menopause
- Hypertension
- Diabetes
- Overweight (50 pounds overweight increases the risk by 10 times)
- Nulliparity

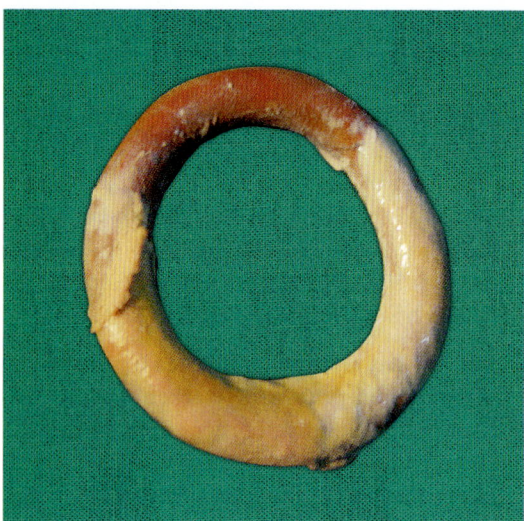

Fig. 1.20: Rubber ring pessary. This had been removed from a 70-year-old woman. She presented with postmenopausal bleeding. She had been using this for last 20 years. This forgotten pessary caused ulceration and infection in the vagina. Crust had been formed on its surface due to its prolonged stay in the vagina.

- Polycystic ovary syndrome (PCOS)
- Tamoxifen therapy
- Family history of endometrial, breast, ovary or colon carcinoma.

Q.142 What is the significance of family history?

Ans. Lynch II syndrome is observed in about 2% of all such cases of hereditary cancers. Such families display high incidence of hereditary nonpolyposis colorectal cancer (HNPCC), adenocarcinoma of ovary, endometrium, stomach, small bowel and the urinary tract. It is associated with mutations in the DNA mismatch repair (MMR) genes (*MSH2, MLH1, PMS1* or *MSH6*).

Q.143 What is the current change in the trends of diagnosis of endometrial cancer?

Ans. Most gynecologists recommend outpatient endometrial biopsy to confirm the diagnosis. Diagnostic accuracy of outpatient endometrial biopsy using pipelle endometrial sampler is 90–98%. Besides pipelle endometrial sampler, Sherman curette, transvaginal ultrasonography, sonohysterography, hysteroscopy and directed biopsy are also used.

Q.144 What is the place of different procedures in the diagnosis of endometrial carcinoma?

Ans. Fractional curettage is a definite diagnostic procedure for endometrial cancer but it is invasive. Role of hysteroscopy in the diagnosis has certain advantages. To date, there is no universal agreement to the cut-off measurement of endometrial thickness to diagnose endometrial cancer. Endometrial thickness less than or equal to mm in a postmenopausal woman is commonly due to atrophy.

- Hysteroscopy is more accurate in detecting polyps or submucous fibroids. It helps to see the pathologic lesion as to take direct biopsy. It also helps to evaluate the endocervical canal.
- Saline infusion sonography (SIS) is helpful in differentiating patients with minimal endometrial tissue from patients with thickened endometrium or polyps.
- Fractional curettage is mandatory if endometrial sampling procedures fail to provide sufficient material for diagnostic evaluation or when the symptoms are persistent in spite of negative endometrial sampling.
- Considering the benefits most clinics prefer to do outpatient (office) endometrial biopsy as a first diagnostic step. When biopsy result is negative and further evaluation is needed, hysteroscopy and biopsy is done.

Q.145 What are the characteristics of type I and type II endometrial carcinoma?

Ans. *Differentiating features of type I and II endometrial carcinoma*

Clinical characters	Type I	Type II
Risk factor	Unopposed estrogen	Age
Occurrence	Common (85%)	Less common
Predisposing factor	Hyperestrogenic state	No such
Precursor endometrium	Atypical hyperplasia	May be atrophic
Age	Young (perimenopause)	Older (postmenopause)
Endometrial hyperplasia	Present	Absent
Tissue differentiation	Well	Poor
Myometrial invasion	Minimal	Deep
Histology	Endometrioid	Serous, clear
Molecular characters		
Ploidy	Polyploid	Aneuploid
HER2/neu overexpression	No	Yes
P-53	No	Yes
PTEN mutations	Yes	No
Prognosis	Favorable	Not favorable

Q.146 Are all endometrial cancers due to estrogenic stimulation?

Ans. Currently, two pathogenic types of endometrial carcinoma are being observed.

Type I: The majority (75–85%) belong to this group. Women having a persistent stimulation of endometrium with unopposed estrogen either endogenous or exogenous, run the risk of developing type I endometrial carcinoma.

Type II: Women with type II develop endometrial carcinoma without any estrogenic stimulation. Carcinoma develops not from the background of endometrial hyperplasia but may arise from an atrophic endometrium.

Estrogen dependent tumors develop in relatively younger perimenopausal women as opposed to the estrogen independent tumors that occur in older postmenopausal women. Tumors that are estrogen dependent have favorable prognosis compared to estrogen independent tumors. Based on molecular genetic studies, these two types of tumors have different pathogenetic pathways.

Q.147 What is the current situation of TVS, CT and MRI in the evaluation of endometrial cancer?

Ans. MRI is found to be superior to conventional CT in the assessment of depth of myometrial invasion. Studies have shown diagnostic accuracy of TVS is about the same (68–69%) compared to T_2-weighted MRI (68–74%) in evaluating myometrial invasion. However, contrast enhanced MRI is always superior to TVS and is found to be better when compared to CT even.

The accuracy of MRI in staging endometrial carcinoma has been reported to be 85% overall. Gadolinium enhanced images significantly improve accuracy.

There are certain clinical situations where assessment of endometrial carcinoma may be difficult (e.g., obesity) or may not be possible (e.g., contraindications for surgical staging or because of tumor spread). In such situations MRI has got distinct advantages to evaluate the disease.

Suggested Reading

1. Walker JL, Piedmonte MR, Spirots NM, et. al. Laparoscopy compared with laparotomy for comprehensive surgical staging of uterine cancer: Gynecologic Oncology Group Study LAP2. JClin Oncol. 2009;27:5331–6.

CASE 15: CARCINOMA CERVIX—A

Case Summary

A 47-year-old woman presented with the complaints of postcoital vaginal bleeding and persistent offensive vaginal discharge, pelvic examination revealed an ulcerated tumor arising from the cervix (Fig. 1.21). Biopsy revealed squamous cell carcinoma of the cervix.

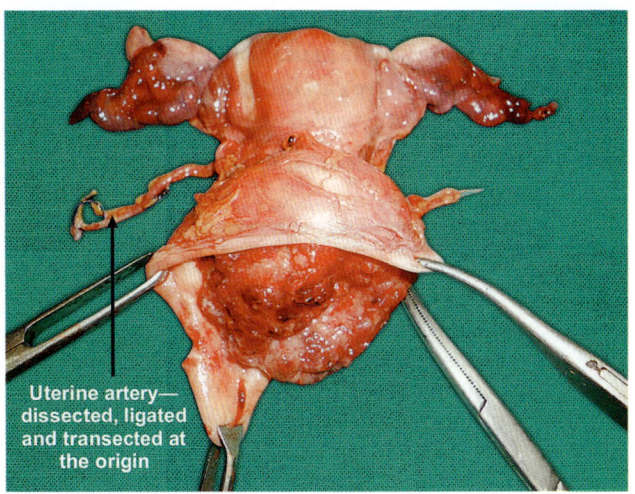

Fig. 1.21: Carcinoma cervix showing an exophytic growth with ulceration.

Q.148 Clinically, what are the different types of the lesion?

Ans. (i) Exophytic, (ii) Ulcerative, and (iii) Infiltrative.

Q.149 Histopathologically, what are the different types of carcinoma cervix?

Ans. (i) Squamous cell carcinoma (75–80%), (ii) Adenocarcinoma (20–25%), (iii) Adenosquamous carcinoma, (iv) Neuroendocrine tumors, and (v) Others: Lymphomas.

Q.150 What are the different modes of spread in carcinoma cervix?

Ans.
- Direct extension (parametrium, endocervix, vagina, bladder)
- Lymphatics (pelvic and para-aortic)
- Direct implantation
- Bloodstream (lung, mediastinum, bone, liver).

Q.151 What are the complications that may arise in a case with carcinoma cervix?

Ans.
- Hemorrhage
- Pain in the loin due to pyelitis, pyelonephritis
- Vesicovaginal fistula
- Rectovaginal fistula
- Uremia
- Sepsis.

Q.152 What are the advantages of radiotherapy as a primary modality of therapy?

Ans.
- Wider applicability in all stages of carcinoma cervix.
- Survival rate of radiotherapy (85%) is comparable to that of surgery in early stages.
- Less primary mortality or morbidity.

Q.153 Mention the different types of hysterectomy that can be done for the management of microinvasive and early invasive carcinoma cervix?

Ans. Classification of extended hysterectomy (ACOG–1974).

Rutledge's classification of extended hysterectomy (1974)

Class	Description	Indication
I	Extrafascial hysterectomy; pubocervical ligament is incised, allowing lateral deflection of the ureter	CIN, early stromal invasion
II	Removal of the medial half of the cardinal and uterosacral ligaments; upper third of the vagina	Microcarcinoma post-irradiation
III	Removal of the entire cardinal and uterosacral ligaments; upper third of the vagina removed	Stage IB and stage IIA tumors
IV	Removal of all periureteral tissue, superior vesical artery and three-fourths of the vagina	Anteriorly occurring central recurrences
V	Removal of portions of the distal ureter and bladder	Central recurrent cancer involving bladder and ureter

Q.154 What are the preventive measures against carcinoma cervix?

Ans. *Primary prevention*
- *Identifying and preventing the high-risk factors:* Preventing human papillomavirus (HPV) infection with HPV vaccine to all school girls (9–15 years).

Other risk factors (cofactors) to avoid are:
- Early sexual intercourse
- Early age of first pregnancy
- Multiple partners
- Too many births and too frequent births
- Poor local hygiene.

Secondary prevention:
- Screening against carcinoma cervix: cytology (liquid-based cytology), HPV testing (hybrid capture II), visual inspection with acetic acid (VIA), colposcopy and biopsy.
- 'Down staging screening' by WHO—intends to diagnose the disease early and to minimize cancer death.

Q.155 What is the role of HPV in the pathogenesis of carcinoma cervix?

Ans. HPV is a DNA virus which is epitheliotropic. High oncogenic risk HPV (types 16, 18, 31, 33, 35, 45, 56) types are responsible in the etiopathogenesis of cancer cervix (Fig. 1.22).

Over 99.7% of patients with CIN and invasive cancer are found to be positive with HPV-DNA. Infection always starts at the transformation zone (TZ) of the squamocolumnar junction (SCJ). Once the high-risk oncogenic HPV-DNA integration occurs within human (host) genome (infection), there is overexpression of E6 and E7 oncoproteins. These oncoproteins suppress the tumor suppressor genes [P-53 and retinoblastoma (Rb)]. This results in neoplastic transformation of the mitotically active metaplastic epithelium of the 'transformation zone' at

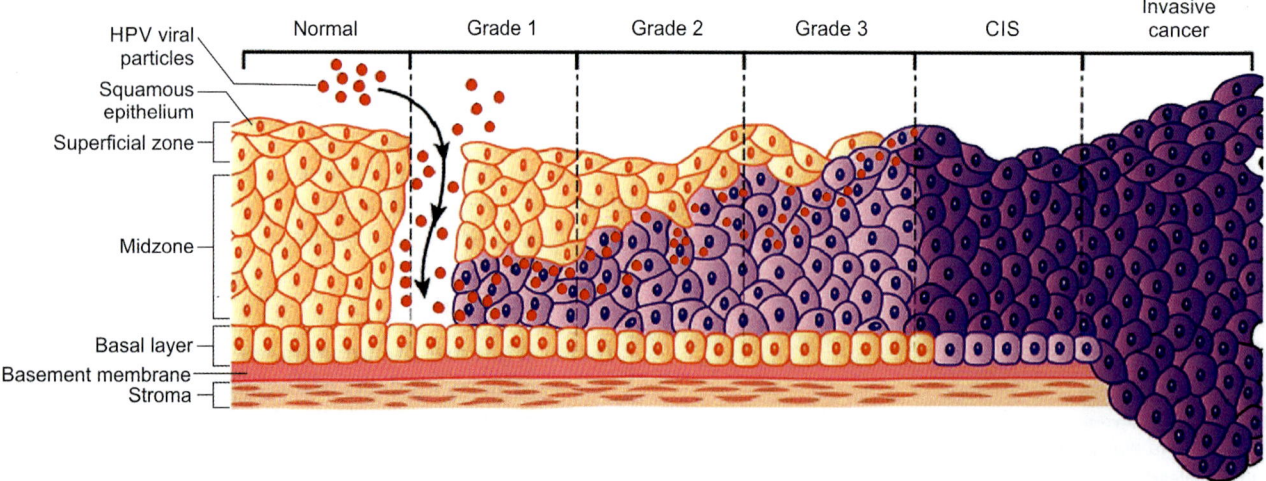

Fig. 1.22: Pathogenesis of HPV infection showing normal stratified squamous epithelium on the left and its progression to CIN/CIS and invasive on the right. The grades of CIN (I to III), CIS and the invasive carcinoma are shown.

the level of SCJ (*See* Dutta's Textbook of Gynecology, 8th Edition, p. 269). Normally the tumor suppressor gene P-53 will cause infected cell death by apoptosis and thus halting the viral multiplication. But these oncoproteins cause proteolytic degradation of P-53, resulting in cell immortalization and viral multiplication. Currently, HPV vaccines are available. Vaccines are very effective in preventing infection with HPV. Vaccines (Cervarix, Gardasil) are approved to all school girls (9–15 years) and women (16–26 years). Immunity persists for about 5–7.5 years. Vaccines are type specific and effective only when used prophylactically. Currently nonvalent vaccines are available. Single dose vaccine may be used and is found to be effective (61.6%).

Q.156 What are the advantages of surgery in the management of carcinoma cervix, over radiotherapy?

Ans.
- Thorough surgicopathological staging during surgery.
- Accurate prediction of survival rate by para-aortic and pelvic node assessment surgically.
- Preservation of ovarian function when desired.
- Retention of more functional and pliable vagina.
- Transposition of ovaries when needed for consideration of future radiotherapy.
- Psychological benefit of the woman.

Q.157 What is neoadjuvant chemotherapy and what are the benefits?

Ans. Platinum-based combination chemotherapy is given for three cycles. This is followed by radical hyterectomy and pelvic lymphadenectomy. Neoadjuvant chemotherapy improves the resectibility of bulky (4 cm) disease (stage IB2 and stage IIA).

Q.158 What is concurrent chemoradiation?

Ans. It is the combined therapy with radiation and weekly cisplatin-based combination chemotherapy. This therapy is found helpful as a primary treatment for stage IB, IIA or advanced stage (IIB to IVA) disease.

Q.159 How the radiation dose is calculated in the management of cancer cervix?

Ans. Radiation dose is calculated with respect of radiation received at two arbitary points—point A and point B.
- **Point A** is 2 cm cephalic and 2 cm lateral to the external os. It is the point of crossing of the uterine artery and ureter.
- **Point B** is 2 cm cephalic and 5 cm lateral at the same plane. It is approximately the site of obturator node.
- **Point A** gets about 7000–8000 cGy and point B 2000 cgy from radium (brachytherapy). Cancerolytic dose is approximately 7000–75000 cGy. The rest of the dose at point B is supplemented by external beam radiation.

Q.160 What is the overall 5 years survival rate following therapy in a woman with carcinoma cervix?

Ans.

Stages	5 years survival rate (%) (International Federation of Gynecology and Obstetrics)	
IA1	98.7	The overall 5 years survival for all the stages is 1.9%
IA2	95.9	
IB1	88.0	
IB2	78.8	
IIA	68.8	Important prognostic factors are: tumor volume, lymph node metastasis, parametrial invasion and lymphovasular space invasion
IIB	64.7	
IIIA	40.4	
IIIB	43.3	
IVA	19.5	
IVB	15	

Q.161 How cervical cancer screening could be organized in a low-resource setting?

Ans. Cytology based cervical cancer screening program (India, Pacific islands) could not be successful, in many countries of the world, as it requires a number of procedures. Alternative cervical cancer screening strategies in low resource settings can have a consistent and significant impact to improve upon the burden of cancer deaths.

Recommendations (ACOG-2015): The following are the acceptable alternatives where cytology based screening is not feasible or practical.
- HPV testing and follow-up treatment for woman with positive test results.
- In settings where HPV-DNA is not available, visual inspection with acetic acid followed by treatment with cryotherapy to be done. Cryotherapy should not be done in women where squamocolumnar junction is not entirely visualized. It has been established with a prospective randomized study in rural India that a single life time HPV-DNA screening test can reduce cervical cancer mortality and late stage disease by about 50%.

Q.162 Discuss the sensitivity of different screening procedures to detect CIN2$^+$.

Ans. **Sensitivity of screening to detect CIN2$^+$**

Test	Sensitivity (%)
1. Conventional pap	55–82 (63)
2. Liquid-based cytology	57–90 (74)
3. VIA	41–79 (60)
4. HPV	94–98 (96)
5. HPV + Pap test	99–100 (99+)

Q.163 What is the strategy of WHO for the elimination of cervical cancer by 2030?
Ans.

ROAD TO 'ELIMINATE' CERVICAL CANCER				
THRESHOLD: All countries to reach < 4 cases 100,000 women-years				
2030 control targets				
90% of girls fully vaccinated with HPV vaccine by 15 years of age		70% of women screened with an high precision test at 35 and 45 years of age	90% of women identified with cervical disease receive treatment and care	30% reduction in mortality from cervical cancer
SDG 2030: Target 30% reduction in mortality from cervical cancer				
The 2030 targets and elimination threshold are subject to revision depending on the outcomes of the modeling and the WHO approval process.				

Q.164 What are the aims of palliative treatment? What different palliative treatments can be given to a woman with carcinoma cervix?

Ans. Palliative treatment is aimed to provide comprehensive care for relief of symptoms along with treatment of the cancer, in the advanced stage.

Palliative treatment is given:
- To control vaginal discharge
- To control hemorrhage
- To relief pain.

Discussion continued: Case 16.

Suggested Reading

1. Clavel C, Masure M, Bory JP, Putaud I, Mangeonjean C, Lorenzato M, et al. Human papillomavirus testing in primary screening for the detection of high-grade cervical lesions: a study of 7932 women. BJC. 2001;89:616.
2. Cuzick J, Clavel C, Petry KU, et al. Overview of the European and North American studies on HPV testing in primary cervical cancer screening. IJC. 2006;119:1095-101.
3. Ronco G, Segnan N, Giorgi-Rossi P, et al. Human papillomavirus testing and liquid-based cytology: results at recruitment from the new technologies for cervical cancer randomized controlled trial. JNCL. 2006;98:765-74.
4. Sangrajrang S, Laowahutanont P, Wongsena M, Muwonge R, Karalak A, et al. Comparative accuracy of Pap smear and HPV screening in Ubon Ratchathani in Thailand. Papillomavirus Res. 2017;3:30-35.
5. Sankaranarayanan R, Gaffikin L, Jacob M, Sellors J, Robles S. A critical assessment of screening methods for cervical neoplasia. Int J Gynaecol Obstet. 2005;89(Suppl 2):S4-S12.
6. Sankaranarayan R, Nene BM, Shastri SS, et al. HPV screening for cervical cancer in rural India. N Engl J Med. 2009;360:1385-94.
7. Srivastava AN, Misra JS, Srivastava S, Das BC, Gupta S. Cervical cancer screening in rural India: Status and current concepts. IJMR. 2018;148(6):687-96.

CASE 16: CARCINOMA CERVIX—B

Case Summary

Mrs LM, 42-year-old lady was diagnosed to have squamous cell carcinoma of the cervix, stage IIA. She underwent radical hysterectomy with pelvic lymphadenectomy (Fig. 1.23). Before the operation she wanted to have the following information.

Q.165 What is the stage IIA carcinoma cervix?

Ans. Carcinoma of the cervix extending downwards up to upper two-third of the vagina but not laterally (without parametrial invasion).

It is subdivided into:
IIA1: Clinically visible lesion less than or equal to 4.0 cm in greatest dimension.
IIA2: Clinically visible lesion greater than 4 cm in greatest dimension.

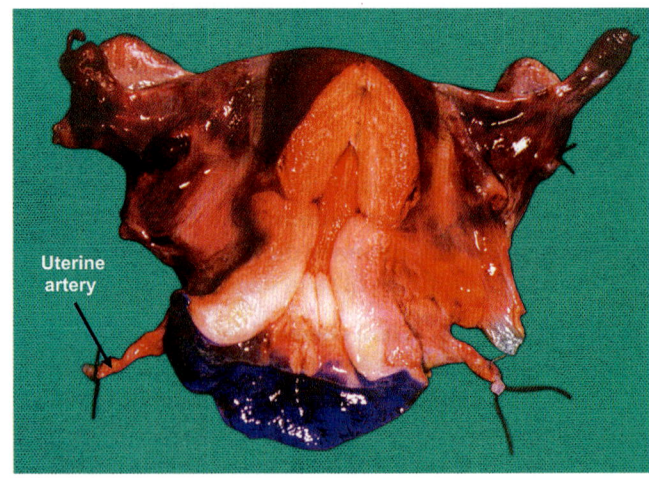

Fig. 1.23: Carcinoma cervix—radical hysterectomy done. Tied ends of uterine arteries are seen as they were dissected out and severed from the origin.

Q.166 What does this radical hysterectomy mean?

Ans. Removal of the uterus, cervix, upper vagina, parametrium, pelvic lymph nodes. Para-aortic node sampling is also done.

Q.167 What are the important complications of the operation?

Ans. Anesthetic complications and complications due to surgery: hemorrhage, injury to bladder, bowel, ureters, infection, intestinal obstruction and lately fistula and lymphocyst formation.

Q.168 What are the consequences if she refuses the operation?

Ans. Progression of the disease and the problems of bleeding, sepsis, metastases, cachexia and renal failure (uremia).

Q.169 What is the long-term outcome following the operation?

Ans. If the nodes are not involved, 5-year survival rate is about 80%. On the other hand 5-year survival rate is about 50% if nodes are involved.

Q.170 Is there any alternative method of treatment?

Ans. Radiotherapy (combined teletherapy and brachytherapy) has got equal survival rate for this stage. Chemoradiation therapy is also effective. (*See* Dutta's Textbook of Gynecology, 8th Edition, p. 295).

Q.171 What is the place of fertility sparing surgery for carcinoma cervix?

Ans. Fertility-preserving surgery for carcinoma cervix is done in highly selected women (*See* Ch 39).

Indication: Woman keen to preserve her fertility and has no other factor for infertility.

Case selection criteria
- Early stage disease (*See* Dutta's Textbook of Gynecology, 8th Edition, p. 295)
- Woman is strongly motivated for follow-up
- Invasive disease has been excluded on thorough examination
- Tumor is not a highly aggressive histologic subtype (neuroendocrine tumor).

Stage (FIGO) of the disease and the type of operation

Stage (FIGO)	Operation (fertility preservation)
• Microinvasive carcinoma stage 1A1 (no LVSI) • Stage 1A1 with ♦ Lymphovascular space involvement (LVSI) ♦ Stage 1A2 ♦ Stage 1A (adenocarcinoma) ♦ Stage IB1 (tumor volume ≤ 2 cm)	• Cervical conization (cold knife cone) • Radical trachelectomy with lymphadenectomy (laparoscopic robotic assisted) • Radical trachelectomy removes most of the cervix, bilateral parametria and upper vagina • Uterus is preserved for child-bearing function. It can be done vaginally or abdominally (laparoscopically or a robotic-assisted laparoscopy)

Q.172 What are the serum tumor markers of carcinoma cervix?

Ans. Serum tumor markers are valuable for predicting the prognosis, the response to treatment and also the risk of recurrence. In carcinoma cervix, the role of serum tumor markers in predicting 5-year survival rate is limited.

The most commonly studied tumor markers are:
- Squamus cell carcinoma antigen (SCCA)
- Cancer antigen 125 (CA 125)
- Cytokeratin fragment 19 (CYFRA 21.1).
- Raised levels of SCCA, CYFRA 21.1 and CA 125 have been observed in 20–88% of women with cervical cancer. Raised levels are correlated with tumor stage, tumor volume, cervical stromal invasion, lymphovascular space invasion, parametrial involvement and lymph node metastasis.

Q.173 What is the role of radiographic studies in tumor evaluation?

Ans. According to FIGO, radiographical studies such as CT, PET, combined PET/CT and MRI may be used to determine the extent of the disease within the pelvis, lymph nodes, for evaluation of prognosis and risk of recurrence following of initial treatment. However, imaging and pathology can be used, where available. In that case, adding notation of r (imaging) and p (pathology) has to be made.
- MRI is more accurate to determine tumor diameter, uterine extension and parametrial involvement compared to CT or clinical examination.
- PET/CT is more valuable to evaluate nodal metastases.
- Dynamic contrast-enhanced MRI can evaluate tumor vascularity and perfusion. [18F] fluorodeoxyglucose PET: PET/CT can evaluate intratumoral metabolic actively. All these can predict response to therapy. Discussion continued: Case 17.

CASE 17: CARCINOMA CERVIX—C

Case Summary

Mrs LK, a 34-year-old woman $P_{1+0+0+1'}$ diagnosed to have carcinoma cervix stage IA. She is admitted for subsequent management. Before that she desired to be counseled with the following information.

Q.174 What is stage IA carcinoma cervix?

Ans. Carcinoma strictly confined to the cervix and that is in the preclinical stage. It is diagnosed by biopsy only.

Q.175 Is there any subdivisions of the stage?

Ans. Yes, stage IA1: When there is minimal microscopically evident stromal invasion < 3.0 mm in depth.

Stage IA2: Microscopically measured stromal invasion > 3 mm but < 5 mm.

Q.176 What is the significance of such classification?
Ans. It is entirely related to spread of the disease and hence directly related to the prognosis and survival outcome.

Q.177 What is the approximate rate of lymph node involvement in this stage and 5-year survival rate?
Ans. Pelvic nodes involvement for stage IA1 (< 3 mm) is 0–0.5% and for stage IA2 (3–5 mm) is 5–6%. The risk of para-aortic nodes involvement is 0 and 1%, respectively. 5-year survival rate for stage IA1 is 98.7% and for stage IA2 is 95.9% respectively. (*See* Dutta's Textbook of Gynecology, 8th Edition, p. 296).

Q.178 What are the treatment options for this woman?
Ans. Either extrafascial hysterectomy (type I) or modified radical hysterectomy (type II) should be optimum for her depending on whether she belongs to stage IA1 or stage IA2.

Q.179 What is meant by type I and type II hysterectomy?
Ans. *Type I:* Extrafascial hysterectomy; the pubocervical ligament is incised allowing lateral deflection of the ureter.
Type II (modified radical): Here medial half of the Mackenrodt's and uterosacral ligaments along with selective (clinically enlarged and palpable) lymph nodes are removed. Upper third of vagina is also removed.

Q.180 Can she have any surgery preserving her fertility status?
Ans. Yes, such treatment can be provided in exceptional circumstances only. Therapeutic conization is the option that she can have. In that case, she must realize the need of long-term follow-up. She should be followed up with cytology and colposcopy regularly.
Laparoscopic-assisted radical vaginal trachelectomy with pelvic and aortic lymphadenectomy (LARVT) is also recommended currently for early stage (IA2 and IB1) disease. This is done only for a strongly motivated woman who wants to preserve her fertility (*See* Dutta's Textbook of Gynecology, 8th Edition, p. 295).
In either of the above treatment options, the surgical margin must be free of disease.

Q.181 What is radical trachelectomy?
Ans. It involves removing the cervix, parametria and cuff of vagina. Body of the uterus is preserved for fertility. This procedure is combined with either extraperitoneal or laparoscopic pelvic lymphadenectomy.

Q.182 What is concurrent chemoradiation?
Ans. Cisplatin-based concurrent chemoradiation is currently recommended as a treatment option of carcinoma cervix. It acts as a radiosensitizer and reduces disease progression. The appropriate cases for this treatment are: (i) Early stage (stages IA2, IB, IIA) disease after radical hysterectomy, (ii) Locally advanced (stages IIB to IVA) disease as a primary therapy.

CASE 18: CARCINOMA ENDOMETRIUM

Case Summary

A 55-year-old obese, hypertensive woman presented with postmenopausal bleeding. Hysteroscopy showed an irregular polypoid mass at the fundus. Biopsy revealed adenocarcinoma of the endometrium [moderately differentiated, Grade 2 (Fig. 1.24)].

Q.183 What are the important etiological factors for endometrial carcinoma?
Ans.
- Unapposed estrogen stimulation
- Age: 50–60 years
- Parity—nulliparity
- Late menopause
- Corpus cancer syndrome (obesity, hypertension and diabetes)
- Overweight (21–50 pounds overweight increases the risk 3 times)
- Tamoxifen therapy
- Positive family history
- Endometrial hyperplasia.

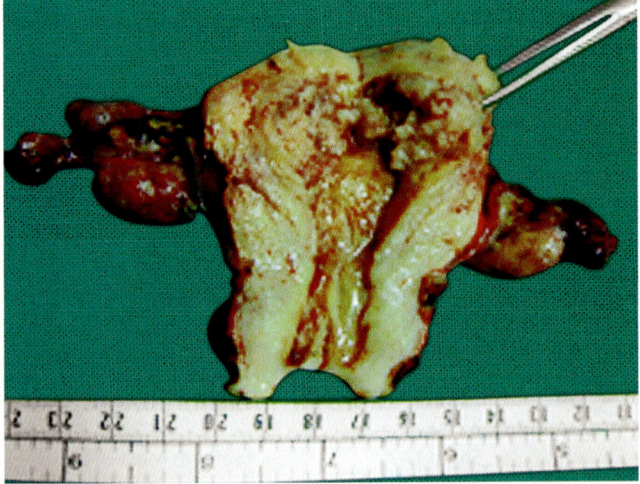

Fig. 1.24: Following surgery, uterus of the same woman is cut open to show a diffused and ulcerated growth at the fundus. The growth is seen to invade the myometrium. Histology confirmed adenocarcinoma

Q.184 What is the common histological type of endometrial carcinoma?
Ans. Adenocarcinoma.

Q.185 What are the high-risk factors for endometrial carcinoma?

Ans.
- Persistent and unopposed estrogen stimulation of endometrium
- Corpus cancer syndrome—obesity, hypertension and diabetes
- Endometrial hyperplasia
- Family history of colon, ovarian or breast cancer.

Q.186 How can be endometrial carcinoma diagnosed?

Ans.
- History and clinical examination: A case of postmenopausal bleeding is considered due to endometrial carcinoma unless proved otherwise.
- Endometrial biopsy (pipelle) diagnostic accuracy is 90–98%.
- Papanicolaou smear (unreliable) as diagnosis accuracy is only 30%.
- Ultrasonography (TVS) including color Doppler, endometrial thickness > 4 mm with increased vascularity is suggestive.
- Endometrial thickness ≥ 13 mm is strongly suggestive.
- Hysteroscopy helps in detecting polyps or submucous myomas.
- Fractional curettage is the definitive method of diagnosis in case where adequate evaluation is not possible with pipelle biopsy specimen or where bleeding recurs after a negative endometrial biopsy.
- CT and MRI, both can detect myometrial invasion, lymph node involvement and also the spread of the disease. MRI is superior to CT (Figs. 1.25A and B).

Q.187 Describe orderly the steps of fractional curettage.

Ans.
- Endocervical curettage
- Dilatation of internal os
- Introduction of a polyp forceps to remove any polyp
- Uterine curettage (1) Uterine fundus, and (2) body of the uterus
- Specimens, so obtained are sent for histology separately.

Q.188 Mention the important surgical procedures for the management of a case of endometrial carcinoma.

Ans. *In stage I:* Extrafascial hysterectomy, bilateral salpingo-oophorectomy.

Procedures
- Incision—longitudinal
- Peritoneal washings for cytology
- Thorough exploration of pelvic and abdominal organs including the pelvic and para-aortic lymph nodes
- Extrafascial hysterectomy (TAH and BSO) is done
- Uterus is cut open in the theater for tumor evaluation (gross examination or frozen section)
- Lymph node sampling—pelvic and para-aortic nodes are done when there is myometrial invasion (*See* Ch 33 and 34).

CASE 19: CARCINOMA OF THE OVARY

Q.189 What are the reasons for failure to improve the outcome of ovarian cancer?

Ans.
- No high-risk factor is known
- Deep-seated organs—diagnosis is often late
- No effective preventive measures
- No preinvasive stage of the disease
- No effective screening procedure for early detection
- Spread of the disease is unrelated to the size of the mass and or symptoms of the woman

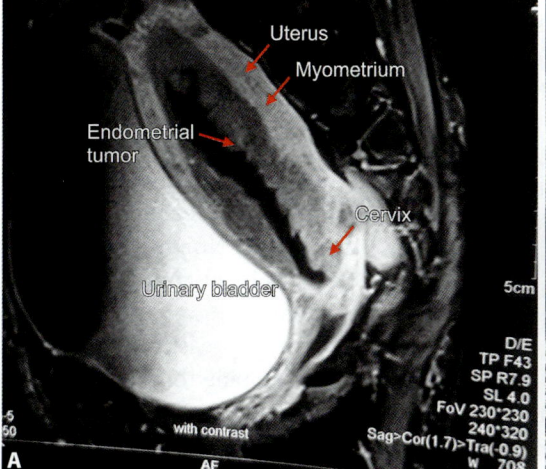 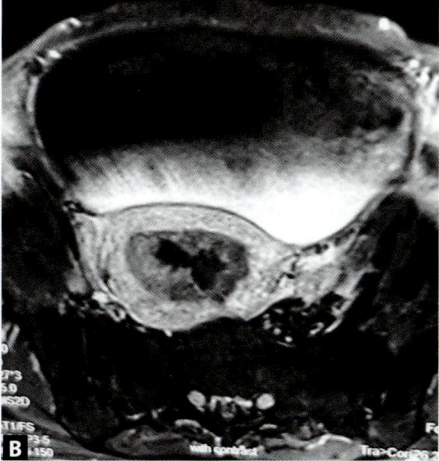

Figs. 1.25A and B: (A) Magnetic resonance image (MRI) in the sagittal plane of a 55-year-old woman with endometrial carcinoma. Sagittal T_1-weighted image shows endometrial tumor with invasion to the myometrium, more than 50%. There is extension of the cancer to the cervix (*see* arrows); (B) Magnetic resonance image (MRI) in the axial view of the same woman with endometrial carcinoma. Invasion to the myometrium, more than 50% is seen.

Courtesy: Department of Obstetrics and Gynecology and Department of Radiology, Assam Medical College, Dibrugarh, Assam, India.

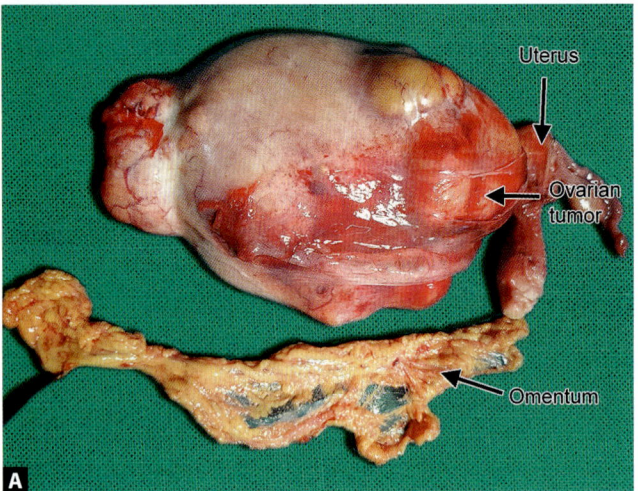 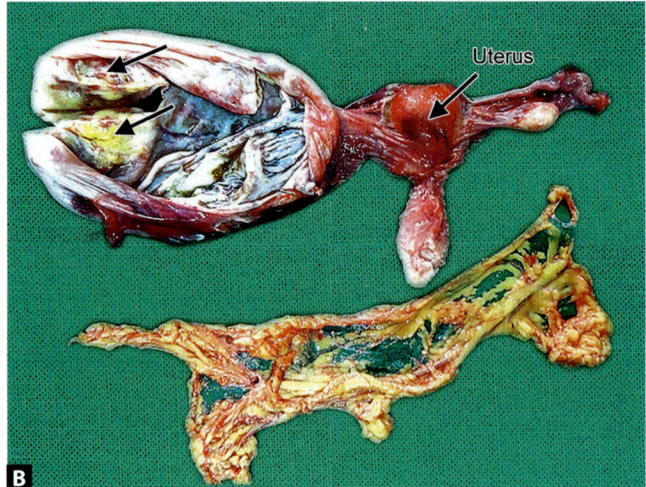

Figs. 1.26A and B: (A) Gross photograph of a surgical specimen showing the uterus with a huge ovarian tumor. The other tube and the ovary are seen. Stretched fallopian tube over the tumor is seen; (B) The cut section of the same ovarian tumor to show the solid areas (see arrows). Histology revealed serous cyst adenocarcinoma.

- Tumor cells move freely within the peritoneal cavity
- Limitations of cytoreductive surgery, chemotherapy and radiation therapy.

Q.190 What is the place of screening for ovarian cancer?

Ans. Unfortunately, till date no specific method of screening for early detection of epithelial ovarian cancer is available.
- ***Clinical methods***—bimanual pelvic examination is neither specific nor helpful.
- ***Tumor markers CA-125*** and HE4 are being done. These are useful but nonspecific (*See* Ch 17).
- ***Ultrasound imaging TVS*** color Doppler imaging has been used to differentiate a benign from a malignant mass. However, it is not specific also.
- ***Risk of malignancy index (RMI)*** is calculated by U × M × CA 125. The risk of cancer is 75% when the RMI value is greater than 250. When RMI is less than 25 the woman is in the low-risk group. RMI: 25–250 is in the moderate-risk category.
- ***Risk of ovarian malignancy algorithm (ROMA):*** ROMA is a quantitative test using CA-125, HE4 concentration and menopausal status to calculate the risk of ovarian cancer (see below).
- No screening procedure is effective for early detection of ovarian cancer.

Tumor Marker (HE4)

Human epididymis 4 (HE4) protein is derived from the distal epithelium of the epididymis. It is essential for sperm maturation as it is a protease inhibitor.

Levels of serum HE4 is found high in women with serous epithelial ovarian cancer. Unlike serum CA-125, serum levels of HE4 are less affected by other benign pelvic conditions like endometriosis. The sensitivity and specificity of detecting ovarian malignancy with HE4 is high in premenopausal women. This is especially beneficial for early stage ovarian cancer.

The use in combination of serum CA-125 and HE4 was found superior when compared with any other marker alone.

Risk of ovarian malignancy algorithm (ROMA): ROMA calculation is based on the combined results of the CA-125 and the HE4. This algorithm classifies women either as low-risk or high-risk for malignant disease. A cut-off value of 2.27 representing a high-risk of malignancy. Overall, it has a sensitivity of 89% and a specificity of 75%. Both the tumor markers are related to tumor stage and histological type of serous epithelial ovarian cancer.

Q.191 What are the other tumor markers?

Ans. CEA, CDX2, CA 72-4, CA19-9, Alpha FP, LDH and beta-hCG. There is not enough evidence to do the panels of multiple markers as there is no added advantage. All these markers have low sensitivity and wide variation in specificity. The routine use of any of these markers is not recommended (RCOG-2016).

Q.192 What are the epidemiology and risk factors for epithelial ovarian cancer?

Ans.
- Women of North America and most of the industrialized countries of Europe have high incidence.
- Pregnancy, breastfeeding reduce the risk.
- Use of combined oral contraceptives are associated with reduced risk.
- Pregnancy in a women after the age of 35 years is more protective against ovarian cancer.
- Use of long-acting progestin only contraceptive (DMPA, Provera) has protective effects similar to COCs.

- Surgery: Tubal ligation (interruption) and hysterectomy can reduce the risk of ovarian cancer.
- Prophylactic/risk reducing salpingectomy in high-risk women is protective (*See* Ch 53).

Q.193 What is the place of imaging studies in the management of ovarian cancer?

Ans. *Computed tomography (CT)/positron emission tomography (PET) scan* has been integrated for the diagnosis of ovarian cancer and evaluation of disease recurrence. PET scan has very high sensitivity but low specificity. There are false positive results due to increased FDG uptake in benign but metabolically active tissues and with inflammatory changes. Combined CT/PET scan had high sensitivity of 100% and specificity of 92%. It can detect recurrent disease which is superior to CA 125 or CT/MRI scans used alone.

Magnetic resonance imaging (MRI) is a nonradioactive imaging modality. It has excellent soft tissue contrast resolution. MRI is better than CT or ultrasonography in the diagnosis of small peritoneal metastases. CT imaging is better in identifying omental metastasis in ovarian cancer.

Q.194 What is the place of lymph node dissection in the managment of ovarian cancer?

Ans. *Lymph node dissection in early* ovarian cancer: Both pelvic and para-aortic lymph nodes should be removed. Lymph node dissection provides important prognostic and staging information for patients with suspected early stage ovarian cancer. This is helpful for the decision of about adjuvant chemotherapy. However, there is no convincing evidence that lymphadenectomy has got any therapeutic survival benefit in advanced ovarian cancer. Enlarged nodes may be removed as a part of debulking procedure.

Q.195 What is the place of neoadjuvant chemotherapy?

Ans. *Neoadjuvant chemotherapy:* Women with FIGO IIIC or IV ovarian cancers were treated with neoadjuvant platinum-based chemotherapy followed by primary debulking surgery. Subsequently, they were treated with platinum-based chemotherapy. The blood loss during surgery was less. The largest residual tumor could be reduced to less than 1 cm. The operative time was also shorter. For patients with huge tumor burden, ascites and several comorbidities, neoadjuvant chemotherapy is a very reasonable choice. Surgical debulking procedure is the single most important component in the management of ovarian cancer.

Suggested Reading

1. Moore RG, Brown AK, Miller MC, et al. The use of multiple novel tumor biomarkers for the detection of ovarian carcinoma in patients with a pelvic mass. Gynecol Oncol. 2008;108(2): 402-8.
2. Rafael Malina, Jose M, Jose Auge, et al. HE4 a novel tumor marker for ovarian cancer: Comparison with CA125 and ROMA algorithm in patients with gynecological diseases. International Society of Oncology and Biomarkers 2011.

CASE 20: INHERITED CANCERS AND THE MANAGEMENT

Case Summary

Ms RT, 44-year-old lecturer, nulligravida was seen for her abnormal uterine bleeding for last 8 months. Family history revealed cancers in the first-degree relatives for three generations. Family cancers included ovarian cancer, endometrial cancer and colorectal cancer—all are confirmed histologically. Her grandmother, mother, maternal uncles, sisters, brothers all are affected. Her thorough investigation including hysteroscopy and biopsy revealed endometrial adenocarcinoma (G-I). Total abdominal hysterectomy (extrafascial) with bilateral salpingo-oophorectomy was done. Para-aortic lymph node sampling was done. Histology revealed stage IA GI adenocarcinoma of the endometrium. Sampled nodes were negative.

Q.196 Ms RT is keen to know what is inherited or familial cancers. How it could be prevented?

Ans. Familial or inherited cancers are well known. They are more common in relation to ovarian, endometrial, breast and colon cancers. Unfortunately, as regard the diagnosis and prevention, no such specific guidelines are there as yet.

Q.197 What are the diagnostic criteria for familial cancers?

Ans. Till date no such specific guidelines are there. Amsterdam criteria (1999) has considered the following:
- At least three relations with breast, ovarian cancer and hereditary nonpolyposis colorectal cancer must be there.
- One affected person is a first-degree relative of the other two.
- At least two successive generations are affected.
- At least one person was diagnosed before the age of 50 years.
- Familial adenomatous polyposis had been excluded.
- Tumors have been verified by histopathological examination.

Q.198 How do BRCA-1, BRCA-2 and mismatch repair genes protect us?

Ans. *BRCA-1* and *BRCA-2* are the tumor suppressor genes. Others: *MLH-1, MSH-2* and *MSH-6* are the mismatch repair genes. These genes repair the single base pair mismatches that occur during DNA replication. Mutations in these genes cause cell immortalization, neoplastic proliferation and ultimately cancers.

Q.199 How familial cancers could be prevented?

Ans. At the moment there are no such guidelines. But following measures could be adopted:
- Family history must be enquired and recorded in all positive cases.
- Clinical geneticist must be consulted and family tree should be drawn in a positive case (Amsterdam criteria).
- Molecular screening for detection of gene mutation is not possible at the moment. This is very expensive, time consuming and also labor intensive.
- Screening procedure may be initiated wherever available (e.g., breast cancer, colon cancer).
- Combined oral contraceptives are chemopreventive against ovarian cancer and endometrial cancer. Tamoxifen is chemopreventive against breast cancer.
- Place of prophylactic surgery may be considered. Prophylactic salpingo-oophorectomy/salpingectomy may be done especially while doing hysterectomy for some other reason. This is an alternative in the high-risk group of women for ovarian cancer.
- Human fertilization and embryology authority (HFEA), UK, has recommended preimplantation genetic diagnosis in cases with familial cancers. Affected blastocysts are removed from the transfer in ART. This may be one way to eliminate the risk of inherited cancers.
- As a prophylaxis to endometrial cancer, LNG-IUS is currently being used. Long-term reports are awaited.
- Resequencing chips are being tried, once available molecular diagnosis of gene mutation would be helpful.

Q.200 Who are the women that may be considered for molecular screening?

Ans. At the moment there is no such established criteria. However, women fulfilling the following criteria are the high-risk group for consideration:
- Positive family history following Amsterdam criteria.
- Risk scoring more than 10 (Manchester scoring system).
- Tumors positive for microsatellite instability by immunohistochemistry method.

Q.201 What is the significance of family history?

Ans. This is often observed in early age onset (around 45 years).

Lifetime risk of endometrial cancer in women with Lynch II syndrome is 32–60% and that of ovarian cancer is 10–12%.

Chapter 2: Self-Assessment in Gynecology

SINGLE BEST ANSWER (SBA) AND MULTIPLE CHOICE QUESTIONS (MCQs)

Q.1 The following are hormonal changes during a normal 28 days menstrual cycle, *except*:
 a. The rising LH in the first part of the cycle stimulates estrogen production from theca cells
 b. FSH begins to fall after 7th day
 c. There is sudden rise of estrogen few days prior to ovulation
 d. The estrogen surge results in LH surge and prostaglandin F2α secretion

Ans. a. In the early follicular phase, FSH initiates the appearance of LH receptors on the theca cells. These receptors are activated by LH to produce primarily androstenedione and testosterone. These steroids diffuse into the granulosa cells and are aromatized to estradiol under the influence of FSH.

Q.2 The following are related to granulosa cells, *except*:
 a. It has got no blood supply
 b. In the first half of the cycle, it has no steroidogenic function
 c. Granulosa cells produce activin and inhibin
 d. Estrogen stimulates the proliferation of granulosa cells

Ans. b. In the late follicular phase, FSH augmented by estrogen, stimulates the appearance of LH receptors on the granulosa cells. Small amount of progesterone is also produced.

Q.3 The following are related to corpus luteum, *except*:
 a. Luteinized granulosa cells produce progesterone
 b. Estrogen continues to be produced by the luteinized theca cells
 c. Luteolysis is due to estrogen, PGF2α and endothelin
 d. The peak steroid production is between 23rd and 25th day

Ans. d. The peak production is between 18th and 22nd days.

Q.4 Endometrial carcinoma is related to all, *except*:
 a. Feminizing ovarian tumor
 b. Polycystic ovarian disease
 c. Exogenous estrogen therapy
 d. Early menopause

Ans. d.

Q.5 The following statements are related to tuberculous salpingitis, *except*:
 a. The abdominal ostium may be patent with eversion of fimbriae
 b. The early lesion may be confused with adenocarcinoma on histology
 c. Genital tuberculosis is always secondary and the tubes are invariably the primary sites
 d. Salpingitis isthmica nodosa is the exclusive pathology to tuberculosis

Ans. d. It is also observed in endometriosis. a. It is called 'tobacco pouch' appearance.

Q.6 The following statements are related to genital tuberculosis:
 a. Ovarian involvement can occur without tubal affection
 b. Infertility is mainly due to anovulation
 c. Acid-fast bacilli is identified in 100% cases of tuberculous endometritis
 d. A negative Mantoux test reasonably excludes tuberculosis

Ans. d. Ovaries are involved in following tubal affection. b. Infertility is mainly due to tubal and endometrial pathology. (*See* Dutta's Textbook of Gynecology, 8th Edition, p. 203).

Q.7 Follicular cysts of the ovary may undergo all these changes, *except*:
 a. Spontaneous resorption
 b. Malignant change
 c. Intracystic hemorrhage
 d. Rupture

Ans. b.

Q.8 The following are related to staging of pelvic malignancy, as per FIGO, *except*:
 a. Cervical carcinoma staging is based on clinical examination, imaging and pathological studies
 b. Staging of ovarian malignancy should be done from clinical, operative and pathologic consideration
 c. Staging of carcinoma body of the uterus is based both on clinical as well as surgical findings
 d. Vulvar carcinoma staging is based principally on surgery

Ans. d. It is clinical staging.

Q.9 The following statements are related to Krukenberg tumor, *except*:
   a. It is always secondary
   b. The most common primary site is pylorus of the stomach
   c. The tumor is bilateral
   d. 'Signet ring' looking cells are characteristic

Ans. a. The primary site is not uncommon and the prognosis is better.

Q.10 Regarding infertility:
   a. Fecundability in a healthy couple is 80%
   b. Unexplained infertility is about 10-15%
   c. Women with amenorrhea, ↓E2, ↓FSH, belong to WHO group I anovulation
   d. Elevated basal FSH indicates poor ovarian reserve

Ans. b and d. Likelihood of pregnancy in an ovulatory cycle in a healthy young couple (fecundability) is 20%. According to WHO, anovulatory states are: *Group I*—(hypogonadotropic hypogonadism) woman with amenorrhea, ↓E2, ↓FSH, ↓LH and with negative progesterone challenge test (hypothalamic cause). Women in c. belong to *Group I*; *Group III* belongs to hypergonadotropic hypogonadism (ovarian failure group). *Group II* includes women with PCOS (hypothalamic-pituitary dysfunction). Elevated basal FSH (>20%) indicates extremely poor prognosis (or ovarian failure).

Q.11 Cervical intraepithelial (CIN I, II) neoplasia may undergo:
   a. Regression in majority
   b. Persistence in few cases
   c. Progress to invasive carcinoma in majority
   d. Recurrence following local treatment is high

Ans. a, c. Progression to CIS is 10-15%. d. It is 3-5%.

Q.12 The most important clinical feature in the diagnosis of PCOS:
   a. Oligomenorrhea and/or anovulation
   b. Hyperandrogenism (clinical/biochemical)
   c. Polycystic ovaries
   d. Any two of the above

Ans. d. Presence of any two of the above three criteria (a, b and c) has been considered diagnostic (with exclusion of other etiologies) at a joint meeting of the American Society for Reproductive Medicine (ASRM) and the European Society of Human Reproduction and Embryology (ESHRE) in Rotterdam, 2018.

Q.13 The following are the definitive surgeries for microinvasive carcinoma of the cervix:
   a. Hysterectomy with or without removal of vaginal cuff
   b. Radical hysterectomy
   c. Therapeutic conization
   d. All of the above

Ans. d. Microinvasion of less than 3 mm beyond the basement membrane along with colposcopic evidence of presence of carcinoma in situ in the vault requires removal of cuff along with hysterectomy. Involvement of the lymphatic channels or confluence needs radical hysterectomy. In highly motivated cases with rigid follow-up, therapeutic conization can be done.

Q.14 Primary amenorrhea is most commonly associated with:
   a. Developmental defect of the genital tract
   b. Tuberculosis
   c. Endocrine disorders
   d. Chromosomal abnormality

Ans. d.

Q.15 Secondary amenorrhea is most commonly associated with:
   a. Sheehan's syndrome
   b. Premature ovarian failure
   c. Polycystic ovarian disease
   d. Hyperprolactinemia

Ans. c.

Q.16 The most common site of defect in primary amenorrhea:
   a. Pituitary
   b. Ovary
   c. Endometrium
   d. Chromosomal

Ans. d. Chromosomal abnormality is the most common.

Q.17 The most common site of defect in secondary amenorrhea:
   a. Hypothalamus
   b. Pituitary
   c. Ovary
   d. Thyroid

Ans. c.

Q.18 Causes of premature ovarian failure are all, *except*:
   a. Systemic chemotherapy
   b. Resistant ovarian syndrome
   c. Autoimmune response
   d. Androgenic polycystic ovary

Ans. d.

Q.19 Congenital vaginal agenesis is usually associated with all, *except*:
   a. Normal female karyotype
   b. Absence of functioning uterus
   c. Normal secondary sexual characters
   d. Presence of nonfunctional ovaries

Ans. d. Ovaries are not Müllerian structures; so they are normal anatomically and functionally.

Q.20 Agenesis of vagina is usually associated with all, *except*:
a. Presence of urinary tract anomalies in about one-third
b. High incidence of gonadal malignancy
c. Presence of skeletal anomalies of spine in about 10%
d. Absence of uterus

Ans. b.

Q.21 About the embryology of the urogenital system:
a. The trigone of the bladder is mesodermal in origin
b. The rest of the bladder is endodermal in development
c. The urachal fistula is due to patent allantoic diverticulum
d. Most of the females urethra is mesodermal in origin

Ans. a, b and c; d. It is developed from the vesicourethral part of the endodermal cloaca.

Q.22 The following statements are related to genital tuberculosis:
a. Should be treated surgically in the first instance when tubercular tubo-ovarian mass is present
b. Cervical tuberculosis is mainly sexually transmitted
c. Is a cause of infertility
d. Pregnancy outcome is usually successful by following treatment

Ans. c; AT drugs must be started before surgery at best for 6 weeks; b. It is rare; d. Pregnancy is rare; if occurs, chance of ectopic is more; if uterine pregnancy occurs, chance of abortion is more and delivery of a live baby is a remote possibility.

Q.23 Vault prolapse is most commonly due to the following:
a. Vaginal hysterectomy for prolapse
b. Abdominal total hysterectomy
c. Subtotal hysterectomy
d. Extended hysterectomy

Ans. a. The presence of pre-existing anatomical abnormality (laxity of the supporting structures) in spite of effective repair is the responsible factor in recurrence. Pre-existing enterocele, if left uncorrected increases the risk. Vault prolapse is expected to be less following subtotal than total hysterectomy.

Q.24 The following statements are correct in relation to paraovarian cyst, *except*:
a. It is a true broad ligament cyst
b. It usually arises from epoophoron
c. More chance of ureteric injuries during surgical removal
d. Malignant change is frequent

Ans. d. Malignant alteration is rare.

Q.25 The following relations of the ureter are correct, *except*:
a. Ureter lies anterior to internal iliac artery
b. Ureter forms the anterior boundary of the ovarian fossa
c. Ureter crosses the uterine artery from below
d. Because of dextrorotation of the uterus, the left ureter is more close to the cervix

Ans. b. Ureter forms the posterior boundary.

Q.26 Testicular feminization syndrome has got the following features, *except*:
a. Poorly developed breasts
b. Scanty axillary and pubic hair
c. Short and blind vagina
d. Karyotype—46XY

Ans. a. Breasts are large with less glandular tissue.

Q.27 Regarding sterilization by the Pomeroy method all are correct, *except*:
a. Is performed with absorbable suture material
b. Includes crushing of the fallopian tube
c. Results in two separate ends of the fallopian tubes several months later
d. Has a higher failure rate, if performed at the time of cesarean section

Ans. b.

Q.28 Regarding placenta accreta:
a. Ultrasonography can diagnose it antenatally
b. Color Doppler USG has a specificity > 90%
c. MRI is reliable to the diagnosis
d. Internal iliac ligation is effective to control hemorrhage in majority

Ans. b. Sensitivity and specificity of color Doppler are found to be 82% and 97%, respectively. Internal iliac ligation has been shown to fail in 40–60% cases.

Q.29 Accidental injury of the ureter during abdominal operation should be managed by all, *except*:
a. Deligation
b. End-to-end anastomosis through a ureteric catheter
c. Implantation into the bladder
d. Colonic implantation

Ans. d.

Q.30 Laparoscopic ovarian drilling (LOD) for a woman with PCOS who is clomiphene-resistant:
a. Results in higher pregnancy rates compared to that of gonadotropin use
b. Four punctures per ovary is considered optimum

c. The women ovulate spontaneously for several years following LOD
d. Incidence of multiple pregnancy is not changed

Ans. b, c and d.

Q.31 Regarding the sling procedure for urodynamic stress incontinence (USI):
a. Tension-free vaginal tape (TVT) elevates the bladder neck to a retropubic position
b. TVT is an autologous sling material
c. Recurrent USI, intrinsic sphincter deficiency are the common indications
d. Success rate of TVT is low than other retropubic procedures

Ans. c; a. TVT acts by increasing urethral coaptation, kinking the urethra with the rise in abdominal pressure; b. TVT is made from polypropylene (marlex) or polytetrafluoroethylene (Gore tex). Natural sling materials are made from rectus fascia or porcine dermis. These are less antigenic; d. Success rate of sling procedure is over 80% and it can be performed under local anesthetic.

Q.32 Ureter is commonly injured directly during operation of hysterectomy for all, *except*:
a. Broad ligament fibroid
b. Cervical fibroid
c. Radical hysterectomy
d. Endometriosis

Ans. c. In radical hysterectomy, ureter is dissected under direct vision all through. As such, direct injury during operation is a rarity. But avascular necrosis with fistula formation may occur at a later date.

Q.33 Ureteric injury can be prevented during total hysterectomy by the following procedures:
a. Using a lighted ureteral catheter
b. Enucleation followed by hysterectomy in cervical fibroid
c. Direct visualization rather than ureteric catheterization during pelvic surgery
d. Utmost care during clamping the uterine artery in simple hysterectomy

Ans. b and c. Ureter is not injured during clamping of the uterine artery. It is commonly injured while clamping the Mackenrodt's ligament along with descending cervical artery near the vaginal angle. a. It is cumbersome and of no added advantage.

Q.34 Granulosa cell tumor of the ovary has the following features:
a. It may present as postmenopausal bleeding
b. Known to cause true precocious puberty
c. Call-Exner bodies are pathognomonic.
d. Follow-up is needed even after hysterectomy and bilateral salpingo-oophorectomy

Ans. a, c and d; a. It is due to unopposed estrogen causing endometrial hyperplasia or endometrial carcinoma; b. It causes precocious pseudopuberty; d. It is of low-grade malignancy and late recurrences (even up to 20 years) have been noted.

Q.35 Diagnosis of Sheehan's syndrome is made by all, *except*:
a. Secondary amenorrhea following a turmoil childbirth
b. Lactation is not affected
c. Falling pubic hair
d. Evidences of hypogonadotropic hypogonadism

Ans. b. Failure of lactation is a constant and important feature.

Q.36 The essential substitution therapy in Sheehan's syndrome is by:
a. Combined estrogen and progestogen preparations
b. Cortisone followed by thyroid hormone
c. Gonadotropins for fertility improvement
d. Combination of all the above drugs

Ans. b. Although there is plurideficiency state, essential substitution therapy includes cortisone and thyroid.

Q.37 Regarding Fitz-Hugh-Curtis syndrome:
a. Characterized by violin string adhesions in the perihepatic region
b. Primary pathology is hepatitis
c. Pain is felt in the suprapubic region
d. Organisms involved are *N. gonorrhoeae* and/or *C. trachomatis*

Ans. a and d; b. Acute salpingitis → acute perihepatitis → perihepatic adhesions; c. Chronic right upper quadrant pain. (*See* Dutta's Textbook of Gynecology, 8th Edition, p. 124).

Q.38 Menstrual pattern preceding menopause are all, *except*:
a. Sudden stoppage following normal periods
b. Gradual hypomenorrhea
c. Increasing oligomenorrhea
d. Period of shorter cycles

Ans. d. Anovulation becomes more prevalent and menstrual cycle length increases.

Q.39 Withdrawal bleeding following administration of progesterone in a case of secondary amenorrhea indicates all, *except*:
a. Absence of pregnancy
b. Production of endogenous estrogen
c. Endometrium is responsive to estrogen
d. Defect in pituitary gonadal axis

Ans. d.

Q.40 Surest laboratory test to confirm the onset of menopause:
a. Estriol assay
b. Endometrial biopsy

c. Cytohormonal study
d. Serum gonadotropin assay

Ans. d. Serum FSH and LH > 40 mIU/mL, three values at weeks interval are needed. Persistent serum estradiol < 20 pg/mL along with raised FSH is also diagnostic.

Q.41 Regarding tubal sterilization procedure:
a. A pregnancy test should be performed, when there is a missed period
b. Routine curettage should be done during the procedure to prevent luteal phase pregnancy
c. Failure rate is the same as in interval procedure done during MTP
d. A negative pregnancy test cannot exclude pregnancy reliably

Ans. d. RCOG guidelines recommend universal pregnancy testing for women undergoing tubal occlusion. b. Routine curettage does not reduce luteal phase pregnancy. c. Failure rate is high when sterilization is done during MTP.

Q.42 Regarding reversal of tubal sterilization:
a. Falope rings damage the tube less compared to Pomeroy method
b. Filshie clips damage the tube more than the Falope rings
c. The rate of ectopic pregnancy is 10%
d. Chance of successful pregnancy is over 70%

Ans. a and d. Filshie clips damage less (5 mm) compared to Falope rings (2 cm). Rate of ectopic pregnancy is about 3–4%. Success rate following reversal has increased with the use of rings, clips and also due to new surgical procedures for reversal (microsurgery).

Q.43 The following are related to adrenal gland:
a. Adrenal medulla secretes epinephrine and norepinephrine
b. Zona glomerulosa produces steroid hormone, testosterone
c. Zona fasciculata mainly produces aldosterone
d. Zona reticularis produces glucocorticoids

Ans. a. Zona glomerulosa produces aldosterone; zona fasciculata produces glucocorticoids and zona reticularis produces sex steroids, predominantly androgens.

Q.44 Laparoscopic ovarian surgery (LOS) in women with PCOS:
a. All women, who are resistant to clomiphene citrate respond to LOS
b. Failure of ovulation within 6–8 weeks or conception within 12 months is considered as the failure of LOS
c. LOS makes intrafollicular microenvironment from androgenic to estrogenic
d. The cautery needle should preferably be put close to the ovarian hilum

Ans. b and c. Women resistant to LOS are: BMI > 35 kg/m^2, serum testosterone > 4.5 nmol/L, free androgen index (FAI) >15 and infertility for > 3 years. The cautery needle should be away from the ovarian hilum to avoid damage to ovarian vessels. Otherwise risk of premature ovarian failure is there.

Q.45 Ovarian causes of hirsutism are all, *except*:
a. Polycystic ovarian disease (PCOS)
b. Sertoli-Leydig cell tumor
c. Luteoma of pregnancy
d. Brenner tumor

Ans. d.

Q.46 Testicular biopsy is indicated in:
a. Azoospermia
b. Oligospermia with high FSH
c. Oligospermia with normal FSH level
d. All of the above

Ans. a and c. It can differentiate obstructive cause of azoospermia from testicular failure. Raised FSH level indicates testicular failure. But in Sertoli cell, only syndrome, focal areas of spermatogenesis may be present. This can help in intracytoplasmic sperm injection (ICSI).

Q.47 The cause of adrenal hyperplasia is due to:
a. Defect in cortisol synthesis
b. Defect in ACTH synthesis
c. Defect in testosterone synthesis
d. None of the above

Ans. a. An enzyme 21-hydroxylase deficiency leads to inadequate cortisol synthesis → by negative feedback leads to excessive secretion of ACTH → excessive stimulation of adrenal → adrenal hyperplasia → excessive secretion of adrenal androgen → virilization.

Q.48 The following statements are related to choriocarcinoma:
a. It is not a tumor of the uterus but the uterus is secondarily involved
b. Histologic confirmation of diagnosis is a must before chemotherapy
c. The most common site of metastasis is in the anterior wall of the vagina
d. 1–5% of hydatidiform mole develops persistent gestational trophoblastic neoplasia (GTN)

Ans. a. Histological confirmation is neither essential to the diagnosis nor a prerequisite to treatment. A new pregnancy must be excluded, as serum β-hCG is important. The most common site of metastasis is lungs. 15–20% of hydatidiform mole develop persistent GTN.

Q.49 The most common cause of precocious puberty:
a. Constitutional
b. Endocrinal
c. Intracranial lesion
d. Iatrogenic
Ans. a.

Q.50 Ovarian tumor producing features of thyrotoxicosis:
a. Carcinoid tumor
b. Struma ovarii
c. Dermoid
d. Lipid cell tumor
Ans. b.

Q.51 The following are related to bromocriptine, *except*:
a. It is dopamine agonist
b. It may cause multiple pregnancy
c. Cabergoline (dopamine agonist) can be administered vaginally
d. It restores menstruation earlier than stoppage of galactorrhea
Ans. b. It is not associated with multiple pregnancy. Cabergoline, an ergot derivative has low side effects and oral dose is 0.5–3 mg once a week.

Q.52 Position of the patient should be as described, *except*:
a. Diagnostic laparoscopy—Trendelenburg with about 30° tilt
b. Colposcopy—lithotomy
c. Transvaginal sonography in gynecology—lithotomy with full bladder
d. Hysteroscopy—lithotomy
Ans. c. The position is dorsal with legs drawn up, full bladder is not needed.

Q.53 Major sources of androgen in females are all, *except*:
a. Adrenals
b. Ovaries
c. Peripheral conversion to androgen precursors in the liver, gastrointestinal tract and adipose tissue
d. Corpus luteum
Ans. d.

Q.54 The biochemical changes in established cases of Stein-Leventhal syndrome are as mentioned, *except*:
a. Marked elevation of LH in contrast to FSH
b. Insulin resistance
c. Elevation of plasma testosterone
d. Elevation in the level of sex hormone binding globulin (SHBG) level
Ans. d. SHBG level is low in PCOS.

Q.55 The following are related with vasectomy, *except*:
a. Leads to immediate sterility
b. Failure rate is 0.1%
c. Involves ligation and division of spermatic cord
d. Partner (wife) may be given DMPA for 3 months
Ans. a. DMPA may be used as an interim contraception before vasectomy is effective.

Q.56 Regarding puberty and primary amenorrhea:
a. Precocious puberty is diagnosed when secondary sexual characters appear before the age of ten
b. Congenital absence of vagina is associated with renal tract abnormality in about 10% of cases
c. Primary amenorrhea is defined as the absence of menstruation by 14 years of age
d. Precocious puberty may be due to congenital adrenal hyperplasia
Ans. d. b. Renal tract abnormality in association with the absence of vagina is 30%.

Q.57 Sex cord stromal tumors of the ovary include all, *except*:
a. Luteomas
b. Gynandroblastomas
c. Sertoli-Leydig cell tumors of the ovary
d. Theca-fibroma
Ans. a.

Q.58 The following are related to carcinoma fallopian tube:
a. It is usually primary
b. Papanicolaou smear is always negative
c. Should be primarily treated by radiotherapy
d. 'Hydrops tubae profluens'—may be a presentation
Ans. d. The carcinoma of the fallopian tube is usually secondary following carcinoma of the uterine body or ovary. Histologically, it is always adenocarcinoma. The diagnosed case should be treated by surgery. Papanicolaou smear may be positive without any cervical or endometrial pathology.

Q.59 The following are related to theca cell tumor, *except*:
a. It is a cause for postmenopausal bleeding
b. It is usually associated with Brenner tumor
c. It may be associated with ascites and hydrothorax
d. Either conservative or radical surgery gives excellent result
Ans. b. It is usually associated by granulosa cell tumor.

Q.60 Regarding the surgical treatment for urodynamic stress incontinence (USI) all are correct, *except*:
a. Burch colposuspension is superior to Marshall-Marchetti-Krantz (MMK) on 5-year follow-up
b. Midurethral tape procedures (TOT) are considered as Grade A

c. Following colposuspension long-term voiding disorders are seen in about 10% of women
d. Enterocele is more common after the suburethral sling procedures

Ans. d. It is more common with following colposuspension.

Q.61 The following statements are related to congenital adrenogenital syndrome in the female newborn, *except*:
a. The most common variety is due to 21-hydroxylation deficiency
b. Palpable gonads in the inguinal canal or labial fold excludes the diagnosis
c. Karyotype is 46 XX
d. Normal excretion of urinary pregnanetriol

Ans. d. In adrenogenital syndrome, the gonads are placed in normal position. Urinary pregnanetriol excretion is markedly elevated.

Q.62 Fetal testis has got the following functions, *except*:
a. Masculinization of the external genitalia
b. Suppression of the Müllerian structures
c. Enhancement of Wolffian structures
d. Differentiation of the gonad

Ans. d. Differentiation of the biopotential gonad is done by SRY gene, located on the Y chromosome.

Q.63 The following are related to Paget's disease of vulva, *except*:
a. It arises from the apocrine glands of labia majora
b. Paget's disease of the vulva is much more common than its breast counterpart
c. The presence of Paget's cells (large cells with clear cytoplasm) within the epidermis is diagnostic
d. Simple vulvectomy is the optimum treatment

Ans. b. Paget's disease of the breast is more common than its vulvar counterpart. Multiple biopsies must be taken to exclude associated adenocarcinoma, which if present needs bilateral lymph node dissection.

Q.64 The following statements are related to bromocriptine therapy, *except*:
a. It is used in cases with galactorrhea and amenorrhea
b. Resumption of ovulation is earlier than cessation of galactorrhea
c. Galactorrhea is commonly observed with irregular menses and with high prolactin level
d. In most of the cases, there is reduction in prolactin level and pituitary adenoma size

Ans. c. Galactorrhea is commonly observed with regular menses and with normal prolactin level.

Q.65 Endometrial curettage in a suspected case of genital tuberculosis should be done:
a. In the proliferative phase
b. In the secretory phase
c. Following antitubercular drug for 1 week in secretory phase
d. All of the above

Ans. b. The tubercle bacilli are expected to come more towards the surface with the thickness of the endometrium as in secretory phase. Prior antitubercular therapy prevents dissemination.

Q.66 The following are related to ectopy, *except*:
a. It is due to the downward movement of the squamocolumnar junction with high level of estrogen
b. It is not in the true sense, an ulcer
c. It is only cured by cauterization or cryotherapy of the cervix
d. Nabothian follicles are formed during the process of healing

Ans. c. The physiological erosion is too often cured spontaneously.

Q.67 Pick up the correct statements:
a. "Strawberry" look of the ectocervix in monilial cervicitis
b. "Tobacco pouch" appearance of the fallopian tube is due to tubercular salpingitis
c. "Matchstick spots" in the pelvic peritoneum is in toxic shock syndrome
d. "Retort shape" fallopian tube is due to unruptured tubal ectopic

Ans. b. Strawberry look is peculiar to trichomonal vaginitis. Retort shape is due to large hydrosalpinx of the tube. 'Matchstick spots' are characteristic of pelvic endometriosis.

Q.68 Causes of deep dyspareunia are all, *except*:
a. Fixed retroverted uterus
b. Prolapsed ovary
c. Endometriosis on rectovaginal septum
d. Vaginal atrophy in menopause

Ans. d. It causes superficial dyspareunia.

Q.69 As regard the PCOS and hyperinsulinemia:
a. Hyperinsulinemia is observed in about 40–80% of women with PCOS
b. Hyperinsulinemia stimulates hepatic synthesis of SHBG
c. Metformin causes hypoglycemia in normoglycemic women
d. Metformin has many other health benefits

Ans. a and d. Insulin resistance and compensatory hyperinsulinemia is observed in about 40% of women with normal weight and 80% obese women with PCOS. Hyperinsulinemia results in decreased hepatic synthesis of SHBG and increased ovarian androgen biosynthesis. Metformin reduces fasting insulin levels, blood pressure and LDL cholesterol. Metformin does not cause hypoglycemia either with normoglycemic or with diabetic individuals.

Q.70 The following are the contraindications of tubal reconstructive surgery:
a. Tubal damage following sterilization operation
b. Patients over 30 years of age
c. Pelvic tuberculosis
d. Active pelvic inflammatory disease

Ans. c and d. Reversal of tubal sterilization is more successful where tubal damage is less as following laparoscopic procedures. Age over 30, is not a contraindication, though age-related fertility is reduced.

Q.71 The following are related to estrogen secretion from the ovary:
a. Theca cells and granulosa cells are interlinked in the secretion of estrogen
b. Granulosa cells takes no part in the secretion
c. Estrogen is solely secreted from theca cells
d. Luteinized granulosa cells are the source

Ans. a. LH acts on theca cells to produce androgen precursors. When activated by FSH and IGF-II, the receptors on the granulosa induces aromatase enzyme activity. This converts thecal androstenedione and testosterone to estradiol. A small amount of progesterone is also produced by the granulosa cells in the proliferative phase. IGF-II stimulates granulosa cell proliferation, aromatase activity and progesterone synthesis.

Q.72 The following are the ovarian cancer markers—match them appropriately:
a. CA 125   1. Ovarian germ cell tumor
b. Carcinoembryonic 2. Choriocarcinoma of antigen   ovary
c. Alpha fetoprotein 3. Serous, endometrioid cancer
d. High serum hCG   4. Epithelial malignancy

Ans. a = 4; b = 3; c = 1; d = 2.

Q.73 The following are related to cloaca:
a. The gut caudal to the allantois widens to form the cloaca
b. The cloaca divides into a dorsal hindgut and a ventral urogenital sinus
c. The external opening of the ventral cloaca is the urogenital ostium
d. All of the above

Ans. d.

Q.74 In the female, the following structures are developed from the urogenital sinus:
a. Urinary bladder and urethra
b. Lower part of vagina
c. Bartholin's glands
d. All of the above

Ans. d.

Q.75 The contents of the mesosalpinx are:
a. Fallopian tube
b. Utero-ovarian anastomosis vessels
c. Parovarium—a vestigial structure derived from the mesonephros
d. All of the above

Ans. d. Parovarium derived from Wolffian duct (mesonephros).

Q.76 The following are related to differentiation of external genitalia, *except*:
a. Dihydrotestosterone from fetal testis cause male differentiation of external genital organs from cloaca
b. In the absence of fetal testosterone, external genitalia of either sex fails to differentiate
c. Once the female genitalia develop, even a heavy dose of exogenous testosterone cannot alter the genital structure to male
d. Differentiation in male is earlier than female

Ans. b. In the absence of fetal testosterone, the female external genitalia will form.

Q.77 Causes of isosexual (true) precocious puberty are all, *except*:
a. Constitutional
b. Juvenile hypothyroidism
c. Albright's syndrome
d. Granulosa cell tumor

Ans. d. Isosexual is synonymous with true precocious puberty. In this condition, sexual maturation occurs due to premature precocious maturation of hypothalamo-pituitary-ovarian axis. Granulosa cell tumor produces pseudoprecocious puberty. There is no premature ovarian maturation and the serum gonadotropins are not elevated.

Q.78 Regarding primary peritoneal adenocarcinoma (PPA):
a. In PPA, the ovaries are either absent or normal in size
b. The tumor is predominantly of the serous type histologically
c. FIGO staging for ovarian carcinoma is currently being used for PPA
d. Prophylactic oophorectomy is protective against PPA

Ans. a, b and c. PPA is thought to be a separate clinical entity from papillary serous ovarian carcinoma (PSOC). Clinical presentation of cases with PPA and PSOC are similar and the prognosis of patients with PPA is poor. Prophylactic oophorectomy is not protective against PPA.

Q.79 The refrigerants used in cryosurgery include:
a. Freon (– 60° C)
b. Carbon dioxide (– 60° C)
c. Nitrous oxide (– 80° C)
d. All of the above

Ans. d.

Q.80 Female genital tuberculosis:
a. Genital tract involvement results from lymphatic spread
b. Premenstrual endometrial biopsy is diagnostic
c. Polymerase chain reaction (PCR) techniques have got higher sensitivity in detection
d. Reproductive outcome following antituberculous chemotherapy is satisfactory

Ans. c. Genital tuberculosis is usually secondary to primary infection (lungs, bones, lymph nodes). It is by hematogenous spread leading to endosalpingitis. Caseous granulomatous lesions with giant cells on histology are suggestive of TB but is not diagnostic as it can be seen in fungal infection and sarcoidosis. PCR can detect even less than 10 organisms in a clinical specimen compared to 10,000 necessary for smear positivity. Reproductive outcome even after treatment is poor. Pregnancy rate is about 20%, livebirth rate is only 7%. Risk of miscarriage and ectopic pregnancy are high.

Q.81 All the statements are correct, *except*:
a. Presence of the ovary is essential for female genital tract differentiation
b. Two normal "X" chromosomes seem to be essential for normal ovarian function
c. A loss of even a portion of one of the "X" chromosomes results in gonadal dysgenesis
d. Apart from SRY, autosomal genes are essential for gonadal differentiation

Ans. a. Ovaries do not play any part in the embryological development of the genital tract.

Q.82 Definite diagnostic procedure to detect invasive carcinoma cervix:
a. Colposcopy
b. Wedge biopsy
c. Cone biopsy
d. Cervical cytology

Ans. c.

Q.83 Absolute contraindications of laparoscopy are:
a. Diaphragmatic hernia
b. Generalized peritonitis
c. Patient on anticoagulant therapy
d. Previous incomplete laparoscopy

Ans. a, b and c. Previous incomplete laparoscopy is an indication for repeat laparoscopy for detailed evaluation.

Q.84 For operative hysteroscopy, the preferred substance to distend the uterine cavity:
a. Carbon dioxide at the rate of 80–150 mL/minute
b. Saline or dextrose solution in rapid drip
c. Heavy dextran (70%)
d. Glycine 1.5%

Ans. d. Glycine is commonly used because blood is not miscible with glycine. As such, the view is better and it does not conduct electricity.

Q.85 The following are related to androgen:
a. The term hyperandrogenemia implies virilism and hirsutism
b. The most potent androgen is dihydrotestosterone followed by testosterone
c. In normal women, about 1% of testosterone is free
d. Pilosebaceous units in the skin are sensitive to androgens and their number increases with androgen level

Ans. b and c. Sebaceous glands and hair follicles together comprise pilosebaceous unit. Total number of hair follicle per unit area of skin is fixed by 22 weeks of gestational age.

Q.86 The following statements are related to development of female genital organs, *except*:
a. In the absence of anti-Müllerian hormone (AMH), the urogenital sinus develops towards female
b. The development of the female genital tract organs is due to the absence of testis
c. AMH gene mutation may cause persistence of uterus and tubes in a male
d. AMH is secreted by the Leydig cells

Ans. d. AMH is secreted by the Sertoli cells.

Q.87 The following are related to pelvic ureter, *except*:
a. The ureter enters the pelvis behind the root of the mesentery on the right side
b. Its length is about 13 cm
c. The mucus layer is lined by columnar epithelium
d. It is crossed by uterine artery anteriorly

Ans. c. The mucus coat is lined by transitional epithelium.

Q.88 The following are the contents of deep perineal pouch, *except*:
a. Deep transverse perinei (paired)
b. Sphincter urethrae
c. Blood vessels and nerves
d. Bartholin's gland

Ans. d. Bartholin's gland is situated in the superficial perineal pouch.

Q.89 The following are related to round ligament, *except*:
a. Developmentally, it corresponds to the gubernaculum testis
b. It is attached to the uterine cornu anterior to uterine tube
c. It courses medial to the inferior epigastric artery
d. It terminates at the upper border of labium majus

Ans. c. Round ligament courses lateral to the artery and through the deep ring.

Q.90 Lymphatics of the body of the uterus drain primarily into the following glands, *except*:
a. Para-aortic
b. Deep inguinal
c. Internal iliac
d. External iliac

Ans. b. Lymphatics from the cornu of the uterus drain into the superficial group of inguinal glands.

Q.91 Superficial inguinal glands receive lymphatics from the following, *except*:
a. Cornu of the uterus
b. Labia majora
c. Glans of clitoris
d. Bartholin's gland

Ans. c. Glans of the clitoris directly drains into the pelvic nodes.

Q.92 Sensory component of pudendal nerve supplies the following structures, *except*:
a. Skin of the vulva
b. Lower half of the anal canal
c. Clitoris
d. Whole of urethra

Ans. d.

Q.93 The following are related to the course of pudendal nerve, *except*:
a. The nerve leaves the pelvis through greater sciatic foramen between piriformis and coccygeus muscle
b. The nerve re-enters the pelvis curling the ischial spine through lesser sciatic foramen
c. Pudendal canal is at the medial wall of the ischiorectal fossa
d. The dorsal nerve to the clitoris is a content of the deep perineal pouch

Ans. c. The pudendal canal, which is a fascial tunnel, is situated at the lateral wall of the ischiorectal fossa about 2.5 cm above the ischial tuberosity.

Q.94 Regarding pneumoperitoneum during laparoscopic surgery:
a. CO_2 is less soluble in blood than air
b. CO_2 is not easily excreted by the lungs
c. CO_2 is buffered by formation of bicarbonate
d. Insufflation pressures of 10–15 mm Hg are well-tolerated

Ans. c and d. CO_2 is twenty times more soluble in blood than air and it is easily excreted by the lungs. It is nontoxic and does not support combustion. It is thus preferred in laparoscopic surgery.

Q.95 The following are in relation to Bartholin's gland, *except*:
a. It is a compound racemose gland
b. It measures about 5 mm
c. It lies deep to the urogenital diaphragm
d. Its duct measures about 20 mm

Ans. c. Bartholin's gland lies superficial to urogenital diaphragm, in the superficial perineal pouch.

Q.96 The following are few branches of anterior division of internal iliac artery, *except*:
a. Uterine
b. Vaginal
c. Superior gluteal
d. Middle rectal

Ans. c. Superior gluteal artery is a branch of posterior division of internal iliac artery.

Q.97 The following are related to fallopian tube, *except*:
a. It is developed from paramesonephric duct
b. Its widest part is infundibulum and the longest part is the isthmus
c. The mucus lining is columnar
d. The blood supply is from uterine and ovarian

Ans. b. The maximum diameter of the infundibulum measures about 6 mm and the ampulla is the longest part, measuring 5 cm.

Q.98 The following are related to levator ani, *except*:
a. Viewed from above, it slopes downwards, forwards and medially
b. The inferior surface is related to the anatomical perineum
c. It is entirely innervated by pudendal nerve
d. Its important function is to support the pelvic organs

Ans. c. Apart from the pudendal nerve (S2, S3), the levator ani is supplied directly by the S4 from the pelvic surface.

Q.99 The following are related to internal iliac artery, *except*:
a. It measures about 2 cm
b. Internal iliac vein lies anteriorly
c. One of its visceral branches is middle rectal
d. One of its parietal branches is inferior gluteal

Ans. b. Internal iliac vein lies posterior to the artery.

Q.100 The following are related to development of genital organs, *except*:
   a. Bartholin's gland is developed from the urogenital sinus
   b. Clitoris is developed from genital tubercle
   c. Labia minora is developed from the urogenital sinus
   d. Endometrium is developed from the coelomic epithelium

Ans. c. Labia minora is developed from the urogenital folds.

Q.101 The following are related to development of ovary, *except*:
   a. Ovary is developed from the gonadal ridge
   b. The germ cells are endodermal in origin from the yolk sac
   c. The bipotential gonad develops into an ovary about two weeks before the testicular development
   d. At birth, the ovaries are situated at or above the pelvic brim

Ans. c. The bipotential gonad develops into an ovary about two weeks after the testicular development.

Q.102 In female, the following structures are developed from the urogenital sinus, *except*:
   a. Urethrovesical unit
   b. Vestibule
   c. Bartholin's gland
   d. Anal canal

Ans. d. The anal canal is not developed from the urogenital sinus. It develops from the cloaca—an endodermal structure.

Q.103 Regarding oligoasthenoteratozoospermia (OAT) syndrome:
   a. Testicular biopsy can differentiate obstructive from testicular cause of oligospermia
   b. The biopsied tissue should be sent in formal saline
   c. Congenital absence of vas deferens is observed in Young's syndrome
   d. The number of sperms required for IVF and ICSI are the same

Ans. a. Testicular biopsy can detect spermatogenic disorder; the tissue should be sent in either Bouin's, Zenker's or in buffered glutaraldehyde solution. Formaline solution is avoided because it causes destruction of seminiferous tubular structures. 95% of men with cystic fibrosis have congenital absence of vas. IVF needs 50,000–100,000 sperm for insemination of the eggs, whereas ICSI is performed with essentially one sperm for one egg.

Q.104 The following are related to hypothalamopituitary secretions, *except*:
   a. Gonadotropin-releasing hormone (GnRH) is a decapeptide
   b. Thyrotropin-releasing hormone (TRH) is a tridecapeptide
   c. Corticotropin-releasing hormone (CRH) is a tetradecapeptide
   d. Oxytocin is a nonpeptide

Ans. b. TRH is a tripeptide and not tridecapeptide.

Q.105 Regarding ovarian cancer:
   a. Combined oral contraceptive pill reduces the risk of ovarian cancer
   b. Mutation in BRCA genes account for about 80% of all ovarian cancers
   c. Prophylactic salpingo-oophorectomy has no effect on the risk of breast cancer
   d. Prophylactic salpingo-oophorectomy reduces the risk of ovarian cancer

Ans. a and d. BRCA gene mutation group account for only 10% of all ovarian cancers. Prophylactic oophorectomy reduces the incidence of breast cancer by 50%.

Q.106 The following subjects may be excluded from routine cervical cancer screening program, *except*:
   a. Women who had never been sexually active
   b. Women over the age of 65 who had negative smears in the past
   c. Women who had hysterectomy for benign lesion
   d. Women on oral pill

Ans. d. Oral pill users should be included in the routine screening program.

Q.107 The following embryonic and adult structures are related:
   a. Mesonephric tubules   1. Labia minora
   b. Mesonephric duct   2. Urethra
   c. Urogenital sinus   3. Duct of Gartner
   d. Urogenital folds   4. Epoophoron

Ans. a = 4; b = 3; c = 2; d = 1.

Q.108 The following are the clinical presentations of genital tuberculosis in Indian context, *except*:
   a. Infertility is present in about 70% cases of pelvic tuberculosis
   b. About 10% infertile women have got genital tuberculosis
   c. There may not be any menstrual abnormality
   d. Menorrhagia is the late manifestation

Ans. d. Menorrhagia is the early manifestation due to endometrial hyperemia.

Q.109 The following are related to function of testis, *except*:
   a. Seminiferous tubules are the site of spermatogenesis
   b. Leydig cells are the site of production of testosterone

c. Sertoli cells produce androgen binding protein
d. Inhibin is synthesized by the leydig cells

Ans. d. Inhibin is synthesized from the sertoli cells of the testis in response to FSH.

Q.110 Regarding uterine artery embolization (UAE) for the treatment of uterine fibroids:
a. Polyvinyl particles are used for the procedure
b. It is an alternative to myomectomy in infertile women
c. It causes amenorrhea in 25% of the women
d. Pregnancy outcome is uneventful following the procedure

Ans. a. RCOG and NICE have stated that UAE should not be offered to women who desirous of future childbearing. Avascular necrosis of myometrium makes it prone to rupture during pregnancy. Amenorrhea occurs in 1% of women and often it is transient.

Q.111 The following are related to SHBG, *except*:
a. It is a glycoprotein
b. The circulatory level is directly related to weight
c. Increased circulatory levels of insulin lower its level
d. Danazol decreases its level

Ans. b. The circulatory level of SHBG is inversely related to weight. In obese, the SHBG level decreases.

Q.112 The following are related to increased circulatory SHBG, *except*:
a. Pregnancy
b. Hyperthyroidism
c. Combined steroidal contraceptives users
d. Hirsutism

Ans. d. In hirsutism, SHBG is decreased resulting in increased free testosterone to act on the target cells—hair follicles. SHBG is a glycoprotein. 69% of estradiol and 80% of testosterone are bound to SHBG and only 30% and 19% respectively, are bound to albumin, only about 1% of testosterone are unbound and free. Hyperthyroidism, pregnancy and estrogen administration increase SHBG levels whereas corticosteroids, androgens and progestogens decrease SHBG. The circulatory level of SHBG is inversely related to weight. Hyperinsulinemia lowers the SHBG levels.

Q.113 The following are related to inhibin, *except*:
a. It is secreted from the granulosa cells
b. FSH controls its secretion
c. It preferentially stimulates FSH
d. When the follicle grows—level of activin declines and levels of inhibin and follistatin increase

Ans. c. Inhibin inhibits FSH.

Q.114 Regarding the viral infections true statements are:
a. Human papillomavirus (HPV) infection is associated with koilocytic atypia on cervical cytology
b. Nosocomial exposure is a mode of spread for HIV
c. The carrier neonate of hepatitis B virus may suffer from hepatocellular carcinoma
d. Patients with anti-HBe ('e' antibodies) are of high-risk for transmitting the infection

Ans. a and c. Patients with HBeAg ('e' antigen) are high-risk for transmitting the infection, but presence of 'e' antibodies is protective against transmission. Koilocytes have irregular hyperchromatic cells surrounded by clear cytoplasm. Certain HPV types are strongly associated with some genital cancers.

Q.115 The major contribution to the human seminal fluid is from:
a. Testes
b. Seminal vesicles
c. Prostate
d. Bulbourethral and urethral glands

Ans. b. The seminal vesicle contributes 60% and prostate about 30% of the seminal fluid.

Q.116 As regard the use of laser in gynecology, all are correct, *except*:
a. Management of CIN, VIN, VaIN
b. Laser laparoscopy for ectopic pregnancy
c. Laser hysteroscopy for presacral neurectomy
d. It acts by tissue cutting, vaporization or coagulation

Ans. c. Laser hysteroscopy is used for endometrial ablation and septum resection. Presacral neurectomy is done by laser laparoscopy.

Q.117 Regarding Asherman's syndrome all are true, *except*:
a. May occur following myomectomy
b. Always associated with amenorrhea
c. Progesterone challenge test is negative
d. Hysteroscopy or hysterography can be diagnostic

Ans. b. There may also be hypomenorrhea or Oligomenorrhea depending on the extent.

Q.118 Genuine stress incontinence (GSI) is due to all of these, *except*:
a. Dysfunction of the intrinsic bladder sphincter
b. Descent of the bladder neck and proximal urethra below the urogenital diaphragm
c. Hypermobility of the urethra
d. Increase in intraurethral pressure

Ans. d. There is decrease in intraurethral pressure.

Q.119 As regard ovulation all are correct, *except*:
a. Ovulation occurs 24–36 hours after the estradiol peak
b. Ovulation occurs 24 hours after the LH peak
c. Ovulation occurs 32–36 hours after the onset of LH surge
d. A threshold of LH surge should persist for 24 hours

Ans. b. It is 10–16 hours after the LH peak.

Q.120 Indications of diagnostic conization are all, *except*:
   a. Entire squamocolumnar junction is not seen
   b. Normal colposcopy with persistent abnormal cytology
   c. Cytology, colposcopy and biopsy revealed CIN lesion
   d. Colposcopically directed biopsy revealed microinvasion

Ans. c.

Q.121 In microinvasive cancer of the cervix all are true, *except*:
   a. Belongs to Stage IA
   b. Microscopically measured depth of invasion should not be more than 5 mm
   c. Can be diagnosed by colposcopy
   d. Can be treated by cone biopsy

Ans. c. Depth of invasion is measured only by biopsy.

Q.122 As regard to endometrial carcinoma all are correct, *except*:
   a. Serous cell histology has poorer prognosis compared to endometrioid type
   b. Prognostically depth of myometrial invasion is important
   c. Squamous metaplasia on histology has worst prognosis
   d. Ovarian metastasis is about 3–5%

Ans. c. Adenoacanthoma has similar prognosis as that of adenocarcinoma. Serous cell type has worst prognosis.

Q.123 Increased incidence of endometrial carcinoma is observed in women with:
   a. Cigarette smoking
   b. Premature menopause
   c. Members of the Lynch type-II family
   d. Women using DMPA as contraception

Ans. c.

Q.124 Regarding sarcoma botryoides:
   a. Usually occurs around the age of 18
   b. It is an embryonal rhabdomyosarcoma
   c. It is not sensitive to chemotherapy
   d. It is a tumor of the uterine body

Ans. b. Embryonal rhabdomyosarcoma is a highly malignant tumor, seen commonly below the age of 5, arising from the cervix or vagina (lower end of Müllerian tubercle) and is sensitive to chemotherapy.

Q.125 Regarding neoplasms of the ovary:
   a. Stromal invasion is commonly present in ovarian tumors of borderline malignancy
   b. Lymphocytic infiltration is characteristic to dysgerminoma
   c. Presence of ascites and pleural effusion in Brenner tumor indicates poor prognosis
   d. Endometrioid carcinoma of the ovary may coexist with endometrial adenocarcinoma

Ans. b and d. Stromal invasion is absent. The epithelium shows multilayering, cellular atypia, pleomorphism and mitotic activity. Brenner tumor may present with the features of Meigs syndrome and treatment prognosis is satisfactory. 20% of ovarian endometrioid carcinoma is associated with endometrial carcinoma.

Q.126 Concerning PCOS:
   a. PCOS increases the risk of type I diabetes mellitus
   b. Levonorgestrel-releasing IUS is a management option
   c. Metformin decreases insulin secretion
   d. Insulin therapy is a management option

Ans. b. Women with PCOS have an increased risk of developing type-2 diabetes and gestational diabetes. LNG-IUS gives endometrial protection against hyperplasia and carcinoma due to unopposed estrogen action. Such women are insulin resistant due to abnormalities of the insulin receptor. Metformin is used to improve sensitivity to insulin like other strategies that includes diet, exercise, lifestyle changes. Metformin improves hyperandrogenism, fertility and lipid profile. However, it has some gastrointestinal adverse effects (anorexia, nausea, diarrhea, flatulence).

Q.127 Regarding bacterial vaginosis, all are true, *except*:
   a. Homogeneous vaginal discharge with pH 5.0–6.0
   b. Positive KOH—with fishy odor
   c. Positive clue cells in 100% of cases
   d. It is due to *Gardnerella vaginalis*

Ans. c. Clue cells are diagnostic but about 40% patients may not have clue cells.

Q.128 These organisms cause vaginitis—match them appropriately:

a. *Trichomonas vaginalis*	1.	Gram-negative rod
b. *Candida albicans*	2.	Stippled desquamated epithelial cells
c. *Gardnerella vaginalis*	3.	Gram-positive fungus
d. *Mobiluncus*	4.	'Strawberry' cervix

Ans. a = 4; b = 3; c = 2; d = 1.

Q.129 Regarding prolactinomas:
   a. Often progresses from microadenoma to macroadenoma
   b. In men, it causes oligospermia
   c. Surgical excision completely cures the patient on long-term basis
   d. Women with normal prolactin level can have prolactinomas

Ans. d; a. Not necessarily all microadenomas progress to macroadenoma. b. In men it causes impotence, decreased libido. c. Cases may recur even following surgery or may develop panhypopituitarism.

Q.130 Regarding sex hormone binding globulin (SHBG):
 a. 25% of circulating testosterone in female is bound to SHBG
 b. Combined oral pill lowers its level
 c. Low level predicts development of type II diabetes mellitus
 d. SHBG binds 70% of circulating progesterone

Ans. c. SHBG is a glycoprotein. 69% of E2 and 80% of T are bound to SHBG and only 30% and 19% respectively are bound to albumin leaving only about 1% unbound and free. Hyperthyroidism, pregnancy and estrogen administration increase SHBG levels whereas corticosteroids, androgens and progestins decrease SHBG. The level of SHBG is inversely related to weight. Hyperinsulinemia lowers the SHBG levels; d. 79% progesterone is bound to albumin.

Q.131 Regarding craniopharyngioma all are correct, *except*:
 a. May cause secondary amenorrhea
 b. Leads to hypogonadotropic hypogonadism
 c. May cause hyperprolactinemia
 d. It is a tumor of the meninges

Ans. d. It is a cyst derived from the remnants of Rathke's pouch. Severity of pathology varies depending upon the extent of pituitary stalk involvement.

Q.132 Hypogonadism is observed in all, *except*:
 a. Savage's syndrome
 b. Turner's syndrome
 c. Stein-Leventhal syndrome
 d. Laurence-Moon-Bardet-Biedl syndrome

Ans. c.

Q.133 Kallmann's syndrome is characterized by all, *except*:
 a. State of hypogonadotropic hypogonadism
 b. Anosmia, color blindness are associated
 c. Deficient secretion of GnRH
 d. Abnormal female karyotype

Ans. d.

Q.134 Regarding follicle stimulating hormone and luteinizing hormone (FSH and LH) all are correct, *except*:
 a. LH is high in androgen insensitivity syndrome
 b. FSH stimulates spermatogenesis from sertoli cells of the testis
 c. FSH level is raised when long-term GnRH agonist is used
 d. LH stimulates testosterone secretion from leydig cells of the testis

Ans. c. Level is suppressed.

Q.135 In relation to precocious puberty in girls all are true, *except*:
 a. It is the development of secondary sexual characters before the age of 8
 b. Most common cause is idiopathic
 c. GnRH analogs is a useful treatment for all cases
 d. Premature adrenarche is a cause

Ans. c. It is useful only when it is gonadotropin dependent.

Q.136 Regarding GnRH analogs all are correct, *except*:
 a. Plasma half-life is about 10 minutes
 b. There is significant reduction of trabecular bone density after 6 months of use
 c. Benefits of antagonists are the same as that of agonists
 d. Can be used as a diagnostic test for premenstrual tension syndrome

Ans. a. Plasma half-life is more than 2 hours.

Q.137 As regard the gonadotropin releasing hormone all are true, *except*:
 a. It is a decapeptide
 b. It is secreted from the arcuate nucleus of the hypothalamus
 c. Plasma half-life is about 30–40 min
 d. Endogenous opioids suppress its release

Ans. c. It is 2–4 minutes.

Q.138 Regarding adrenogenital syndrome:
 a. Treated by low-dose combined oral pill
 b. It is inherited as an autosomal dominant mode
 c. 17-OHP is elevated in 3β hydroxysteroid dehydrogenase deficiency
 d. Majority of the IIβ hydroxylase deficient patients become hypertensive

Ans. d; a. Treatment is low-dose dexamethasone; b. It is an autosomal recessive condition; c. Blood levels of DHA and DHES are markedly increased.

Q.139 Regarding Asherman's syndrome all are correct, *except*:
 a. Is a cause of recurrent miscarriage
 b. May be due to uterine schistosomiasis
 c. Despite treatment, prospect of pregnancy is poor
 d. Hysteroscopic adhesiolysis is preferred to D and C

Ans. c. Successful pregnancy following treatment is approximately 70–80%.

Q.140 Regarding male pseudohermaphroditism all are true, *except*:
 a. It is due to failure of virilization
 b. The individual is a male genetically (46 XY)
 c. Testosterone level is within normal female range

d. The individual is reared up as a female and the gonads are removed

Ans. c. It is normal or slightly elevated male range.

Q.141 Regarding congenital adrenal hyperplasia all are true, *except*:
a. Characterized by masculinized external genitalia
b. Enzyme defects in cortisol synthesis is 21-hydroxylase P450c21 mainly (95%)
c. Prenatal diagnosis and treatment is yet to develop
d. Testosterone is the major circulating androgen

Ans. c. Chorionic villus biopsy and DNA probe can make the diagnosis. Treatment includes pregnancy termination or dexamethasone therapy.

Q.142 Regarding luteal phase defect (LPD):
a. Is an established cause of infertility
b. Is diagnosed by ultrasonography
c. Defective follicular maturation may be a cause
d. The basal body temperature (BBT) chart is monophasic

Ans. c. LPD is due to deficient function of the corpus luteum with insufficient progesterone production. Whether it is an established cause of infertility, remains controversial. BBT can be biphasic but the duration of temperature rise is short. Diagnosis of luteal phase defect is made by BBT chart, estimation of serum progesterone and accurate dating of endometrial sampling is extremely important. USG is not helpful in this regard.

Q.143 Concerning female sexual development all are correct, *except*:
a. Lack of SRY gene
b. Absence of testosterone
c. Absence of anti-Müllerian hormone (AMH)
d. SRY gene is located on the long arm of Y chromosome

Ans. d. SRY gene is located on the short arm of the Y chromosome.

Q.144 Regarding transcervical resection of endometrium (TCRE):
a. Resectoscope must remove the basal layer of endometrium
b. Prior hysteroscopic assessment is recommended
c. Uterine size is not a consideration
d. Success rate is nearly 100%

Ans. a and b; c. Large uterine size is a contraindication; d. Success rate is about 80%.

Q.145 Effectiveness of combined oral pills is reduced by all, *except*:
a. Phenobarbitone
b. Rifampicin
c. Sodium valproate
d. Spironolactone

Ans. c.

Q.146 Regarding Mifepristone:
a. It is an antiestrogen
b. Used for medical termination of pregnancy
c. Can be used up to 63 days of pregnancy
d. Failure rate is about 5%

Ans. b and c; a. Antiprogesterone; d. It is only 1%.

Q.147 In relation to pelvic infection:
a. Laparoscopy should be used for diagnosis in all cases
b. 'Violin string' adhesions suggest chlamydial infection
c. Ultrasonography is superior to laparoscopy
d. Salpingitis isthmica nodosa is one form of tubal endometriosis

Ans. b and d.

Q.148 The ovarian ligament has the following characteristics:
a. Is attached medially to the uterus
b. Contains the ovarian vessels
c. Is attached laterally to the pelvic wall
d. Is homologous to the gubernaculum testis in male

Ans. a and d.

Q.149 The following are the correlations with the types of epithelium and the organ:
a. Cervix and the columnar epithelium
b. Urethral meatus and the transitional epithelium
c. Vagina and the stratified squamous epithelium
d. Uterine body and the ciliated epithelium

Ans. c.

Q.150 As regard the karyotype and the diagnosis—match the following:
a. 45 XO   1. Androgen insensitivity syndrome
b. 46 XY   2. Turner's syndrome
c. 47 XXY   3. Super female
d. 47 XXX   4. Klinefelter's syndrome

Ans. a = 2; b = 1; c = 4; d = 3.

Q.151 The following ovarian tumors are malignant:
a. Brenner tumor
b. Dermoid cyst
c. Krukenberg tumor
d. Granulosa cell tumor

Ans. c and d.

Q.152 Regarding cervical cytology screening:
a. Primary aim of cytology is to detect cervical cancer
b. It is preferred to screen all the high risk types of HPV
c. There is a significant difference in the reduction of cervical cancer between 3 and 5 yearly screening
d. Liquid-based cytology is superior to conventional smears

Ans. c and d; a. The primary aim of cervical cytology screening is to prevent deaths from cervical cancer by preventing the disease. This is done by **detecting and treating the precancerous condition**; b. Currently screening is limited to only the high risks 16 and 18 HPV types; c. Five yearly screening of women (aged between 20 and 65 years) could reduce the incidence of cervical cancer by 84%, whereas by 3 yearly it is 91% and by annual screening it is 93%; d. Liquid-based cytology can reduce the number of unsatisfactory smears and false-negative smears. It increases the sensitivity. **Liquid-based cytology (LBC):** Smear is taken with a plastic device. The device is rinsed in a buffered methanol solution. Cells are separated by centrifugation. Thin layer smears are then made. LBC can reduce the number of unsatisfactory and false-negative smears. It increases the sensitivity also.

Q.153 Regarding postmenopausal osteoporosis:
  a. Bone density in the proximal forearm is generally measured to assess the bone mineral content
  b. Single photon absorptiometry is the investigation of choice to detect lumbar spine mineral content
  c. Average bone mineral loss every year is 5%, postmenopausally
  d. Estrogen therapy even after fracture, prevents further bone loss

Ans. a and d; b. Dual energy X-ray absorptiometry (DEXA) is the most accurate method; c. Average bone mineral loss in the first year is 3%, thereafter it is 1% annually.

Q.154 Hormone replacement therapy (HRT) and menopause:
  a. Estrogen is ideal for a woman who has intact uterus
  b. Progestins in HRT should be given for 12–14 days per cycle
  c. Continuous estrogen and progestin therapy protects bone loss equally
  d. HRT is to be continued for 10 years or more as desired

Ans. b and c; a. Women with intact uterus should have combined HRT either cyclical or continuous; d. HRT is currently recommended for a short period of time, preferably for 5 years.

Q.155 As regard the three swab test for urinary fistula—match the following:

a. Uppermost swab soaked but unstained with dye and lower two swabs remain dry	1. Vesicovaginal fistula
b. Lower swab stained with dye and upper two swabs dry	2. Ureterovaginal fistula
c. Middle swab stained with dye and upper and lower swab dry	3. Stress incontinence
d. Swabs dry but dye leaks from urethral meatus	4. Urethrovaginal fistula

Ans. a = 2; b = 4; c = 1; d = 3.

Q.156 The first choice of surgical treatment for stress urinary incontinence is:
  a. Cystourethroplasty or MMK procedure
  b. Sling procedure (TVT, TVT-O)
  c. Salvage procedure
  d. Raj or Stamey procedure especially in a young woman

Ans. b.

Q.157 Regarding interstitial cystitis all are true, *except*:
  a. It presents with dysuria, frequency, hematuria
  b. Cause is obscure
  c. Cystoscopy reveals normal bladder mucosa
  d. Management is unsatisfactory

Ans. c. Bladder mucosa is ulcerated.

Q.158 Urge incontinence is characterized by:
  a. Absence of urge prior to urine leak
  b. Amount of urine loss is always small
  c. Detrusor is hypersensitive to infection or calculi
  d. Cystourethroscopy is always normal

Ans. c; a. Urge is always present; b. Amount of loss is large; d. Usually informative. (*See* Dutta's Textbook of Gynecology, 8th Edition, p. 341).

Q.159 Genuine stress urinary incontinence (GSI) is characterized by all, *except*:
  a. Occurs usually in parous woman
  b. Escape of urine occurs during coughing, laughing (stress)
  c. Amount is always large
  d. Micturition is normal

Ans. c. It is always small in amount.

Q.160 Detrusor overactivity is characterized by:
  a. Leakage of urine due to detrusor overactivity
  b. Patient can voluntarily inhibit it
  c. Cystometry reveals normal detrusor pressure
  d. It is usually observed when the bladder is full.

Ans. a; b. Patient cannot control it; c. Detrusor pressure is increased on cystometry; d. It occurs at a much lower bladder filling.

Q.161 Regarding urinary incontinence and urodynamic investigation all are correct, *except*:
  a. Normal bladder capacity is in the range of 400–600 mL
  b. Detrusor overactivity can be accurately diagnosed by these investigations
  c. Midstream specimen of urine must be cultured in all cases of incontinence
  d. Normal voiding is affected by sympathetic control of bladder

Ans. d. It is the parasympathetic nerve control.

Q.162 The Burch colposuspension includes all, *except*:
  a. Is the operation for genuine stress incontinence
  b. 5 years success rate is about 90%

c. May be complicated by detrusor instability after the operation
d. Involves suturing the vagina to the rectus sheath

Ans. d. Suturing is done to the ipsilateral iliopectineal ligament.

Q.163 Regarding ovarian follicular development:
a. Time required for a follicle to achieve preovulatory status is about 120 days
b. Dominant follicle is selected by 5–7 days of the cycle
c. Midfollicular rise in estradiol exerts a negative feedback to FSH and positive feedback to LH
d. FSH stimulates activin and inhibin production by granulosa cells

Ans. b, c and d; a. Time required is about 85 days. (*See* Dutta's Textbook of Gynecology, 8th Edition, p. 72).

Q.164 Regarding spermatogenesis:
a. FSH stimulates leydig cells
b. Sertoli cells produce androgen binding protein (ABP) and inhibin B
c. Spermatogenesis requires very high local androgen concentration
d. Sertoli cells are analogous to theca cells of the ovary

Ans. b and c; a. FSH stimulates spermatogenesis and sertoli cells. d. Sertoli cells are analogous to granulosa cells and the leydig cells to theca cells of the ovary.

Q.165 Regarding gestational trophoblastic disease (GTD):
a. Complete moles show chromosomal pattern 46 XY in majority
b. Any plateau or re-elevation of hCG level during follow-up, suggests persistent GTD
c. Presence of pre-eclampsia increases the risk for persistent GTD
d. While on chemotherapy, drop of hCG < 25%, suggests a repeat course of the drug

Ans. b and c. Complete moles have a chromosomal complement of 46 XX in majority (90%) and both are paternally derived. Partial moles are often with a fetus and triploidy (69 XXX or XXY); b. This condition is for careful review and for chemotherapy; c. Risk is as high as 80%; d. This suggests resistance and change in the chemotherapeutic regimen and not to repeat the same drug.

Q.166 Concerning thyroid function and reproduction:
a. Elevated TSH with normal T_4 level suggests a subclinical hypothyroid state
b. Patients on long-term thyroid hormone should not stop taking the drug
c. Subclinical hypothyroidism should not be treated
d. Response to TSH with thyroid hormone therapy is slow

Ans. a. and d; b. Patient may stop taking medication as there is chance of recovery of hypothalamic-pituitary axis; c. This state should be treated to prevent development of goiter.

Q.167 Regarding toxic shock syndrome:
a. May occur at any age group
b. Often the patient presents with hypothermia
c. Exotoxin liberated by *Staphylococcus aureus* is the causative factor
d. Mortality may be as high as 30%

Ans. c; a. Common in menstruating women (15–30 years of age); b. Fever is common; d. Mortality is 5–10%.

Q.168 Regarding ectopic pregnancy:
a. The incidence of ectopic pregnancy is declining
b. The use of IUD is protective against ectopic pregnancy
c. It may coexist with an intrauterine pregnancy
d. The use of low-dose combined pills increases the risk

Ans. c; a. Incidence is rising; b. IUDs increases the risk; d. It is protective.

Q.169 Regarding cancer of the female genital organs:
a. Combined oral pills reduces the risk of ovarian carcinoma
b. Obesity increases the risk of endometrial carcinoma
c. Breastfeeding increases the risk of ovarian cancer
d. Late menopause increases the risk of breast carcinomas

Ans. a, b and d; c. It is protective.

Q.170 Carcinoma of the vagina:
a. Commonly occurs as a primary lesion
b. Most common site is the anterior and upper third vaginal wall
c. Usually is an adenocarcinoma
d. Inguinofemoral lymph nodes are involved

Ans. d; a. Primary vaginal carcinoma is rare 1–2% of all genital malignancies; spread from adjacent organs or metastasis is common; b. It is posterior and upper third vaginal wall; c. Common site is squamous cell carcinoma in 90% of cases.

Q.171 Regarding choriocarcinoma:
a. Characterized by snowstorm pattern on uterine ultrasonography
b. Histological examination reveals absence of chorionic villi
c. Lymph node metastases are common
d. Commonly, it is preceded by a hydatidiform mole or miscarriage

Ans. b and d; a. It is common in hydatidiform moles. Estimation of hCG, is the most reliable parameter for diagnosis and therapy; c. Lymph node and bone metastases are rare. Metastasis of lungs (60–95%), vagina (40–50%), vulva/cervix (10–15%), brain (5–15%) and liver (5–15%) are common; d. Choriocarcinoma develops following hydatidiform mole (50%), term pregnancy (15%) and following abortion or ectopic pregnancy (25%). Trophoblastic disease following a normal pregnancy is either choriocarcinoma or PSTT and not a benign mole.

Q.172 **Vulvodynia:**
 a. It is commonly due to fungal infection
 b. Associated with dyspareunia
 c. Clinical examination reveals vulvar erythema
 d. Amitriptyline is the first choice of treatment
Ans. d.

Q.173 **Regarding androgen metabolism in female:**
 a. Rapid progression of hirsutism suggests Cushing's syndrome
 b. 90% of dehydroepiandrosterone sulfate is of adrenal origin
 c. GnRH analogs decrease hepatic synthesis of SHBG
 d. GnRH analogs can inhibit adrenal androgen secretion
Ans. b. Rapid progression of hirsutism suggests ovarian or adrenal tumor. GnRH analogs neither affect hepatic synthesis of SHBG nor can inhibit adrenal androgen synthesis.

Q.174 **Regarding endometriosis:**
 a. Endometriosis is always a progressive disease
 b. Minimal or mild endometriosis must be treated when diagnosed in any subfertile patient
 c. Danazol acts by increasing the hepatic synthesis of SHBG
 d. Powder burn areas are not the active lesions
Ans. d. Endometriosis is usually progressive but spontaneous regression may occur. Danazol suppresses the midcycle LH and FSH surges and inhibits ovarian steroidogenesis. It inhibits the hepatic synthesis of SHBG. Management (conservative laparoscopic or medical) of minimal or mild endometriosis is controversial. In minimal or mild endometriosis, there is no place of ovulation suppression by medical treatment. During diagnostic laparoscopy, ablation of endometriotic lesion may be considered (Marcoux, et al. 1997). Treatment should be individualized depending on woman's age and duration of infertility.

Q.175 **The endometrium of a normal menstrual cycle:**
 a. Regeneration of endometrium starts after the menstruation ceases
 b. Subnuclear vacuolation indicates ovulation is imminent
 c. The endometrium regresses 1 or 2 days prior to menstruation
 d. The postovulatory endometrial changes are due to estrogen
Ans. c. Subnuclear vacuolation of gland epithelium usually occurs 24–36 hours after ovulation.

Q.176 **About the inguinal canal:**
 a. The anterior wall is formed by the external oblique aponeurosis
 b. Posterior wall is formed by the internal oblique muscle
 c. The deep ring is situated in transversus abdominis muscle
 d. The superficial ring is situated on the pubic crest
Ans. d. Inguinal canal is oblique and extends from deep inguinal ring, a gap in the fascia transversal to the superficial inguinal ring, a gap in the external oblique aponeurosis. Anterior wall is formed also by internal oblique laterally. So, also the posterior wall by fascia transversalis and conjoint tendon.

Q.177 **In relation to labia majora all are correct, *except*:**
 a. Developmentally, it is homologous to scrotum in male
 b. Lymphatic systems are separate on each side
 c. It is supplied by the branches of internal and external pudendal arteries
 d. Abnormal fusion is most commonly seen in testicular feminization
Ans. d. Abnormal fusion of labioscrotal swelling is most common due to congenital adrenal hyperplasia.

Q.178 **The femoral triangle:**
 a. Femoral nerve lies in the lateral compartment of the femoral sheath
 b. Base of the femoral triangle is formed by fascia transversalis
 c. Branch of genitofemoral nerve is a content of femoral sheath
 d. Femoral ring lies between the artery and the vein
Ans. c. Base of femoral triangle formed by the inguinal ligament. Femoral sheath is formed by the fascia transversalis in front and fascia iliaca behind. The femoral sheath has three compartments.
 1. Femoral artery, femoral branch of the genitofemoral nerve
 2. Femoral vein in the intermediate compartment
 3. Femoral canal lies in the medial compartment. Mouth of the femoral canal is called femoral ring.

Q.179 **The labia minora:**
 a. Contains sebaceous glands
 b. The lower ends fuse to form the posterior commissure

c. Developmentally similar to labia majora
d. Contains few hair follicles

Ans. a. The lower end fuse each other to form fourchette. Labia minora is developed from the genital folds whereas labia majora from the genital swellings. Labia minora do not contain hair follicles.

Q.180 Primary dysmenorrhea:
a. Usually, there is a primary cause underneath
b. Often associated with anovulation
c. Pain usually begins a week before the menstruation
d. Oral contraceptive pills are effective to relieve the pain

Ans. d.

Q.181 McCune-Albright syndrome:
a. Puberty is delayed but menarche is early
b. Associated with endocrinopathies
c. It is GnRH dependent
d. The condition affects boys more than the girls

Ans. b. *See* Dutta's Textbook of Gynecology, 8th Edition, p. 41. There is precocious puberty including premature menarche. Girls are affected more than the boys.

Q.182 Regarding ovulation in a normal menstrual cycle:
a. Biphasic BBT indicates ovulation is imminent
b. LH surge occurs immediately following ovulation
c. Disappearance of cervical mucus ferning is suggestive of ovulation
d. Vaginal cytology, shift of maturation index (MI) to the right indicates ovulation

Ans. c. Biphasic BBT indicates ovulation in retrospect. LH surge is prior to ovulation and secretion of progesterone from corpus luteum following ovulation causes shift of MI to the left in vaginal cytology.

Q.183 Regarding ambiguous genitalia [Disorder of sex development (DSD)]:
a. In a girl with congenital adrenal hyperplasia—uterus will be absent
b. Uterus will be present in a case with 'testicular feminization syndrome (46 XY)'
c. Ovaries are absent in a case with Mayer-Rokitansky-Küster-Hauser syndrome
d. In Turner's syndrome, secondary sex characters are poor

Ans. d.

Q.184 Regarding Turner's syndrome all are correct, *except*:
a. The patient usually presents with primary amenorrhea
b. The Karyotype is 45 XO
c. The patient usually have mental retardation
d. Breast development is poor

Ans. c. Usually there is no mental retardation.

Q.185 Regarding development of gonads all are correct, *except*:
a. The bipotential gonad differentiate by 6–7 weeks time
b. Ovarian differentiation occurs 2 weeks later than the testis
c. SRY gene of Y chromosome controls the differentiation of ovary
d. The germ cell number in the ovary is maximum at 20th week

Ans. c.

Q.186 Regarding development of genital organs all are correct, *except*:
a. The Müllerian tubercle is formed at the dorsal wall of the urogenital sinus
b. The hymen is developed at the junction of the sinovaginal bulbs and the urogenital sinus
c. The paramesonephric duct crosses the mesonephric duct anteriorly
d. The paramesonephric ducts begin to fuse with each other at 12th week

Ans. d. The paramesonephric ducts begin to fuse each other by 7–8 weeks and it is completed by 12th week.

Q.187 Indications of prophylactic chemotherapy in molar pregnancy are all, *except*:
a. When hCG level following evacuation fails to become normal by 6–9 weeks time
b. In a woman with number of high-risk factors for malignant change
c. Preferably as a routine to all cases following evacuation
d. In cases where there is re-elevation of hCG level following its initial normalization

Ans. c. Routine use of cytotoxic drugs prophylactically is not recommended considering their toxicity.

Q.188 Choriocarcinoma:
a. Antecedent term pregnancy is a low-risk factor
b. About 25% develop following hydatidiform mole
c. Villus pattern is usually present
d. May follow an ectopic pregnancy

Ans. d.

Q.189 Regarding hCG all are correct, *except*:
a. Reaches its peak level between 60 and 70 days of pregnancy
b. Level is increased in hydatidiform mole
c. It can be used as a tumor marker
d. It is needed for the differentiation of female external genitalia

Ans. d. hCG stimulate leydig cells of the male fetus to produce testosterone. It is helpful for the development of male external genitalia.

Q.190 Granulosa cell tumors of the ovary:
a. Is a common germ cell tumor of younger age
b. May cause true isosexual precocious puberty
c. Characterized histologically by Call-Exner bodies
d. May cause endometrial carcinoma in about 50% cases

Ans. c. Risk of endometrial carcinoma is 5–10%.

Q.191 The round ligament:
a. It measures 24 cm in length
b. It is attached to the cornu of the uterus below and behind the fallopian tube
c. It runs posterior to the obturator artery
d. It traverses through the inguinal canal

Ans. d.

Q.192 The round ligament:
a. It contains striated muscle
b. It passes medial to the inferior epigastric artery
c. It is homologous to the gubernaculum testis
d. It is inserted in the inguinal ligament

Ans. c.

Q.193 The uterine artery:
a. Purely supplies the uterus
b. Is a branch of the posterior division of internal iliac artery
c. Passes below the ureter in the tunnel of the Mackenrodt's ligament
d. It supplies the round ligament through utero-ovarian anastomosis

Ans. d.

Q.194 The ovary:
a. Receives its blood supply mainly from the internal iliac artery
b. Ovarian veins drain into the inferior vena cava
c. Ligament of ovary is attached at its lateral pole
d. It is attached to posterior leaf of the broad ligament

Ans. d.

Q.195 Regarding the fallopian tube the correct statement is:
a. It is entirely lined by ciliated columnar epithelium
b. The abdominal ostium is narrower than the uterine ostium
c. It undergoes cyclical changes during the menstrual cycle
d. Fimbria ovarica is attached to the lateral pole of the ovary

Ans. d. The abdominal ostium is 2 mm whereas uterine ostium is 1 mm in diameter.

Q.196 The vagina:
a. Is lined by single layer of squamous epithelium
b. Is endodermal in origin
c. Is developed from the mesonephric duct
d. Complete agenesis of vagina is often associated with absence of uterus

Ans. d.

Q.197 Germ cell tumors of the ovary:
a. Majority are malignant
b. Dysgerminoma is the most common malignant germ cell tumor
c. Endodermal sinus tumor is the least common malignant germ cell tumor
d. Dysgerminomas are usually bilateral

Ans. b. Germ cell tumors constitute about 15–20% of all ovarian neoplasm and around 2–3% of them are malignant. Cystic teratomas or dermoids are the most common benign germ cell tumor. Dysgerminoma is the most common malignant germ cell tumor. Endodermal sinus tumor is the second common malignant germ cell tumor. Dysgerminomas are bilateral in 10–15% cases only.

Q.198 Regarding arterial supply of the pelvis all are true, *except*:
a. Posterior trunk of the internal iliac supplies the gluteal muscles
b. Median sacral artery arises from the aorta
c. Inferior vesical artery arises from the posterior trunk of internal iliac artery
d. Inferior rectal artery is a branch of internal pudendal artery

Ans. c.

Q.199 All are true about acquired immunodeficiency syndrome (AIDS), *except*:
a. The infection is caused by DNA virus
b. The virus binds to the CD4 molecule of the T cells
c. Transplacental transmission to fetus is about 14–25%
d. The virus can be transmitted by artificial insemination

Ans. a.

Q.200 Regarding Müllerian duct:
a. Develops medial to the Wolffian duct
b. Is also known as mesonephric duct
c. Starts to differentiate at 5–6 weeks of embryonic life
d. The blind end projects into the urogenital sinus as Müllerian tubercle

Ans. d; c. Differentiation starts after 8 weeks. Before that, both the Müllerian and Wolffian ducts coexist in all embryos.

Q.201 Laparoscopic ovarian drilling (LOD) for a woman with PCOS:
a. Monopolar coagulation current is used for 5 seconds
b. Power setting is at 30 W
c. The needle is pushed within the capsule to a depth of 6–8 mm
d. The ovary is irrigated with normal saline at the end of the procedure

Ans. a, b, c and d.

Q.202 Laparoscopic ovarian surgery (LOS) for a woman with PCOS:
a. For LOS, laser is found superior to electrocautery
b. LOS restores regular ovulation in about 70% cases
c. Cumulative rates of conception and miscarriage are high
d. There is persistent fall in circulating androgens and continued improvement in insulin sensitivity.

Ans. b. Electrocautery is found more effective in achieving ovulation and pregnancy. Cumulative rates of conception are high (75%) but miscarriage rates are similar to general population. Following LOS, the levels of androgens (testosterone, androsterone) fall rapidly. But there is no improvement of insulin sensitivity and lipid abnormalities.

Q.203 Failure rates of different contraceptive methods per 100 women year:

Ans.

Intrauterine contraceptive devices (IUCDs)		Laparoscopic sterilization electrocoagulation	
■ CuT 380 A	0.8–0.6	■ Unipolar method	0.75%
■ LNG-IUS	0.1	■ Bipolar method	2.1%
Implanon	0.01		
Tubal sterilization (Pomeroy)	0.15–0.5	**Ring**	
		■ Falope ring	1.77%
		■ Filshie clip	0.1%

Q.204 Unsatisfactory colposcopy means:
a. Failure to visualize cervix
b. Failure to visualize transformation zone
c. Failure to visualize squamous epithelium
d. Failure to visualize columnar epithelium

Ans. b. See Dutta's Textbook of Gynecology, 8th Edition, p. 272, 273.

Q.205 Virilizing tumors of the ovary are:
a. Arrhenoblastoma
b. Adrenal tumors of the ovary
c. Leydig cell tumor
d. Gynandroblastoma
e. All of the above

Ans. e. See Dutta's Textbook of Gynecology, 8th Edition, p. 324.

Hormone producing tumors of the ovary (See Dutta's Textbook of Gynecology, 8th Edition, p. 324)

Male hormone	Female hormone	Mixed tumor
■ Sertoli cell tumor ■ Leydig cell tumor	■ Granulosa cell tumor ■ Theca cell tumor	Gynandroblastoma contains both Sertoli-Leydig cell (androgenic) and granulosa cell (estrogenic component)

Q.206 Feminizing tumors of the ovary are:
a. Granulosa cell tumor
b. Theca cell tumor
c. Dermoid cyst
d. Serous cystadenoma

Ans. a and b.

Q.207 Anencephaly is best diagnosed at 12 weeks by:
a. Serum alpha fetoprotein
b. Ultrasonography
c. Radiography
d. Amniography

Ans. b.

Conditions associated with elevated maternal serum alpha fetoprotein level

■ Neural tube defects	■ Retroplacental hemorrhage
■ IUFD	■ Placental abruption
■ Multiple pregnancy	■ Gastroschisis
■ Renal agenesis	■ Omphalocele
■ Polycystic kidney disease	■ Esophageal or duodenal atresia
■ Placental abnormalities	■ Fetal hydrops or ascites
■ Hemangiomas of placenta	■ Cystic hygroma
	■ Sacrococcygeal teratoma
	■ Oligohydramnios

Low levels of maternal serum alpha fetoprotein

■ Chromosomal trisomies	■ Gestational trophoblastic neoplasia	■ Inaccurate gestational age

Q.208 Call-Exner bodies is seen with:
a. Granulosa cell tumor
b. Pseudomucinous cystadenoma
c. Papillary cystadenoma
d. Dermoid

Ans. a. See Dutta's Textbook of Gynecology, 8th Edition, p. 323.

Specific histological features that are used as in the diagnostic criteria
- ***Psammoma bodies*** in papillary serous cystadenoma of the ovary
- ***Signet ring cells*** for Krukenberg tumor (metastatic ovarian carcinoma)
- ***Call-Exner body*** in granulosa cell tumor of the ovary
- ***Reinke's crystal*** in hilus cell ovarian tumor
- ***Hobnail cells*** in clear cell carcinoma of the ovary
- ***Keratin pearls*** in squamous cell carcinoma of the cervix
- ***Struma ovarii,*** presence of thyroid tissue in ovarian teratoma
- ***Schiller-Duval body*** in endodermal sinus cell tumor of the ovary
- ***'Coffee bean' nuclei*** in granulosa cell tumor of the ovary

Q.209 Which of the following feature of second trimester ultrasound is not a marker of Down's syndrome?
   a. Single umbilical artery
   b. Choroid plexus cyst
   c. Aplasia cutis
   d. Duodenal atresia

Ans. c.
Abnormalities associated with Down's syndrome (Trisomy 21)
It is the most common autosomal chromosomal syndrome. Its relationship with maternal age is: 1 in 952 by the age of 30 and 1 in 106 by the age of 40 years. 95% cases are due to maternal nondisjunction, usually in meiosis-I.
The characteristic features are: Brachycephaly, epicanthal folds, broad nasal bridge, a protruding tongue, small and low set ears, hypotonia, broad short fingers, clinodactyly, wide space between the first two toes (sandle gap), single palmar crease (30%), cardiac lesions, duodenal atresia, diaphragmatic hernia, single umbilical artery. Cardiac defects (ASD, VSD), hypoechoic bowel, short humerus and femur, thickened nuchal fold and hydrocephalus. The risk of recurrence in subsequent pregnancy is 1%. Females with Down's syndrome are fertile and the risk of having Down baby for them is about 30%. Males are usually sterile.

Q.210 Chorionic villus sampling done before 10 weeks may result in:
   a. Fetal loss
   b. Fetomaternal hemorrhage
   c. Oromandibular limb defects
   d. Sufficient material not obtained

Ans. c.
CVS of the developing trophoblast is done in the first trimester of pregnancy. Indications are similar to amniocentesis for the purpose of molecular (DNA analysis), cytogenetic and biochemical studies.
CVS is done between 10 and 12 completed weeks of pregnancy. Chorion frondosum is sampled as it contains the most mitotically active cells. CVS is done either by transcervical or transabdominal route. Prior ultrasound evaluation is done to detect fetal viability gestational age and placental location.

Procedure
- ***Transcervical CVS:*** A polythene catheter with a malleable obturator is passed through the cervix under ultrasound guidance. Placental trophoblast is aspirated into a 20 mL syringe containing the tissue culture medium.
- ***Transabdominal CVS:*** A 19 or 20 gauge needle with a stylet is directed into the thickest part of the placenta under the ultrasound guidance. The stylet is withdrawn and a syringe containing tissue culture medium is attached to the hub of the needle and suction is applied as the needle is moved up and down until an adequate amount of tissue is obtained. The sample is inspected to ensure that 20–40 mg of villus material is obtained.

Selection of method for CVS: CVS can be performed by any of the two routes and it is safe and effective. ***Transcervical approach*** is preferred when the placenta is located posteriorly and the uterus is retroverted. ***Transabdominal route*** is preferable in anterior location of placenta, anteverted uterus and with fundal position.

Contraindication of transcervical approach: Local infection (cervix and vagina), genital tract bleeding, uterine fibroid, cervical polyps (mechanical hindrance), and markedly retroverted uterus.

Q.211 Congenital anomalies are most severe in:
   a. Rubella infection
   b. Mumps
   c. CMV
   d. Toxoplasma

Ans. a. Fetal *malformations with maternal rubella infection:* Risks of congenital rubella infection is about 54% in first trimester, 25% at the end of second trimester. The *common manifestations of congenital rubella syndrome (CRS) are:* IUGR, sensorineural hearing loss, hepatosplenomegaly, cardiac lesion (ductus arteriosus), eye defects (cataracts, glaucoma, retinitis, microphthalmia), microcephaly, cerebral palsy, mental retardation. Following congenital rubella infection, infant may shed virus up to 1 year after birth.

Q.212 Chorionic villus sampling is not done before 9 weeks of gestation age because of:
   a. Fetomaternal hemorrhage
   b. Fetal limb defect
   c. Inadequate tissue is obtained for diagnosis
   d. High incidence of abortion

Ans. b.

Safety of CVS

Pregnancy loss: CVS is a safe and effective procedure provided properly done by an experienced person. Pregnancy loss presently has decreased from 2.35 to 1.16%. The pregnancy loss rates between CVS and amniocentesis are not significantly different at present. Limb reduction defects are not observed when CVS was done after 9 weeks of gestation. Confined placental mosaicism may be observed in some cases where the fetus does not carry the mosaic cell line but it is present in the placenta. In such a case, amniocentesis should be performed to determine whether the fetus is affected or not.

Q.213 Most common ovarian tumor below 20 years of age is:
   a. Epithelial cell tumor
   b. Sertoli cell tumor
   c. Leydig cell tumor
   d. Germ cell tumor

Ans. d.

Occurrence of ovarian tumors
- *Common in all ages:* Epithelial tumors of the ovary
- *Common in young woman:* Germ cell tumors
- *Common epithelial ovarian tumor:* Serous cystadenoma
- *Pseudomyxoma peritonei:* Mucinous cyst tumor
- *Tumor causing Meigs syndrome:* Fibroma, thecoma, Brenner and granulosa cell tumor of ovary
- *Common germ cell tumor:* Dermoid
- *Common malignant germ cell tumor:* Dysgerminoma.

Q.214 All are used in treatment of endometriosis, *except*:
   a. Progesterone
   b. Dienogest
   c. GnRH analogue
   d. Estrogen

Ans. d. Uses of GnRH analogues: (i) Pelvic endometriosis, (ii) Dysfunctional uterine bleeding, (iii) Fibrocystic breast disease, (iv) Gynecomastia, (v) Precocious puberty, (vi) Symptomatic fibroid uterus, (vii) Premenstrual tension syndrome, (viii) Prior to hysteroscopic endometrial ablation (to suppress endometrial growth).

Q.215 Regarding bilateral ligation of internal iliac arteries:
   a. Ligation is done on the main trunk of the artery
   b. Artery is transected between the ties
   c. Collateral circulation established between superior rectal with middle and inferior rectal arteries
   d. Bleeding is always controlled with this procedure

Ans. c; a. Ligation should be done on its anterior division; b. Artery should not be transected; d. At times, bleeding may fail to stop even after ligation due to venous bleeding or presence of aberrant vessels. (*See* Clinical in Obstetrics, Ch 47 and 48)

Q.216 The pudendal nerve:
   a. Derives its fibers from the 2nd, 3rd and 4th sacral segments
   b. Leaves the pelvis below the pyriformis through the greater sciatic foramen
   c. The pudendal artery lies on its lateral side when it lies on the ischial spine
   d. The inferior rectal nerve arises from it
   e. Dorsal nerve of the clitoris is a branch

Ans. a, b, d, e = True; c = False.

Q.217 In a postmenopausal woman:
   a. Vaginal pH is increased
   b. Level of total estradiol falls
   c. Level of gonadotropin falls
   d. Treatment with GnRH is often beneficial
   e. Occasional vaginal bleeding is common

Ans. a, b = True; c, d, e = False.

Q.218 The following substances are safe in pregnancy:
   a. Aspirin
   b. Rubella vaccination
   c. Varicella vaccination
   d. ACE inhibitors
   e. Paracetamol

Ans. a, e = True; b, c, d = false.

Q.219 The urinary bladder:
   a. The trigone develops from the urogenital sinus
   b. The bladder base remains fixed even when the bladder is distended
   c. The mucous membrane is lined by transitional epithelium
   d. Lower end of the mesonephric ducts are incorporated within the bladder

e. The inferolateral surfaces are related to the space of Retzius

Ans. b, c, d, e = True, a = False.

Q.220 The female breast:
a. Is made up of 15–20 lobes
b. Lies over the fascia covering the pectoralis major muscle
c. 30–40 lactiferous ducts open in the nipple
d. Lymphatics drain to the axillary nodes
e. Supplied by the internal mammary arteries

Ans. a, b, d, e = True; c = False.

Q.221 The rectum and the anal canal:
a. The anal canal measures 2.5 cm in length
b. Rectum starts at the level of S_1 vertebra
c. Rectum is covered with peritoneum entirely
d. Uterosacral ligaments are related lateral to the rectum
e. All the lymphatics of the anal canal drain into the internal iliac lymph nodes

Ans. a, d = True; b, c, e = False.

Q.222 Regarding thyroid hormones:
a. Thyrotropin-releasing hormone (TRH) is nonapeptide
b. T3 or T4 is formed by iodination of amino acid tyrosine
c. Nearly, 99.5% of circulating thyroid hormones are bound to thyroxin-binding albumin
d. 90% of T3 is derived by peripheral deiodination of T4
e. The ratio of T4:T3 in blood is approximately 20:1

Ans. a, c = False; b, d, e = True. TRH is a tripeptide. 99.5% of circulating thyroid hormones are protein bound of which 75% are bound to thyroxin-binding globulin.

Q.223 Factors for shifting to the right for oxygen dissociation curve are the followings:
a. Decreased temperature
b. Increased blood pH
c. Increased 2,3-diphosphoglycerate
d. Increased CO_2
e. Higher partial pressure of oxygen

Ans. a, b = False; c, d, e = True.

Q.224 Regarding a sample with a normal distribution:
a. It is described as a Gaussian distribution
b. The mode lies at the center of the distribution
c. The median is the middle value in a ranked set of data
d. Normal distribution may be bimodal also
e. 60% of the data set lies within two standard deviations from the mean

Ans. a, b, c, d, = True; e = False. The standard deviation (SD) is a measure of the spread of the data set around the mean. Approximately 68% of the data set in a Gaussian distribution sits within one SD from the mean. Approximately 95% of the data set sits within two SDs from the mean.

Q.225 Regarding shock:
a. Associated with metabolic alkalosis
b. Cellular hypoxia is characteristic
c. Hypokalemia is common
d. Respiratory distress may be associated
e. Capillary permeability is reduced due to endothelial damage

Ans. a, c, e = False; b, d = True.

Q.226 Thyroid function during pregnancy:
a. Maternal serum iodine levels fall
b. Levels of thyroid-binding globulin is raised
c. Gestational thyrotoxicosis is due to high levels of TSH
d. Maternal free T4 levels are raised
e. Total T3 and T4 levels are unchanged

Ans. a, b = True; c, d, e = False. Gestational transient thyrotoxicosis is due to thyrotropic effect of hCG and there is actually some fall in the level of serum TSH in the first trimester. Total T3 and T4 levels are increased.

Causes of fetal heart rate abnormalities		
Tachycardia	**Bradycardia**	**Reduced baseline variability**

▪ Fetal distress
▪ Fetal infection
▪ Fetal anemia
▪ Drugs to mother
  ◆ β-adrenergic
  ◆ Isoxsuprine
▪ Maternal infection
	▪ Fetal hypoxia
	▪ Fetal acidosis
	▪ Drugs to mother
	  ◆ Pethidine
	  ◆ Methyldopa
	  ◆ $MgSO_4$
	▪ Epidural analgesia
	▪ Fetal heart conduction defects (SLE)
		▪ Fetal hypoxia
		▪ Fetal sleep
		▪ Fetal congenital malformations
		▪ Drugs to mother
		  ◆ Sedatives
		  ◆ $MgSO_4$
		  ◆ Antihypertensives
		▪ Maternal acidosis

Section 2: Gynecology Discussion

Section Outline

- Ch. 3. Recurrent Pregnancy Loss
- Ch. 4. Heavy Menstrual Bleeding
- Ch. 5. Congenital HIV Infection and AIDS
- Ch. 6. Urinary Incontinence
- Ch. 7. Fibroid Uterus: Management Issues
- Ch. 8. Polycystic Ovarian Syndrome
- Ch. 9. Hyperandrogenemia
- Ch. 10. Association of Subfertility with Endometriosis
- Ch. 11. Management of Pain in Endometriosis
- Ch. 12. Adenomyosis Uterus
- Ch. 13. High Intensity Focused Ultrasound in the Management of Leiomyomas and Adenomyosis
- Ch. 14. Menopause and the Management Issues
- Ch. 15. Abnormal Uterine Bleeding
- Ch. 16. Abnormal Uterine Bleeding: Investigations and Management Issues
- Ch. 17. Management of Adnexal Mass in Peri- and Post-menopausal Women
- Ch. 18. Use of Selective Progesterone Receptor Modulators in Gynecology

Chapter 3: Recurrent Pregnancy Loss

Recurrent pregnancy loss (RPL) could be considered after the loss of two or more consecutive pregnancies (ESHRE-2017). Clinicians and the clinics should take care of the psychological needs of the couple.

Pregnancy is a hypercoagulable state. Pregnancy is associated with high-risk of thrombotic complications. It is especially so in women associated with inherited thrombophilias. **However, the association of thrombophilias and adverse pregnancy outcome with cause-and-effect relationship has not yet been exclusively established.**

INHERITED THROMBOPHILIAS

- Activated protein C resistance
- Factor V Leiden mutation
- Prothrombin gene G20210A mutation
- Antithrombin deficiency
- Protein C deficiency
- Protein S deficiency
- Factor XIII mutation

ACQUIRED THROMBOPHILIAS

- Lupus anticoagulant
- Anticardiolipin antibodies
- β_2 glycoprotein antibodies

Routine testing for heritable thrombophilias as part of evaluation for possible causes of stillbirth should not be performed. Most guidelines recommended some form of screening particularly if stillbirth is associated with fetal growth restriction (FGR), pre-eclampsia, maternal thrombosis and/or with maternal positive family history.

Acquired thrombophilias or antiphospholipid syndrome (APS) is defined as manifestation of thrombosis and/or fetal loss or pregnancy morbidity in a woman with positive antiphospholipid serology (lupus anticoagulant, anticardiolipin antibodies and/or β_2 glycoprotein antibodies) on at least two occasions at 12 weeks apart. It is important to note that antiphospholipid antibody syndrome (APAS) may be present in a healthy woman without any disease. *Screening for LA, and ACA (IgG and IgM) and β_2 glycoprotein antibodies are to be done after two pregnancy losses (ESHRE-2021).* Although women with APA had higher rates of low-birth-weight babies and placental infarction. Catastrophic antiphospholipid syndrome (CAPS) is a life-threatening disease conferring 50% mortality. It is observed in <1% of APAS cases. It is characterized by the onset of rapidly progressive and widespread thrombotic microangiopathy and multiorgan failure.

Treatment option in such a case is anticoagulation, LMWH, high-dose steroids and plasma exchange.

RECURRENT MISCARRIAGE (FIRST AND SECOND TRIMESTERS)

Single Best Answer (SBA) and Multiple Choice Questions (MCQs)

Q.1 Antiphospholipid antibody syndrome (APAS):
a. It is an important cause of recurrent miscarriage
b. Presence of antiphospholipid antibodies (APAbs) is a high-risk factor
c. Every woman with APA needs pharmacological intervention
d. APAS inhibit trophoblast function and inhibition

Ans. a. T   b. F
      c. F   d. T

Q.2 Genetic factors for recurrent miscarriage:
a. Overall prevalence is 2–5% in couples with recurrent miscarriage
b. Most commonly is reciprocal or Robertsonian translocation
c. Risk of miscarriage due to fetal aneuploidy increases with increasing number of pregnancy losses
d. Risk of euploid pregnancy loss increases as the number of miscarriage increases

Ans. a. T   b. T
      c. F   d. T

Q.3 Immunological factors for recurrent miscarriage:
a. Human leukocyte antigen (HLA) incompatibility among couples is a known factor
b. Altered peripheral blood natural killer (NK) cells is an important factor
c. Uterine natural killer (uNK) cells are raised in these women
d. The response of T helper-1 (Th-1) cytokine is mounting in these women

Ans. a. F   b. F
      c. F   d. T

Q.4 Antiphospholipid antibody syndrome:
  a. All women with recurrent miscarriage should be screened for APAbs
  b. One clinical criteria is diagnostic
  c. One laboratory criteria is confirmatory
  d. Corticosteroid therapy improves the live birth rate

Ans. a. T   b. F
        c. F   d. F

One of the two clinical criteria in addition to at least one laboratory criteria must be present (see below).

Q.5 Management of an unexplained case of recurrent miscarriage should be done by:
  a. Paternal cell immunization
  b. Third party donor leukocyte infusion
  c. Trophoblast membranes infusion
  d. Immunoglobulin IV

Ans. a. F   b. F
        c. F   d. F

Management Issues

Miscarriage is defined as the spontaneous loss of pregnancy before the fetus reaches the period of viability (24 weeks) (RCOG, 2011). It varies from 24 to 28 weeks depending on the country.

Recurrent miscarriage is defined as the loss of three or more consecutive pregnancies. It is about 1% of all couples trying to conceive.

Q.6 What are the important risk factors for recurrent miscarriage?

Ans.
  A. *Advanced maternal age*
  B. *Antiphospholipid antibody syndrome*
  C. *Genetic factors*
     ♦ Parental chromosomal factors
     ♦ Embryonic/fetal chromosomal abnormalities
  D. *Anatomical factors*
     ♦ Congenital uterine malformations
     ♦ Cervical weakness (incompetence/insufficiency)
  E. *Endocrine factors*
     ♦ Diabetes mellitus
     ♦ Thyroid dysfunction
     ♦ Polycystic ovarian syndrome (PCOS)
     ♦ Insulin resistance, hyperinsulinemia
  F. *Immune factors*
  G. *Infective agents:* Bacterial vaginosis, genital tuberculosis
  H. *Inherited thrombophilias*
     ♦ Activated protein C resistance (factor V Leiden mutation)
     ♦ Antithrombin III
     ♦ Prothrombin gene mutation

A. Advanced Maternal Age

It is associated with a reduction in both the number and quality of the remaining oocytes. Age-related risk of miscarriage is as follows:

12–19 years	=	13%
30–34 years	=	15%
35–39 years	=	25%
40–44 years	=	51%
>45 years	=	93%

Advanced paternal age has also been identified as a risk factor. Risk of miscarriage increases after each successive pregnancy loss.

Other environmental factors such as smoking, excess caffeine and alcohol consumption increase the risk. Effects of anesthetic gases for theater workers are conflicting. Obesity is a factor for both sporadic and recurrent miscarriage.

B. Antiphospholipid Antibody Syndrome

Antiphospholipid antibody syndrome is the most important treatable cause (15%) of recurrent miscarriage. Antiphospholipid antibodies are:
- Lupus anticoagulant (LAC)
- Anticardiolipin antibodies (ACA)
- β_2 glycoprotein-1 (β_2 GP-1) antibodies

Q.7 What are the mechanisms of pregnancy loss in association with antiphospholipid antibodies (APAS)?

Ans. The probable mechanisms are:
- Activation of complement pathway
- Release of local inflammatory mediators (cytokines, interleukins)
- Inhibitions of trophoblastic function and differentiation
- Thrombosis of uteroplacental vasculature

However, the prevalence of APAS in low-risk obstetric women is <2%. Women with APAS having recurrent miscarriage, live birth rate without any pharmacological intervention has been reported only 10%.

C. Genetic Factors

- *Parental chromosomal rearrangements:* Balanced structural chromosomal anomaly is present in about 2–5% of couples, most commonly a **balanced reciprocal** or **Robertsonian translocation**. This may result in live births with multiple congenital malformations and/or mental disability.
- *Embryonic/fetal chromosomal abnormalities* have been observed in about 30–57% of couples with recurrent miscarriage. Risk increases with advanced maternal age.

D. Anatomical Factors

Overall prevalence of uterine anomalies in recurrent miscarriage populations ranges between 2% and 38%. Second trimester miscarriage is commonly observed. This may be due to cervical incompetence and/or different types of uterine malformations (septate, bicornuate or unicornuate uterus).

Cervical incompetence: It is a known cause for second trimester miscarriage. Diagnosis is mainly clinical as the available objective tests have poor sensitivity and poor positive predictive value.

E. Endocrine Factors

Well-controlled diabetes mellitus and treated thyroid dysfunction do not have in any increased risk. Antithyroid antibodies have been linked to recurrent miscarriage. The increased risk of miscarriage in women with PCOS has been attributed to insulin resistance, hyperinsulinemia and hyperandrogenism.

F. Immune Factors

Natural killer cells present in peripheral blood and that present in the uterus is function differently. There is no relationship between uNK cell numbers and future pregnancy outcome. ***HLA*** incompatibility between couples or absence of maternal blocking antibodies is not considered as the cause of recurrent miscarriage.

Cytokines are immune molecules. Cytokine response may be either (1) Th-1 type or (2) Th-2 type. ***Th-1 response*** is the production of proinflammatory cytokines, [interleukin-2, interferon and tumor necrosis factor (TNF)]. On the other hand, ***Th-2 response*** is with production of anti-inflammatory cytokines (interleukins 4, 6 and 10).

Successful pregnancy might be the result of predominantly Th-2 cytokine response. On the other hand, women with recurrent miscarriage have a bias towards Th-1 cytokine response.

G. Infective Agents

TORCH and listeria infections are not associated with recurrent miscarriage. Therefore, routine screening for TORCH infection is not recommended. Bacterial vaginosis is a risk factor for second trimester miscarriage and preterm labor.

H. Inherited Thrombophilias

Thrombophilias are the disorders (acquired or inherited) of hemostatic mechanism that predisposes to intravascular thrombosis (British Committee for Standardization in Hematology, 1990).

Factors for Inherited Thrombophilias

- Activated protein C resistance (factor V Leiden mutation)
- Antithrombin III
- Protein C ⎫
- Protein S ⎬ Deficiency
- Prothrombin gene 20210A mutation
- Hyperhomocysteinemia

Natural Anticoagulants and their Mechanism of Action

- ***Activated protein C resistance:*** It is most commonly due to factor V Leiden gene mutation. This makes factor V resistant to degradation by activated protein C (see below). As a result the unimpeded factor V predisposes to thrombosis due to increased generation of thrombin. Importantly, it is observed in 3–15% of European and 3% of African population but it has not been observed (till date) in the Asians.
- ***Antithrombin III:*** Inactivates factors IXa, Xa, XIa, XIIa, and IIa. It inhibits thrombin generation. Homozygous antithrombin III deficiency is lethal and it is most thrombogenic. Risks of thrombosis varies between 3% and 40% depending upon whether the individual is heterozygous or homozygous.
- ***β_2 glycoprotein-1:*** It is a natural anticoagulant. It inhibits factor XII in the coagulation cascade. It is present with high concentration in the syncytiotrophoblasts. It helps implantation with increased vascularity of the endometrium. Damage to β_2 GP-1 with antibodies or complement activation results in intervillous space thrombosis and early pregnancy loss.
- ***Prothrombin gene 20210A mutation:*** It is observed in 2% of white population and it is uncommon in the Asians. Prothrombin gene mutation leads to excessive production of prothrombin. This is finally converted to thrombin. Pregnant women with prothrombin gene mutation run the higher risk of thromboembolism (3–15 times). Women who also inherit factor V Leiden mutation have the further higher risk of thromboembolism. Carriers of both the genes mutation should have lifelong anticoagulation therapy.
- ***Hyperhomocysteinemia:*** It results from deficiency of folic acid, vitamin B_6 and B_{12}. Folic acid acts as a cofactor in the methylation reaction of homocysteine to methionine. Hyperhomocysteinemia (C677T) is due to mutation of the enzyme 5,10 methylenetetrahydrofolate reductase (MTHFR). It is an autosomal recessive disorder. Serum fasting level of homocysteine value ≥ 12 μmol/L is considered diagnostic. Hyperhomocysteinemia causes decreased activation of protein C. Therefore, it results in increased intravascular thrombosis and poor pregnancy outcome.

Besides this, hyperhomocysteinemia is associated with ***increased risks of neural tube defects (NTD).***

Women with RPL, need not be investigated for inherited thrombophilia unless in the context of research or women with additional risk factors for thrombophilia (ESHRE-2017).

Thrombophilias and Adverse Pregnancy Outcome

- Recurrent fetal loss ≥ 10 weeks
- Severe IUGR (recurrent)
- Severe early-onset pre-eclampsia
- Massive placental abruption
- Preterm labor

Diagnosis of APA Syndrome

Clinical

- Unexplained thrombosis
- Unexplained fetal loss (≥ 1) at ≥ 10 weeks gestation
- Miscarriages (≥ 3) at ≤10 weeks gestation
- Preterm birth ≤ 34 weeks

Laboratory

- Anticardiolipin antibodies (ACA)—IgG/IgM (99th percentile) at least two values 12 weeks apart
- Lupus anticoagulant (LAC)—detected twice 6 weeks apart (ACOG, 2007).

Detection of APAS is subject to considerable interlaboratory variation. It is mandatory that two tests must be positive at least 12 weeks apart for either LAC or ACA (IgG and/or IgM) above 99th percentile (40 g/L). There is also temporal fluctuation of APA titers in an individual woman. It may be positive transiently secondary to infections. Detection of LAC with dilute Russell's viper venom time test together with a platelet neutralization procedure is more sensitive and specific than either APTT test or the Kaolin clotting time test (RCOG, 2011).

Definitive diagnosis of APA syndrome is made when atleast one of the clinical and one of the laboratory criteria are met.

Diagnosis of thrombophilias: There is a consensus on the diagnosis and treatment of antiphospholipid syndrome in pregnancy. But detection and management of inherited thrombophilias remained controversial.

Karyotyping and genetic factors: Cytogenetic analysis should be done with the products of conception of the third and subsequent consecutive miscarriage(s). Parental blood karyotyping of both the partners should be done for recurrent miscarriage where testing of products of conception report an unbalanced structural chromosomal abnormality. Risk of miscarriage as a result of fetal aneuploidy decreases with an increasing number of pregnancy losses. For any single miscarriage, sporadic fetal chromosome abnormality is most common. Array-based comparative genomic hybridization (array CGH) is recommended for genetic analysis of the pregnancy tissue. Parental karyotyping is not routinely recommended in couples with RPL. Abnormal parental karyotype needs referral to a clinical geneticist.

Suspected uterine anomalies require investigations to confirm the diagnosis. These include transvaginal 3D ultrasound (high sensitivity and specificity), hysterosalpingography, hysteroscopy, laparoscopy (Fig. 3.1). The value of MRI in the diagnosis is yet to be determined. MRI is not recommended as the first line option.

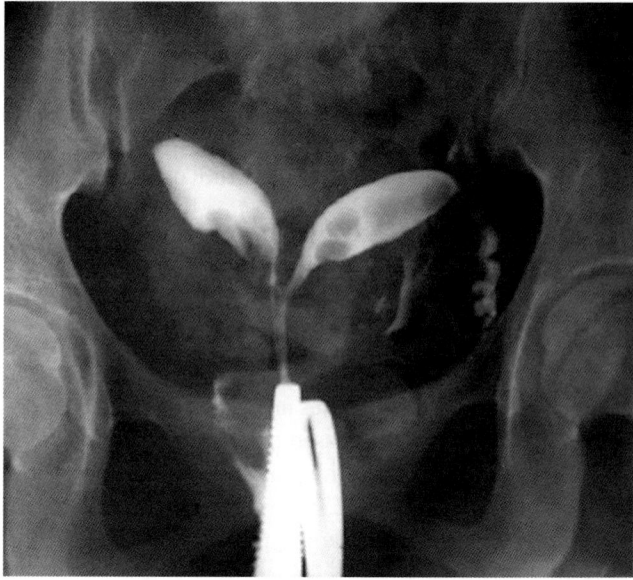

Fig. 3.1: Hysterosalpingography showing septate uterus (confirmed on hysteroscopy and laparoscopy). The woman suffered previous three miscarriages.

Management Options for Recurrent Miscarriage

- ***APAS:*** Pregnant women with APA syndrome should be treated with low dose aspirin plus heparin to prevent further miscarriage. ***Unfractionated heparin and low molecular weight heparin (LMWH) are equally safe and effective in the treatment of APA syndrome. LMWH causes less thrombocytopenia and osteoporosis.*** It is given once daily. This treatment combination improves live birth rate and significantly reduces the miscarriage rate by 54%. Neither corticosteroid nor IV immunoglobulin therapy improve the live birth rate in women with recurrent miscarriage. Women with recurrent first trimester miscarriage associated with inherited thrombophilia, role of heparin therapy is uncertain. Heparin therapy during pregnancy may improve the live birth rate of women with second trimester miscarriage associated with inherited thrombophilia. The live birth rate of women with enoxaparin (LMWH) was 86% compared with 29% in women taking low dose aspirin alone.
- ***Immunotherapy:*** Paternal cell immunization, third party donor leucocytes, trophoblast membranes and intravenous immunoglobulin in women with previous unexplained recurrent miscarriage do not improve the live birth rate. It increases maternal morbidity.
- ***Infection:*** Treatment of bacterial vaginosis with oral clindamycin reduces the risk of miscarriage and preterm birth.

- **Endocrine factors:** Role of progesterone supplementation and/or hCG supplementation in prevention of recurrent miscarriage.

  Progesterone is necessary for successful implantation and maintenance of pregnancy. This is explained due to its immunomodulatory actions. **Progesterone results in inducing a pregnancy protective shift from proinflammatory Th-1 cytokine response to a more favorable anti-inflammatory Th-2 cytokine response. Progesterone treatment reduces miscarriage.** The benefit of therapy with hCG in recurrent miscarriage is still in the context of randomized controlled trials (RCTs). Evidences are still insufficient to recommend the use of progesterone and HCG in the management of RPL. Luteal phase insufficiency testing is not recommended. Bromocriptine can be given in women with RPL and hyperprolactinemia. Prophylactic folic acid and vitamin D supplementation is advised.

- **Women with PCOS:** Increased miscarriage has been attributed to insulin resistance, hyperinsulinemia and hyperandrogenemia.

  Metformin therapy during pregnancy is associated with reduction in miscarriage rate. However, there is no RCT to evaluate the role of metformin in women with recurrent miscarriage. Many uncontrolled studies have shown the benefits of metformin.

- **Anatomical factors:** Surgical correction of uterine anomalies improves pregnancy outcome. Compared to open uterine surgery, endoscopic surgery has got less complications. Hysteroscopic septum resection is effective in achieving successful pregnancy outcome. However, results of prospective RCT are awaited.

  Metroplasty is not recommended for cases with bicornuate uterus. Uterine reconstruction is not recommended for unicornuate uterus (ESHERE-2017).

  Women with second trimester miscarriage due to cervical incompetence can be managed by ultrasound-indicated cerclage if cervical length is 25 mm or less.

- **Unexplained recurrent miscarriage:** Women with unexplained recurrent miscarriage have an excellent prognosis for future pregnancy outcome (75%) without pharmacological intervention. Reassurance, support and tender loving cares are of value.

Suggested Reading

1. Bujold E, Roberge S, Nicolaides KH. Low-dose aspirin for prevention of adverse outcomes related to abnormal placentation. Prenat Diagn. 2014;34:642–8.
2. Empson M, Lassere M, Craig J, et al. Prevention of recurrent miscarriage for women with antiphospholipid antibody or lupus anticoagulant. Cochrane Database Syst Rev. 2005;(2): CD002859.
3. ESHERE Early Pregnancy Guideline Development Group: Recurrent Pregnancy Loss; Version-2, 2017.
4. Farquharson RG, Quenby S, Greaves M. Antiphospholipid syndrome in pregnancy: a randomized, controlled trial of treatment. Obstet Gynecol. 2002;100:408–13.
5. Konar H. Dutta's Textbook of Obstetrics, 9th Edition. New Delhi: Jaypee Brothers Medical Publishers; 2019, p.160.
6. Myers B, Pavord S. Heritable thrombophilias: implications for pregnancy and current evidence for treatment. The Obstetrician and Gynaecologist. 2011;13:225–30.
7. Ogasawara M, Aoki K, Okada S, et al. Embryonic karyotype of abortuses in relation to the number of previous miscarriages. Fertil Steril. 2000;73(2):300–4.
8. Pattison NS, Chamley LW, McKay EJ, et al. Antiphospholipid antibodies in pregnancy: Prevalence and clinical associations. Br J Obstet Gynaecol. 1993;100(10):909–13.
9. Rodger MA, Carrier M, Le Gal G, Martinelli I, Perna A, Rey E, et al. Low-Molecular-Weight Heparin for Placenta-Mediated Pregnancy Complications Study Group. Meta-analysis of low-molecular-weight heparin to prevent recurrent placenta-mediated pregnancy complications. Blood. 2014;123:822–8.
10. Said JM, Higgins JR, Moses EK, Walker SP, Monagle PT, Brennecke SP. Inherited thrombophilias and adverse pregnancy outcomes: a case-control study in an Australian population. Acta Obstet Gynecol Scand. 2012;91:250–5.
11. Skeith L, Carrier M, Kaaja R, Martinelli I, Petroff D, Schleußner E, et al. A meta-analysis of low-molecular-weight heparin to prevent pregnancy loss in women with inherited thrombophilia. Blood. 2016;127:1650–5.

Chapter 4: Heavy Menstrual Bleeding

For clinical purpose, ***heavy menstrual bleeding (HMB) is defined as excessive menstrual blood loss which interferes with women's physical, emotional, social and material quality of life.*** This can occur alone or in combination with other symptoms. Any intervention should aim to improve the quality of life measures.

HISTORY, EXAMINATION AND INVESTIGATIONS FOR HMB

History should cover the nature of bleeding, its duration, cycle interval, and related symptoms like pelvic pain, pelvic pressure, postcoital bleeding, metrorrhagia or any associated comorbidity.

Clinical examination and investigations should be through to reveal any structural (fibroid uterus) or any histological (endometrial carcinoma) abnormality. However, if the history and physical examination suggests HMB without any structural or histological abnormality, treatment (pharmacotherapy) could be started without other investigations. ***Usually, levonorgestrel-releasing intrauterine system (LNG-IUS)*** is recommended. When history and clinical examination suggest any structural or histological abnormality, investigations are carried out.

Measurements of blood loss directly by alkali hematin or indirectly by 'pictorial blood loss chart' are not routinely recommended.

Examination: Physical examination is done to exclude any structural abnormality (fibroid uterus) or any histological abnormality (atypical endometrial hyperplasia) (Figs. 4.1A and B). Women with fibroid uterus that are palpable per abdomen and/or when the uterine length is ≥ 12 cm as measured by ultrasonography or hysteroscopy further investigations are carried out.

Investigations

- A full blood count (Hb%, TLC, DLC, PCV, blood film) should be done on all women with HMB.
- Thyroid hormone testing should be carried out when other signs and symptoms of thyroid disease are suggestive.
- Endometrial biopsy (EB) is taken with pipelle endometrial collection to exclude endometrial hyperplasia.
- Testing for blood coagulation disorders (von Willebrand's disease) should be done in women who have HMB since menarche or have personal or family history suggesting a coagulation disorder.
- Serum ferritin test is not a routine procedure.
- Female hormone (FSH, LH, estradiol) testing is not a routine procedure.

Indications for EB are:
- Women with age ≥ 45 years
- Women having persistent intermenstrual bleeding
- Women not responding to pharmacotherapy.

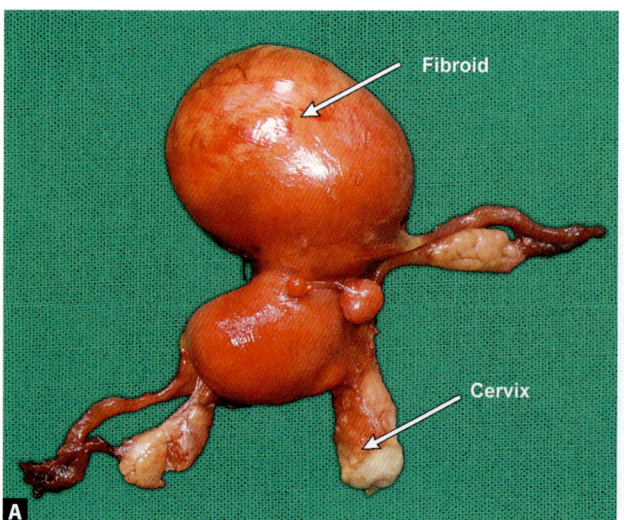
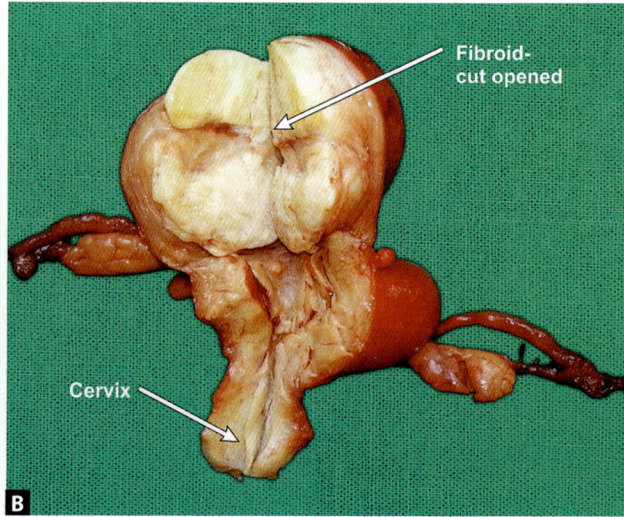

Figs. 4.1A and B: Heavy menstrual bleeding (HMB) due to fibroid uterus.

Indications of imaging study (USG) are:
- Uterus palpable per abdomen or feels bulky on clinical examination
- Vaginal examination reveals a pelvic mass of uncertain origin
- Women not responding to pharmacotherapy (treatment failure).

Special investigations are:
- ***Ultrasound*** is done as a first-line diagnostic tool to detect structural abnormality. Ultrasound should provide the information as regard the location, dimensions and number of fibroids.
- ***Hysteroscopy*** should be used when ultrasound result are inconclusive. Presence of uterine fibroids suggests appropriate treatment to control HMB (see below).
- ***Saline infusion sonography (SIS)*** is not recommended as first-line diagnostic tool.
- ***Magnetic resonance imaging (MRI)*** should not be used as a first-line diagnostic tool.
- ***Dilatation and curettage (D and C)*** is not recommended as a diagnostic tool.

PHARMACOTHERAPY FOR HEAVY MENSTRUAL BLEEDING

Q.1 What are the determinants of treatment?
Ans. *Treatment options depend on the following factors:*
- Presence or absence of uterine structural abnormality (fibroids)
- Presence or absence of histological abnormality (atypical endometrium)
- Women's desire for conception
- Women's desire to use contraception.

Treatment Options
Pharmacotherapy is based on individual woman's need:
- LNG-IUS
- Tranexamic acid
- Nonsteroidal anti-inflammatory drugs (NSAIDs)
- Combined oral contraceptives (COCs)
- Norethisterone 5 mg TID from D5–D26 of the menstrual cycle
- Injectable long-acting progestogens
- Gonadotropin-releasing hormone analog (GnRH analog)
- Women can have either tranexamic acid or NSAIDs when hormonal treatments cannot be recommended
- LNG-IUS takes some time (about 5–6 cycles) to give the therapeutic benefits
- Women with HMB and dysmenorrhea should be offered NSAIDs
- GnRH analog is considered in cases
    - Prior to surgery
    - In cases of having contraindications for surgery or uterine artery embolization (UAE)
- HRT ***add back*** therapy should be recommended when GnRH, the analog therapy is continued for more than 6 months.
- Danazol should not be used routinely for the treatment of HMB
- Oral progesterone in the luteal phase only, should not be used in the treatment of HMB
- Ethamsylate should not be used for the treatment of HMB.

OPERATIVE TREATMENTS FOR HMB

Nonhysterectomy Surgery for HMB
- Endometrial ablation
  Indications
    - When the bleeding is severe enough to affect the quality of life
    - Women does not want to conceive
    - Women with normal uterus or with small uterine fibroids (<3 cm in diameter)
    - Women with uterine size ≤ 10 weeks of pregnant uterus
    - Women should use effective contraception after endometrial ablation. Endometrial ablation techniques should be the ***second generation ones*** (see below).

  Second Generation Endometrial Ablation Methods
    - Impedance-controlled bipolar radiofrequency ablation. A metal fan-shaped device (fabric mesh) is used.
    - Fluid-filled thermal balloon endometrial ablation (TBEA). In this procedure, endometrial thinning is not needed. Therma choice III with silicon balloon at the tip is used.
    - Microwave endometrial ablation (MEA) is done in the postmenstrual phase.
    - Free-fluid thermal endometrial ablation.

  First generation ablation techniques like roller ball endometrial ablation and transcervical resection of endometrium (TCRE) are used when hysteroscopic myomectomy is needed at the same time.
- D and C should be not used as a therapeutic procedure.

Women with HMB due to fibroid uterus (>3 cm in diameter).

Treatment options are:
- Uterine artery embolization (UAE)
- MR-guided focused ultrasound (MRgFUS)
- Myomectomy
- Hysterectomy
- ***UAE:*** It is an option for women, who want to retain their uterus and fertility.
- ***MRgFUS*** is found to be effective. It induces coagulative necrosis in the myoma. It causes less pain compared to UAE. It is safe, effective and minimally invasive. Successful pregnancy following treatment has been observed.
- ***Myomectomy:*** It is an option when preservation of uterus and child-bearing function is desired.

- ***Indication of hysterectomy*** for women with HMB are:
  - When other treatment options have failed or are contraindicated.
  - Women no longer wish to retain her uterus and fertility.
  - Women fully informed about the consequences of hysterectomy like sexual feelings, fertility, bladder function and the complications of the operation.

Route of hysterectomy (abdominal or vaginal) needs the following factors to consider:
- Size of the uterus and fibroids
- Mobility and descent of the uterus
- Size and space in vagina
- Previous surgery.

Place of Oophorectomy during Hysterectomy

- As a routine, oophorectomy during hysterectomy should not be done
- Women's informed consent must be there
- Women with family history of breast or ovarian cancer, need genetic counseling prior to a decision about oophorectomy
- Women with age ≥ 45 years
- Women with premenstrual tension syndrome
- Women should be counseled about the need of hormone replacement therapy (HRT), if oophorectomy is done during hysterectomy.

SIDE EFFECTS/COMPLICATIONS OF DIFFERENT TREATMENT OPTIONS FOR HMB

- ***LNG–IUS:*** Irregular uterine bleeding that may last for about 6 months; breast tenderness, acne or headache, amenorrhea and rarely uterine perforation at the time of insertion.
- ***Tranexamic acid:*** Indigestion, diarrhea, headache.
- ***COCs:*** Mood changes, headache, nausea, fluid retention, breast tenderness, deep vein thrombosis (DVT), stroke, heart attacks (*See* Dutta's Textbook of Gynecology, 8th Edition, p. 405).
- ***NSAIDs:*** Indigestion, diarrhea, deterioration of asthma, peptic ulcer—may cause bleeding, peritonitis.
- ***Oral progestogen:*** Weight gain, bloating, breast tenderness, headache and acne, rarely depression.
- ***Injectable progestogen:*** Weight gain, irregular bleeding, amenorrhea, premenstrual-like syndrome (bloating, fluid retention, breast tenderness), temporary loss of bone mineral density. It is restored once the treatment is discontinued.
- ***GnRH analog:*** Menopausal like symptoms (hot flashes, increased sweating, vaginal dryness). Osteoporosis (trabecular bone) when used more than 6 months.
- ***UAE:*** Persistent vaginal discharge, post-embolization syndrome (pain, nausea, vomiting and fever), need of additional surgery premature ovarian failure (women ≤ 40 years), hematoma, rarely hemorrhage, tissue necrosis and infection causing septicemia (*See* Ch 57).
- ***Myomectomy:*** Hemorrhage; adhesion (causing pain and/or reduced fertility), need for further surgery, recurrence of fibroids, menorrhagia, HMB and infection.
- ***Hysterectomy:*** Hemorrhage, infection, intraoperative hemorrhage, damage to other organs (bladder, ureter), urinary dysfunction, incontinence, DVT and pulmonary embolization.
- ***Oophorectomy during hysterectomy:*** Postmenopausal (surgical menopause) like symptoms.

Q.2 How to exclude underlying hemorrhagic disorder when a woman presents with heavy menstrual bleeding (HMB)?

Ans. Screening (clinical) of a woman with heavy menstrual bleeding to exclude an underlying hemorrhagic disorder (Kouides et al., 2005)

A STRUCTURED HISTORY SHOULD BE RECORDED

Positive Screening

It comprises any of the following parameters:
- **Heavy menstrual bleeding since menarche**
- **One of the following factors**:
  - Postpartum hemorrhage
  - Surgery-related unusual bleeding
  - Bleeding associated with dental work

Two or more of the following symptoms:
■ *Bruising*: 1–2 times per month
■ *Epistaxis*: 1–2 times per month
■ Frequent gum bleeding
■ Family history of bleeding symptoms

Patients with a positive screening test should be considered for evaluation by a hematologist.

SUMMARY OF DIAGNOSTIC EVALUATION FOR ABNORMAL UTERINE BLEEDING

Medical History

■ *Age:* Menarche and menopause
■ Menstrual bleeding patterns
■ Severity of bleeding (passage of clots)
■ Pain (severity)
■ Associated medical disorders (thyroid dysfunction)
■ Surgical history (cesarean delivery)
■ Use of medications (hormones)
■ Symptoms and signs of possible hemostatic disorder

Physical Examination

■ General physical examination
■ Systemic examination
■ Pelvic examination
■ External genitalia
■ Speculum examination with Pap smear test
■ Bimanual pelvic examination
■ Rectal examination (virgins)

Laboratory Tests

- Pregnancy test (blood or urine)
- Complete blood count
- Targeted screening for bleeding disorders (when indicated) (Platelet count, PT, BT, APTT)
- Thyroid stimulating hormone (TSH)—thyroid dysfunction
- *Chlamydia trachomatis* (NAAT)

Diagnostic or Imaging Studies (When Indicated)

- Transvaginal ultrasonography (endometrial thickness)
- Saline infusion sonohysterography (cavitary pathology)
- Hysteroscopy and directed biopsy (endometrial pathology)
- Laparoscopy (pelvic and peritoneal cavity)
- Magnetic resonance imaging (MRI)
- Computed tomography (CT)

Tissue Sampling Methods

- Endometrial sampling (Pipelle sampler)
- Hysteroscopy-directed endometrial sampling
- Dilatation and Curettage (D and C)

Suggested Reading

1. ACOG practice bulletin: Management of anovulatory bleeding. Int J Gynecol Obstet. 2001;72(3):263-71.
2. Heavy menstrual bleeding. [online] NICE guidelines—Gynaecological conditions. Available from "https://www.nice.org.uk/donotdo/measuring-menstrual-blood-loss-indirectly-pictorial-blood-loss-assessment-chart-is-not-routinely-recommended-for-heavy-menstrual-bleeding-hmb-whether-menstrual-blood-loss-is-a-problem-should-be" www.nice.org.uk. [Accessed January 2007].

Chapter 5: Congenital HIV Infection and AIDS

Q.1 What are different modes of MTCT for human immunodeficiency virus (HIV)?

Ans.
- Overall mother to child transmission (MTCT) is 25-40%.
- Only 1.5-2% transplacental.
- Vast majority acquire infection during late pregnancy, parturition and breastfeeding (30-40%).

Q.2 How much is the risk of MTCT for HIV when correct interventions are done?

Ans. With appropriate interventions [highly active antiretroviral therapy (HAART), elective cesarean delivery and absence of breastfeeding], transmission rates can be reduced to less than 1%.

Q.3 What are the risk factor for increased rate of MTCT?

Ans.
- Father with high viral load
- Mother with AIDS
- Previous baby with HIV infection
- First born twin
- Preterm delivery
- Low maternal CD4$^+$ count
- Chorioamnionitis
- Premature rupture of membranes (PROM)
- Breastfeeding.

Q.4 What are the common presentations of the child born with HIV?

Ans. The child presents with the features of impaired cellular immune defense.

Common features are:
- Recurrent bacterial infections, meningitis, pneumonia
- Persistent oral candidiasis that fails to respond with standard therapy
- Recurrent viral infections (e.g. herpes simplex, CMV)
- Unusual infections, e.g. *Mycobacterium avium, Pneumocystis jirovecii*
- Hepatomegaly, splenomegaly, cardiomyopathy.

Q.5 What are the different diagnostic tests for HIV in a childborn to an HIV-positive mother?

Ans.
- An enzyme-linked immunosorbent assay (ELISA) is unreliable for the first 18 months due to transmission of maternal antibodies.
- Polymerase chain reaction (PCR) of viral DNA is to be done at day(s) 0, 2 and 6 weeks and again at 3 months time.
- FDA approved HIV nucleic acid test (NAT).

Second-line confirmatory tests	Additional tests
■ HIV, RNA, PCR	Serology for:
■ CD4 count	■ HBV, HCV
■ HLA B5701	■ CMV, VDRL
	■ Mantoux test

Q.6 What are stages of pediatric HIV (CDC-1994)?

Ans. Stages are:
- ***Category N***—asymptomatic
- ***Category A***—mildly symptomatic, e.g. lymphadenopathy, hepatomegaly, splenomegaly, recurrent respiratory tract infections.
- ***Category B***—moderately symptomatic. These include meningitis, pneumonia, chronic diarrhea, nephropathy, oropharyngeal thrush > 2 months.
- ***Category C***—severely symptomatic with an AIDS-defining illness.

Q.7 What are the different management issues to prevent MTCT?

Ans. Mother is helped to make an informed choice as regard breastfeeding versus bottle feeding. Breastfeeding doubles the risk of MTCT. WHO recommends exclusive breastfeeding in the developing countries for the first 6 months. Exclusive replacement feeding is done only when ***AFASS*** (A = Affordable, F = Feasible, A = Accessible, S = Sustainable and S = Safe) criteria is fulfilled.

Q.8 Describe the management of neonates born to HIV-infected mothers.

Ans.
- Antiretroviral (ARV) therapy to be started within 4 hours of birth.
- Most neonates are treated with zidovudine monotherapy but neonates with higher risk are treated with highly active antiretroviral therapy (HAART). However, single dose nevirapine have been shown to be effective.
- Prophylaxis against pneumocystis pneumonia (PCP) (cotrimoxazole) is to be given.

- Children with confirmed HIV seroconversion should be treated at specialist pediatric infectious disease center.
- Treating with zidovudine 4 mg/kg every 12 hours until 6 weeks of age.
- HIV DNA PCR testing.

WHO and National guideline (2011) for the feeding of HIV-infected infants is exclusive breastfeeding for at least first 6 months. Exclusive replacement feeding may be done on mother's choice or when she fulfills the criteria of AFASS.

Q.9 When should HAART to be started?

Ans. *HAART* can reduce the risk of opportunistic infection significantly. HARRT is to be started in a case where the risk of progression of the disease is more based on CD4 counts and viral load. Serial measurements of these values and clinical assessments are the most useful indicator.

Q.10 What are the toxicities of antiretroviral therapy?

Ans. Major concern is the teratogenesis of drugs when used in the first trimester of pregnancy. Risks of birth defects have been observed with the following drugs:
- Stavudine, abacavir, efavirenz, didanosine, indinavir and darunavir.
- **Common birth defects were:** Anencephaly, anophthalmia, anencephaly, and cleft palate.
- **Maternal toxicities are:** Pancreatitis, neuropathy, hepatitis, mitochondrial toxicity (hyperlactatemia).

Q.11 What is the immunization protocol for such infants?

Ans.
- Routine immunization schedule to be followed.
- Live immunizations (except MMR) are to be avoided.
- Children with AIDS have poor immune response.

Q.12 What is the prognosis of the children born with HIV infection?

Ans.
- Perinatal infection promotes accelerated disease progression compared to adults.
- Approximately 25% of children develop AIDS in the first year of life.
- Mortality is > 50% by 2 years of age.

Suggested Reading

1. Panel on Antiretroviral Therapy and Medical Management of HIV-Infected Children. (2016). Guidelines for the Use of Antiretroviral Agents in Pediatric HIV Infection. [online] Available from http://aidsinfo.nih.gov/contentfiles/lvguidelines/pediatricguidelines.pdf. [Accessed June, 2016]
2. Siegfried N, van der Merwe L, Brocklehurst P, et al. Antiretrovirals for reducing the risk of mother-to-child transmission of HIV infection. Cochrane Database Syste Rev. 2011;(7):CD003510.
3. Volmink J, Siegfried NL, van der Merwe L, et al. Antiretrovirals for reducing the risk of MTCT of HIV infection (review). Cochrane Database Syst Rev. 2007;(1):CD003510.

Chapter 6: Urinary Incontinence

Q.1 Assessment and investigations of a woman with urinary incontinence (UI):
a. Assessment of UI from history alone is often confusing
b. Urodynamic studies should be a routine for all women with UI
c. Multichannel filling and voiding cystometry are recommended before any surgical intervention for UI
d. Carrying out urodynamic studies before any initial treatment of UI improves outcome.

Ans. a. F b. F c. T d. F

Q.2 Regarding the tests and management of UI:
a. Pad tests, Q-tip and Bonney tests are informative
b. Oxybutynin, darifenacin are used for women with overactive bladder (OAB)
c. Duloxetine is helpful for women with stress urinary incontinence (SUI)
d. Midurethral transobturator tape is recommended for OAB.

Ans. a. F b. T c. F d. F

Urinary incontinence may affect physical, social and psychological well-being of the woman.

It is defined as the complaint of any involuntary leakage of urine (International Continence Society).

- **Stress urinary incontinence** is an involuntary leakage of urine on effort, exertion or on sneezing or coughing.
- **Urge urinary incontinence** is an involuntary urine leakage preceded immediately by urgency (a sudden compelling desire to urinate that is difficult to stop).
- **Mixed urinary incontinence** is an involuntary urine leakage associated with both urgency, exertion, efforts, sneezing or coughing.
- **Overactive bladder syndrome** is defined as an involuntary leakage of urine that occurs with or without urge incontinence as usually with frequency and nocturia.

Urinary incontinence (UI) is the involuntary leakage of urine. Woman with UI may be categorized symptomatically based on the history. History is sufficiently reliable to guide initial noninvasive treatment.

Bladder diaries for a period of 3 days, quantifying urinary frequency and incontinence episodes are reliable methods of assessment.

When a woman presents with clearly defined clinical diagnosis of pure SUI, multichannel cystometry is not routinely recommended.

CONSERVATIVE MANAGEMENT FOR SUI OR MIXED UI

- ***Pelvic floor muscle exercise*** (under supervision) for at least 3 months.
- ***Bladder training for a period of 6 weeks*** for woman with urge or mixed UI
- ***Medical management with antimuscarinic drugs***
    ♦ Oxybutynin tablet or transdermal patch
    ♦ Darifenacin
    ♦ Solifenacin
    ♦ Tolterodine
    ♦ Trospium.
- ***Surgical management***
    ♦ Woman with UI due to detrusor overactivity: Sacral nerve stimulation may be done
    ♦ Retropubic midurethral tape procedure:
        • Macroporous tape made of polypropylene are recommended
        • Open colposuspension using rectus sheath (autologous sling) is an alternative procedure.

ASSESSMENT AND INVESTIGATIONS OF A WOMAN WITH UI

- Detailed ***history-taking and physical examination*** is done and the woman is categorized to any of the following groups:
    ♦ Stress urinary incontinence
    ♦ Urge urinary incontinence or overactive bladder
    ♦ Mixed urinary incontinence
  Women having mixed symptoms should be treated with the predominant symptoms first.
- The relevant ***predisposing and precipitating factors*** should be taken care of simultaneously (e.g., cough, prolapsed uterus or obesity).
- ***Urine analysis***
    ♦ Routine urine analysis should be done. Urine dipstick test is done to detect the presence of blood, glucose, protein, leukocytes and nitrites.
    ♦ Women with symptoms suggestive of urinary tract infection (UTI) (dipstick test positive for leukocytes and

nitrites) should have midstream urine sent for culture and sensitivity. The woman should be treated with appropriate course of antibiotics.
- **Assessment of residual urine:** Women with symptoms suggestive of voiding dysfunction or recurrent UTI, should have postvoid residual volume measurement. It may be done with bladder sonography or catheterization.
- **Indications of referral to specialized unit**
  - Presence of hematuria (microscopic or visible)
  - Recurrent or resistant UTI
  - Presence of a pelvic mass
  - Associated neurological disease
- **Bladder diaries:** Minimum for 3 days covering both working and resting days
- **Pad testing:** Not done
- **Urodynamic studies:**
  - Women having clearly defined clinical diagnosis of pure SUI, use of multichannel cystometry is not needed
  - Multichannel cystometry is not needed before starting conservative management.

Urodynamic investigations in all cases of UI as routine before any initial treatment have not been found to improve outcome.

- **Indications of urodynamic studies are:**
  - Women having mixed urinary incontinence (both SUI and OAB)
  - Women with previous surgery for SUI or anterior compartment prolapse
  - Symptoms suggestive of voiding dysfunction.
- **Other tests of urethral competence are:**
  - The Q-tip and Bonney's tests are not recommended
  - Cystoscopy is not recommended in the initial assessment of women with pure SUI
  - Imaging (MRI, CT, X-ray) is not routinely needed. Ultrasound may be needed for the assessment of residual urine volume.

MANAGEMENT OF URINARY INCONTINENCE

Conservative Management
- Reducing intake of caffeine
- Modifying daily intake of fluid
- Obese women (BMI > 30 kg/m^2) should be advised to lose weight.

Treatment
Physical therapy: Supervised pelvic floor muscle exercise for 3 months period is advised. She is advised to perform pelvic floor muscle contraction, three times per day. Electrical stimulation or perineometry is not to be used as a routine.

Drug therapy: See above

Flavoxate, propantheline and imipramine should not be preferably used for the treatment of UI or OAB.
- **Desmopressin:** It may be used in women with UI or OAB with troublesome symptoms.
- **Duloxetine** is not given to women with a predominant stress UI.

Surgical Treatments for Overactive Bladder
- ***Sacral nerve stimulation*** is advised for women with UI due to detrusor overactivity when women are not responding to usual conservative management.
- ***Augmentation cystoplasty*** is done for women who have not responded with conservative management.
  Common complications are metabolic acidosis, mucus production, UTI and urinary retention.
- ***Urinary diversion***
- ***Injection of botulinum toxin*** in the bladder wall.

Surgical Procedures for Stress Urinary Incontinence (SUI)
- Midurethral retropubic tape or tension-free vaginal tape (TVT)
- Transobturator tape (TOT)
- Intramural bulking agents (glutaraldehyde cross-linked collagen) are used by injecting in the periurethral region
- Artificial urinary sphincter: When other surgical methods have failed
- Anterior colporrhaphy, needle suspensions, paravaginal defect repair and Marshall-Marchetti-Krantz procedure are not used for the treatment of stress UI.

Suggested Reading
1. Basu M, Duckett J. A randomized trial of a retropubic tension-free vaginal tape versus a mini-sling for stress incontinence. BJOG. 2010;117(6):730-5.
2. Nygaard IE, Kreder KJ. Pharmacologic therapy of lower urinary tract dysfunction. Clin Obstet Gynecol. 2004;47(1):83-92.
3. Richter HE, Albo ME, Zyczynski HM, et al. Retropubic versus transobturator midurethral slings for stress incontinence. N Engl J Med. 2010;362(22):2066-76.

Chapter 7: Fibroid Uterus: Management Issues

Fibroid uterus is the most common benign tumor of the uterus. Overall prevalence is 30–40%. It is a hormone-dependent tumor. It is due to the neoplastic proliferation of the smooth muscle cells and the fibrous tissues. It has got more of the estrogen receptors.

Risk factors: Nulliparity, age, genetic predisposition, black women, obesity and anovulation.

The **common symptoms for presentation** are: abnormal uterine bleeding, pain during menstruation (dysmenorrhea), pelvic heaviness, pressure symptoms may be there occasionally with urinary retention, incomplete evacuation or problems of defection.

Fibroids may remain asymptomatic for majority of women. The symptoms of presentation depend upon the number, size and location of the fibroid(s) in the uterus.

Location of fibroid(s)	
■ **Corporeal fibroids may be:**	■ **Cervical fibroid may be:**
♦ Intramural (75%)	♦ Anterior
♦ Subserous (15%)	♦ Lateral
♦ Submucous (5%)	♦ Central
	♦ Posterior

Treatment options for the leiomyoma(s)	
■ **Asymptomatic fibroid(s)**	■ **Symptomatic fibroids**
♦ Observation provided diagnosis is certain	♦ Medical management
♦ Periodic examination and assessment at a regular interval (6–12 months)	♦ Surgical management
	♦ Others (see below)

Choice of treatment is tailored for an individual patient depending upon the type, number, location, associated symptoms, availability of resources and also with the desire of the woman.

Nonhormonal treatment for a woman with heavy menstrual period due to fibroid(s).

Women with heavy menstrual bleeding may be treated with tranexamic acid. It is an antifibrinolytic agent. Prostaglandin synthetase inhibitors, mefenamic acid are also helpful. Tranexamic acid therapy combined with mefenamic acid, reduces menorrhagia as well as the severity of dysmenorrhea.

Hormonal treatments: Common medications used are:
a. **Combined oral contraceptives (COCs)** induce endometrial atrophy and result in reduced menstrual blood loss.
b. **Use of progesterone-only pill** or **depot medroxyprogesterone acetate** has also been used and observed to reduce menstrual blood loss as well as volume of fibroid after 6 months of treatment.
c. **Levonorgestrel intrauterine system (LNG-IUS)** has been used as an effective treatment of heavy menstrual bleeding. LNG-IUS improves the symptoms, also increases the hemoglobin levels. It induces endometrial atrophy. Randomized controlled studies have shown LNG-IUS is more effective than combined oral contraceptives in reducing menstrual blood loss and increasing the levels of hemoglobin.

Gonadotropin-releasing Hormone Analog (GnRH-a)

- Reduces the menstrual blood loss as it induces sustained downregulation of the pituitary gland and suppression of the ovarian function.
- GnRH-a treatment induces hypoestrogenic state that cause intolerable side effects and bone loss.
  Add-back therapy is needed to combat hypoestrogenic symptoms. Lower dose estrogen and progestin is given as an add-back therapy.
- GnRH-a treatment causes reduction of fibroid size by 36% and improvement of symptoms. After stoppage of treatment, there is return of menstruation by 4–8 weeks and size of fibroid returned by 4–6 months. Preoperative use of GnRH-a, may facilitate for vaginal hysterectomy or may make abdominal hysterectomy easy with using transverse incision. There is reduction of operative blood loss also.

However, difficulties may be faced during myomectomy as the plane of clearage between the capsule and myoma and the myometrium is obliterated.

Place of Progesterone and Selective Progesterone Receptor Modulators

Progesterone induces myometrial proliferation and increases size of the fibroid. Antiprogestins and the agents that modulate progesterone receptor activity are found to be useful in the treatment of fibroids. The commonly used drug in the category is mifepristone.

Mifepristone is a synthetic steroid. Mifepristone (10 mg) reduces the menstrual blood loss as well as the size of the fibroids. There is also improvement of symptoms in women with fibroid(s). Mifepristone has been associated with changes in the endometrium and its use in treatment of fibroids is currently restricted to research settings.

ANTIESTROGENS

Tamoxifen is an antiestrogen and it blocks the effect of estrogen. Fibroid is an estrogen-dependent tumor, therefore, antiestrogens (tamoxifen or raloxifene) were used to control its growth. Results were inconsistent. It is not recommended at present.

Aromatase inhibitors (AI) have been tried to reduce the size of fibroids. AI inhibit conversion of androgens. However, till date, use of AI is alone in experimental stage and is not recommended for clinical practice presently.

Uterine Artery Embolization (UAE) (See Ch 57)

UAE is an effective method for the treatment of uterine fibroids.

Advantages of UAE	Common side effects of UAE
■ As effective as myomectomy ■ Quicker recovery ■ Early resumption to work ■ Major complications are less ■ Risk of ovarian failure not high	■ Pain ■ Vaginal discharge ■ May need further intervention (23%) within 2–5 years ■ Future fertility outcomes—more information is awaited, though successful pregnancies have been reported

MRI-GUIDED FOCUSED ULTRASONOGRAPHY (MRI-GFUS)

Procedure: High frequency ultrasound waves are used. It produces heat to denature proteins leading to cell death and fibrosis development. This results in shrinkage of fibroids and reduction in size and volume of the uterus. MRI helps to target the fibroid. Tissue temperature needs to be monitored.

Advantages of MRI-GFUS	
■ Effective treatment ■ Safe ■ Less morbidity ■ Ambulatory	■ Preservation of uterus is possible ■ Quick recovery ■ Significant reduction of symptoms related to fibroid

Fibroids with less vascularity (low-signal intensity on MRI) respond to treatment more compared with vascular fibroids (high-signal intensity on MRI). At present, women desiring for pregnancy should not be recommended for this treatment, though successful pregnancies have been reported.

Side Effects of MRI-GFUS	
■ Nausea, vomiting ■ Skin burn ■ Pain in leg or buttock (short-term)	■ Sciatic nerve palsy (transient) ■ About 20% of women may need for the intervention later on

SURGICAL MANAGEMENT OF UTERINE FIBROIDS

Indications of Surgical Management

a. Women with severe symptoms not responding to other modes of therapy
b. Women with severe pressure symptoms
c. Large fibroid(s)
d. Women with infertility or recurrent miscarriage where no cause other than fibroid(s).

Types of Surgery

■ Myomectomy
■ Hysterectomy
■ Myolysis
■ Procedures of myomectomy
  ♦ Laparotomy
  ♦ Laparoscopy
  ♦ Hysteroscopic resection

Hysteroscopic myomectomy is done for submucous and intracavitary fibroids.

Classification Systems of Submucous and Intracavitary Fibroids

The classification systems of submucous fibroid are based on ESGE, FIGO or STEPW.

TABLE 7.1: ESGE and FIGO classifications for submucous myomas.

ESGE classifications	
Type 0: No myometrial involvement, entirely in endometrium (pedunculated)	Submucosal
Type I <50% myometrial extension (sessile) >90% angle of myoma surface to the uterine wall	Others
Type II ≥ 50% myometrial extension (sessile) ≥ 90% angle of myoma surface to the uterine wall	

(ESGE: European Society of Gastrointestinal Endoscopy; FIGO: International Federation of Gynecology and Obstetrics)

FIGO classifications	
0	Pedunculated (Intacavity)
1	<50% intramural
2	≥50% intramural
3	Contact endometrium (100% intramural)
4	Intramural
5	Subserosal ≥50% intramural
6	Subserosal <50% intramural
7	Subserosal pedunculated
8	Others (cervical or parasitic)

Classification system of *European Society of Gynecological Endoscopy (ESGE)* and the *FIGO* are more extensive. They have got some limitations to predict the operative outcome.

Therefore, another classification system has been introduced to improve the outcome in hysteroscopic myomectomy. This is known as **STEPW** (size, topography, extension, penetration and lateral wall).

Grade-0 and Grade-1 fibroids can be easily removed *hysteroscopically.*

Resectoscopic slicing is the gold standard for intracavitary fibroids (Grade-0).

Laparotomy or Laparoscopic Myomectomy

Myomectomy is done for preservation of the uterus.

Measures for reducing blood loss during myomectomy	
■ **Preoperative measures** ♦ Use of GnRH analog ♦ Use of selective progesterone receptor modulators (SPRM)	■ **Measures during operation** ♦ Use of vasoconstrictive agents (Vasopressin) ♦ Use of tourniquets ♦ Use of myomectomy clamp (Boney's)
Laparoscopic myomectomy is considered superior to when compared with open myomectomy	

Advantages of laparoscopic myomectomy

a. Less postoperative pain
b. Shorter hospital stay
c. Operating time may be longer. However, women with multiple fibroids, huge size, may be considered for open myomectomy.

Myolysis

It is an alternative procedure to fibroid resection. Myolysis is done by passing electric current through a needle to destroy the fibroid. Cryomyolysis may be done where a freezing probe is used in the similar manner. These techniques can be used for all types of fibroids using a laparoscope or a hysteroscopy.

Advantages	Disadvantages
■ Simple procedure, less blood loss	■ Increased risk of postoperative adhesions ■ No tissue for histology confirmation ■ Need for further intervention

Hysterectomy is the definitive surgical method of treatment for uterine fibroids. Hysterectomy may be done via abdominal or vaginal route. Else it could be done laparoscopically. Abdominal hysterectomy is a major surgical procedure. It takes longer time, causes more blood loss, longer hospital stay compared with vaginal or laparoscopic method of hysterectomy.

Suggested Reading

1. Bagaria M, Suneja A, Vaid NB, Guleria K, Mishra K. Low-dose mifepristone in treatment of uterine leiomyoma: A randomised double blind placebo-controlled clinical trial. Aust N Z J Obstet Gynaecol. 2009;49:77–83.
2. Flierman PA, Oberye JJ, van der Hulst VP, de Blok S. Rapid reduction of leiomyoma volume during treatment with the GnRH antagonist ganirelix. BJOG. 2005;112:638–42.
3. Lasmar RB, Barrozo PR, Dias R, Oliveira MA. Submuous myomas: a new presurgical classification to evaluate the viability of hysteroscopic surgical treatment–preliminary report. J Minim Invasive Gynecol. 2005;12:308–11.
4. Lethaby A, Vollenhoven B, Sowter M, et al. Preoperative GnRH analogue therapy before hysterectomy or myomectomy for uterine fibroids. Cochrane Database Syst Rev. 2006;(2):CD000547.
5. Munro MG, Critchley HO, Broder MS, Fraser IS. FIGO classification system (PALM-COEIN) for causes of abnormal uterine bleeding in nongravid women in the reproductive years. Int J Gynaecol Obstet. 2011;113:3–13.
6. National Institute for Health and Care Excellence. Uterine artery embolization for fibroids NICE interventional procedure guidance 367. London: NICE; 2011.
7. Sayed GH, Zakherah MS, El-Nashar SA, Shaaban MM. A randomized clinical trial of a levonorgestrel-releasing intrauterine system and a low-dose combined oral contraceptive for fibroid-related menorrhagia. Int J Gynaecol Obstet. 2011;112:126–30.
8. Song H, Lu D, Navaratnam K, Shi G. Aromatase inhibitors for uterine fibroids. Cochrane Database Syst Rev. 2013;(10):CD009505.
9. Wamsteker K, Emanuel MH, de Kruif JH. Transcervical hysteroscopic resection of submucous fibroids for abnormal uterine bleeding: results regarding the degree of intramural extension. Obstet Gynecol. 1993;82:736–40.

Chapter 8: Polycystic Ovarian Syndrome

CARDIOVASCULAR RISK IN CASES WITH PCOS

Cardiovascular risk in polycystic ovarian syndrome (PCOS) is increased significantly. BMI is important. **Android obesity** is a high-risk factor than **gynecoid** obesity.

Measurement of waist circumference important to measure the visceral fat. Visceral fat is metabolically active. Increased visceral fat suggests insulin resistance, type II diabetes mellitus, dyslipidemia, hypertension and left ventricular enlargement, and coronary artery disease. Waist circumference >87 cm suggests high risk. Exercise has a significant effect in reducing the visceral fat and the risk associated with cardiovascular disease. Almost 10% reduction of body weight equates with a 30% reduction of visceral fat.

PCOS HAS BEEN REVIEWED FROM TIME TO TIME

- Irving F Stein and Michael L Leventhal—1935
- NIH Criteria-1991
- ESHRE/ASRM (2003, 2018)
- Heterogeneity of nature
- ESHRE 2018: consensus in diagnosis has not yet been reached.

DIAGNOSIS OF PCOS

- This clinical syndrome was originally described by Stein and Leventhal in 1935. This syndrome was characterized by presence of amenorrhea, hirsutism, obesity, associated with enlarged and polycystic ovaries.
- **NICHD–1990** defined this syndrome with the below mentioned criteria:
    - Hyperandrogenemia
    - Menstruation dysfunction
    - Exclusion of other known similar disorders.

Diagnosis was made with the presence of any two out of total three criteria:
1. Oligo/anovulation
2. Hyperandrogenemia: Clinical or biochemical
3. Polycystic ovaries (USG, Fig. 8.1): Excluding other androgen excess disorders (CAH, thyroid dysfunction, hyperprolactinemia).

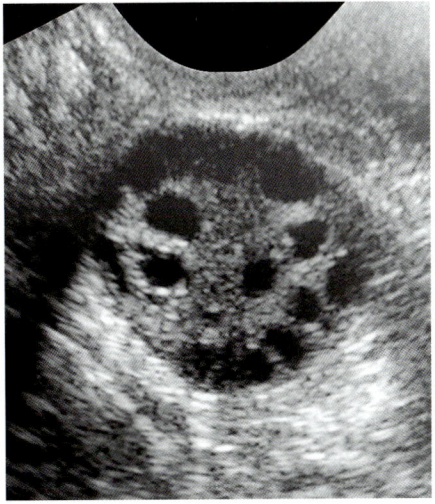

Fig. 8.1: Polycystic changes in the ovary showing multiple small cysts, with increased ovarian stroma.

ETIOPATHOLOGY OF PCOS

- Familial clustering is common in PCOS—50%.
- About 5-10% in general population.
- Clinical and biochemical manifestations of PCOS are expressed at puberty in predisposed individuals.
- Evidences are accumulating that the stigma of PCOS may start long before puberty.
- Excess androgen production by the ovary (genetically determined) starts during intrauterine life.
- This results in programming of hypothalamic pituitary unit.
- There is excess luteinizing hormone (LH) secretion, *preferential abdominal obesity*—predisposes to insulin resistance and anovulation.
- Excess LH secretion is due to genetically determined hyperactive LH pulse generator in hypothalamus.
- Other secondary genetic (multigenic) and environmental factors (dietary) interact to modify the final phenotype.
- This results in heterogeneous nature of the syndrome.

ETIOPATHOLOGY OF PCOS: GENE AND INSULIN

- Insulin receptor gene mutation in the peripheral target tissues

- Post-receptor signaling **(CYP17.20 lyase)** defect:
  - There is increased serine/threonine phosphorylation instead of tyrosine autophosphorylation.
  - High-circulating free fatty acid levels enhance serine phosphorylation. This induces insulin resistance. Ultimately, this leads to increased androgen production.
  - Associated β-cell dysfunction.
  - Increased central obesity leads to increased insulin resistance.

Insulin Resistance (IR) and Increased Androgens are Genetically Determined

Raised fasting insulin levels >25 micro IU/mL and fasting glucose/insulin ratio <4.5 suggests IR. Levels of serum insulin response >300 micro IU/mL at 2 hours post-glucose (75 g), suggests severe IR.

Etiology of insulin resistance is unknown. Mutations of the insulin receptor gene in the peripheral tissues and reduced tyrosine autophosphorylation are thought to be the important cause.

Primarily, it is the tissue insulin resistance and hyperinsulinemia to cause abnormal hypothalamic programming (in utero) and preferential raised LH secretion. This causes hyperandrogenemia.

This hypothesis of fetal tissues reprogramming opens new directions in the management of PCOS.

In general, metformin treatment increases insulin sensitivity and decreases weight and BMI. It also normalizes blood pressure and LDL cholesterol. Above all it reduces the chronic inflammatory state as has been discussed above. Combined oral contraceptives reduce insulin sensitivity and glucose tolerance in some women.

ASSOCIATION OF INSULIN RESISTANCE IN WOMEN WITH PCOS

- **Insulin resistance**: Obese PCOS: 75%, lean PCOS: 50%
- **Impaired GTT**: 35%
- **Type 2 DM**: 10%
- **Insulin resistance and hyperinsulinemia** are the causes of hyperandrogenemia by increased ovarian androgen production. There is decreased hepatic sex hormone binding globulin (SHBG) production. Insulin also potentiates LH action as it acts as a co-gonadotropin.
- Insulin resistance (hyperinsulinemia) is associated with decreased HDL cholesterol and increased LDL cholesterol (see below). **Dyslipidemia** is common in women with PCOS.

OBESITY–INSULIN RESISTANCE

Insulin Resistance and Obesity—Leading to PCOS and Non-insulin-dependent Diabetes Mellitus (NIDDM)

- Recent idea—insulin resistance does not cause obesity
- But obesity causes insulin resistance
- Insulin acts as **co-gonadotropin.**

HOW DOES OBESITY CAUSE INSULIN RESISTANCE?

- Obesity refers to central obesity, i.e., abdominal and visceral obesity.
- Visceral obesity indicates accumulation of omental, mesenteric, retroperitoneal and perinephric fat.

CENTRAL OBESITY AND INSULIN RESISTANCE

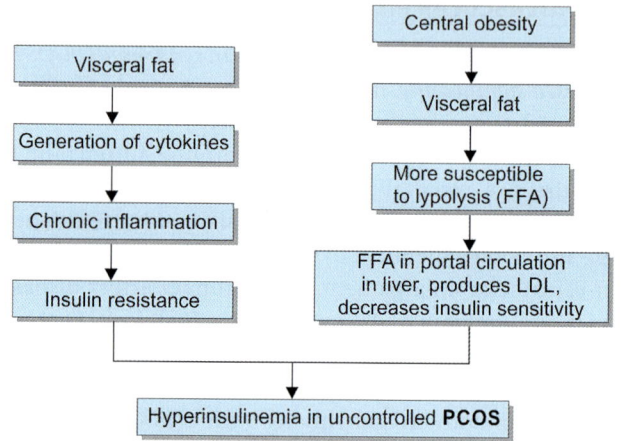

HOW DOES OBESITY CAUSE PCOS?

- Mainly the elevated insulin (hyperinsulinemia), through IGF-1 receptors, amplifies LH-mediated thecal androgen production.
- Elevated insulin also suppresses hepatic synthesis of SHBG and insulin-like growth factor-binding protein (IGFBP)—thereby increases bioavailability of free testosterone.

OBESITY AND PCOS

Hyperandrogenism

E2 is secreted from the ovarian follicles and E1 produced from fat (peripheral) make the blood level of estrogen as static and persistently hyperestrogenic. Chronic nonpulsatile stimulation of GnRH on the receptors of pituitary, cause chronically elevated release of LH which is again not pulsatile. This results in anovulation.

CHRONICALLY ELEVATED GnRH (LHRH)

Chronically elevated GnRH (LHRH) and no LH surge results in anovulation. Numerous stunted follicles (cysts) in ovaries ultimately undergo follicular apoptosis.

There is increase in ovarian stromal elements to produce **androgens**.

Normal or low FSH causes poor follicular growth. Most follicles remain stunted and are the incompetent follicles. There is persistent anovulation.

IMPACT OF PCOS ON HEALTH (ADVERSE EFFECTS)

Short-term	Long-term
■ Menstrual abnormalities ■ Infertility ■ Recurrent miscarriage ■ GDM ■ Acne	**Metabolic syndrome** ■ Insulin resistance (IR)-Dyslipidemia ■ Obesity type 2 DM ■ Hypertension ■ Hyperhomocysteinemia with or without IR **Others** ■ Carcinoma endometrium ■ Thrombophilic disorders ■ Recurrent miscarriage ■ Coronary artery disease (CAD) ■ Sleep disturbances and obstructive sleep apnea (OSA)

SINGLE BEST ANSWER

Q.1 Metabolic abnormalities in women with PCOS:
   a. Hyperandrogenemia is due to excess stimulation with follicle-stimulating hormone (FSH)
   b. Insulin resistance is observed in about 70–80% of women
   c. Obesity is included in the diagnosis of PCOS
   d. Slim PCOS women are more likely to develop type II diabetes.

Ans.   a. F   b. F
            c. F   d. F

Q.2 Metabolic abnormalities in PCOS:
   a. Insulin resistance results in failure of all action of insulin
   b. Estimation of serum insulin level is a routine to treat the PCOS women
   c. Infertility in PCOS women is often due to poor quality of oocyte
   d. Glucose tolerance test should be done in women with positive family history only.

Ans.   a. F   b. F
            c. F   d. F

PCOS and Metformin Therapy

Metabolic functions of metformin are:

- Inhibits hepatic glucose output
- Enhances insulin-mediated glucose utilization
- Decreases fatty acid oxidation
- Improves lipid profile by decreasing triglycerides, fatty acids, low-density lipoprotein (LDL) cholesterol and increases HDL cholesterol
- Does not stimulate insulin secretion
- Does not cause hypoglycemia
- Does not stimulate fetal pancreas to over secrete insulin
- Decreases intestinal absorption of glucose
- Appears to have direct effect on ovarian function
- Lowers serum androgen levels significantly

- Restore menstrual cyclicity (Figs. 8.2 and 8.3)
- Effective in achieving ovulation either alone or when combined with clomiphene citrate
- Cotreatment with metformin improves the response of exogenous gonadotropins or the results of assisted reproductive technology (ART) (IVF pregnancy).
- Appears to reduce body weight.

Q.3 Metformin therapy in PCOS:
   a. It enhances insulin secretion
   b. It is safe in pregnancy as it does not cross the placenta
   c. Once started should be continued in pregnancy
   d. Reduces the risk of significant ovarian hyperstimulation syndrome (OHSS).

Ans.   a. F   b. F
            c. F   d. T

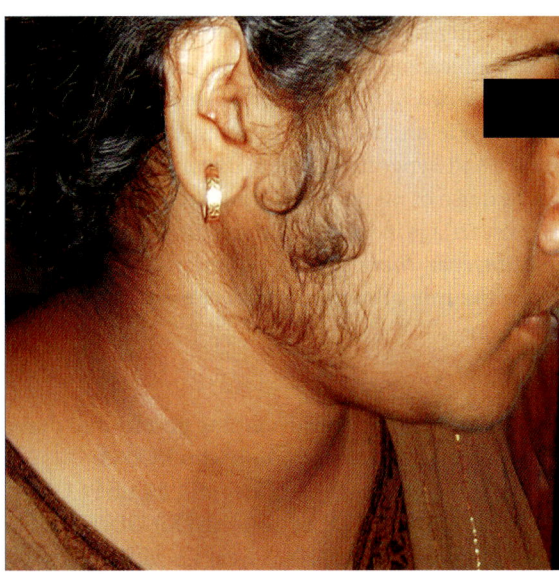

Fig. 8.2: Excess male type of facial hair and acanthosis nigricans in PCOS.

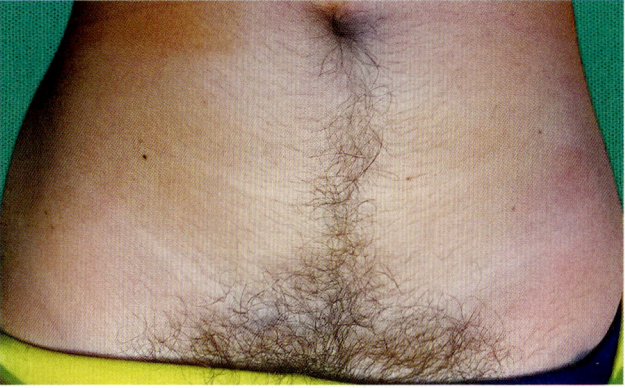

Fig. 8.3: An 18-year-old girl showing male pattern of pubic hair distribution (male escutcheon).

Dose schedule of metformin: 500–3,000 mg/day may be used. Commonly used dose regimens are 500 mg TID or 850 mg BID. Long-acting preparations are associated with less gastrointestinal side effects.

Metformin appears to be safe in pregnancy although it crosses the placenta. There is minimal effect on transplacental flux. However, it is advised to discontinue it, once pregnancy is diagnosed. There is no firm evidence that metformin reduces the risk of miscarriage.

Metformin is found to be less effective in those obese women with BMI ≥ 35 kg/m^2. Combined approach with lifestyle modifications and metformin therapy appear to be effective. Agents such as metformin and thiazolidinediones (rosiglitazone, pioglitazone) improve symptoms and reproductive outcome in women with PCOS either by lowering insulin levels or improving insulin sensitivity at cellular level or both.

Updated Cochrane review concluded that the benefit of therapy with metformin is limited. For young women with PCOS, lifestyle modifications (diet, exercise) remain the mainstay.

Increased risk of miscarriage in women with recurrent miscarriage is attributed to hyperandrogenemia, insulin resistance and hyperinsulinemia. Uncontrolled studies have shown that use of metformin during pregnancy reduces the risk of miscarriage in women with recurrent miscarriage and PCOS. ***However, there is no randomized controlled trials to assess the role of metformin in women with recurrent miscarriage.***

LONG-TERM CONSEQUENCES OF PCOS

Q.4 What is the risk of developing gestational diabetes mellitus (GDM) in women with PCOS?

Ans. Women, who have been diagnosed with PCOS before pregnancy, should be screened for GDM. Screening should be done at 24–28 weeks of gestation. Women who are overweight (BMI ≥ 25 kg/m^2) and who are not overweight (BMI < 25 kg/m^2) but with additional risk factors such as advanced age (>40 years), personal or a family history of GDM should have 2 hours post glucose (75 g) tolerance test is performed.

Q.5 What are the other long-term consequences of PCOS?

Ans. Women with PCOS have the risk of developing sleep apnea.

Q.6 What is the risk of developing cardiovascular disease (CVD) in women with PCOS?

Ans. Women with PCOS have the risks of developing CVD, besides the individual risk factors. Risk factors for CVD are obesity, family history of type II diabetes, dyslipidemia and hypertension.

Q.7 What are the risks of cancer in women with PCOS?

Ans. Women with PCOS suffering from oligo- or amenorrhea, run the risk of developing endometrial hyperplasia and cancer. Women may be screened by transvaginal ultrasound in the absence of withdrawal bleeding. Women with thickened endometrium (>7 mm) or with a polyp should be considered for hysteroscopy and/or endometrial biopsy. Risks of ovarian or breast cancer are not associated.

Q.8 What are the strategies for reduction of risks?

Ans. Important issues are lifestyle modifications with exercises and weight control. First-line approach is diet, exercise and weight loss.

Q.9 Could there be any place for pharmacological treatment?

Ans. Insulin-sensitizing agents are found helpful and safe. But it is uncertain that the use of insulin-sensitizing agents confers any long-term benefit. Weight reduction itself is helpful to control hyperandrogenemia.

Q.10 What is the place of ovarian electrodiathermy (ovarian drilling)?

Ans. It is done in selected women with the problem of anovulation.

Q.11 What is the place of bariatric surgery for women with PCOS?

Ans. PCOS women with morbid obesity (BMI ≥ 40 kg/m^2 or ≥ 35 kg/m^2) with other high-risk factors are considered specially when standard management has failed to reduce weight.

Suggested Reading

1. Amer SA, Laird S, Ledger WL, Li TC. Effect of laparoscopic ovarian diathermy on circulating inhibin B in woman with anovulatory PCOS. Hum Reprod. 2007;22:389-94.
2. Armar NA, McGarrigle HH, Honour J, Holownia P, Jacobs HS, Lachelin GC. Laparoscopic ovarian diathermy in the management of anovulatory infertility in women with polycystic ovaries: endocrine changes and clinical outcome. Fertil Steril. 1990;53:45-9.
3. Asunción M, Calvo RM, San Millán JL, Sancho J, Avila S, Escobar-Morreale HF. A prospective study of the prevalence of the polycystic ovary syndrome in unselected Caucasian women from Spain. J Clin Endocrinol Metab. 2000;85:2434-8.
4. Felemban A, Tan SL, Tulandi T. Laparoscopic treatment of polycystic ovaries with insulated needle cautery—a reappraisal. Fertil Steril. 2000;73:266-9.
5. Gangale MF, Miele L, Lanzone A, Sagnella F, Martinez D, Tropea A, Long-term metformin treatment is able to reduce the prevalence of metabolic syndrome and its hepatic involvement in young hyperinsulinemic overweight patients with polycystic ovarian syndrome. Clin Endocrinol (Oxf). 2011;75(4):520-7.
6. Gjonnaess H. Polycystic ovarian syndrome treated by ovarian electrocautery through the laparoscope. Fertil Steril. 1984;41:20-5.
7. Hull MG. Epidemiology of infertility and polycystic ovarian disease: endocrinological and demographic studies. Gynecol Endocrinol. 1987;1:235-45.
8. Jakubowicz DJ, Iurno MJ, Jakubowiczs, et al. Effects of metformin on early pregnancy loss in the polycystic ovary syndrome. J Clin Endocrinol Metab. 2002;87(2):524-9.

9. Lord JM, Flight IH, Norman RJ. Insulin-sensitizing drugs (metformin, troglitazone, rosiglitazone, pioglitazone, D-chiro-inositol) for polycystic ovary syndrome. Cochrane Database Syst Rev. 2003;(2):CDOO3053.
10. Moran LJ, Hutchison SK, Norman RJ, et al. Lifestyle changes in women with polycystic ovary syndrome. Cochrane Database Syst Rev. 2011;(2):CD007506.
11. Naether OGJ, Fischer R, Weise HC, et al. Laparoscopic electrocoagulation of the ovarian surface in infertile patients with polycystic ovarian disease. Fertil Steril. 1993;60:88-94.
12. Rotterdam ESHRE/ASRM-Sponsored PCOS consensus workshop group. Revised 2003 consensus on diagnostic criteria and long-term health risks related to polycystic ovary syndrome (PCOS). Hum Reprod. 2004;19(1):41-7.
13. Rotterdam ESHRE/ASRM-sponsored PCOS Consensus Workshop Group. Revised 2003 consensus on diagnostic criteria and long-term health risks related to polycystic ovary syndrome. Fertil Steril. 2004.
14. Royal College of Obstetricians and Gynecologists. Diagnosis and Treatment of Gestational Diabetes. Scientific Impact Paper No. 23. London: RCOG; 2011.
15. Tang T, Glanville J, Hayden CJ, et al. Combined lifestyle modification and metformin in obese women with polycystic ovary syndrome (PCOS). A randomized, placebo-controlled, double-blind multicentre study. Hum Reprod. 2006;21(1):80-9.

Chapter 9: Hyperandrogenemia

CLINICAL FEATURES AND DIFFERENTIAL DIAGNOSIS OF HYPERANDROGENEMIA

Clinical Features Associated with Hyperandrogenemia

Clinical features vary depending upon the severity of hyperandrogenemia	
■ Menstrual cycle irregularities ■ Weight gain ■ Hirsutism ■ Acne ■ Alopecia ■ Balding ■ Virilization ■ Enlargement of clitoris	■ Masculinization ■ Rapid and excessive hair growth ■ Change of voice ■ Atrophy of the breasts ■ Skin changes ■ Thinning/bruising of the skin ■ Acanthosis nigricans

Scoring system for hirsutism is done by "**Ferriman-Gallwey**" score board: This system rates hair growth severity from 0 to 4. Total eleven body areas are considered. The different areas are: Upper lip, chest, chin, lower back, upper back, lower abdomen, upper abdomen, forearm, arm, thighs and lower leg (Fig. 9.1). A score of 8 or above defines hirsutism.

Biochemical evaluation of hyperandrogenemia is done by estimating the serum total testosterone level. Serum total testosterone level of hyperandrogenemia is as below:
- 2–5 mol/L = Mild (may be due to PCOS)
- >5 mol/L = Serve (androgen-secreting tumor)

Differential Diagnosis of Hyperandrogenemia
- **Polycystic Ovarian Syndrome**
- **Congenital adrenal hyperplasia** is due to deficiency of 21-hydroxylase (90%), and 11β-hydroxylase or 3β-hydroxysteroid dehydrogenase deficiency.
- **Androgen-producing tumors of the ovary**: Hilus cell tumor, Leydig cell tumor
- **Androgen-producing tumors of the adrenal gland**
- **Iatrogenic**: Use of exogenous androgens. Androgenic-anabolic steroid (AAS) is used by the athletes to increase performances, to increase libido.
- **Cushing's syndrome**
- **Cushing's disease** is due to adrenocortical neoplasm or hyperplasia.

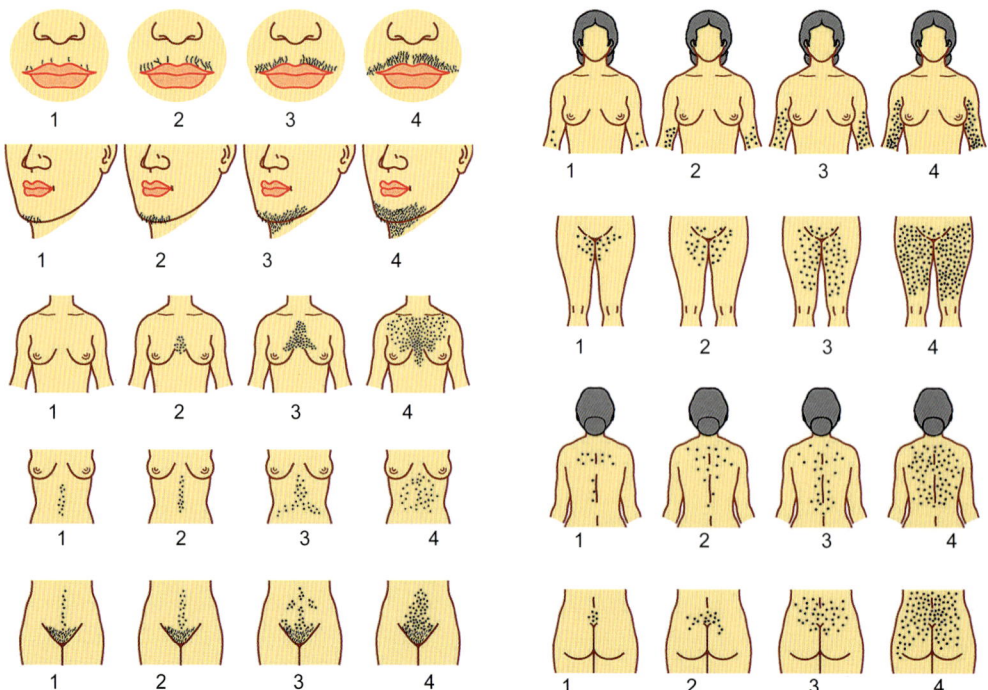

Fig. 9.1: Modified Ferriman-Gallwey score.

Source: Modified from Hatch R, Rosenfield RL, Kim MH, et al. Hirsutism: implications, etiology and management. Am J Obstet Gynecol. 1981;140(7):815-30.

- **Gestational hyperandrogenemia**: It is rare. Serum testosterone level rise slowly in pregnancy and serum sex hormone-binding globulin (SHBG) levels also increase. There is no hyperandrogenemia in a normal pregnancy. However, gestational hyperandrogenemia may be due to luteomas and theca lutein cyst of the ovary.

Suggested Reading

1. Gangale MF, Miele L, Lanzone A, Sagnella F, Martinez D, Tropea A, et al. Long-term metformin treatment is able to reduce the prevalence of metabolic syndrome and its hepatic involvement in young hyperinsulinaemic overweight patients with polycystic ovarian syndrome. Clin Endocrinol (Oxf). 2011;75:520-7.
2. Moran L, Teede H. Metabolic features of the reproductive phenotypes of polycystic ovary syndrome. Hum Reprod Update 2009;15:477-88.
3. Moran LJ, Misso ML, Wild RA, Norman RJ. Impaired glucose tolerance, type 2 diabetes and metabolic syndrome in polycystic ovary syndrome: a systematic review and meta-analysis. Hum Reprod Update. 2010;16:347-63.
4. Rotterdam ESHRE/ASRM-Sponsored PCOS Consensus Workshop Group. Revised 2003 consensus on diagnostic criteria and long-term health risks related to polycystic ovary syndrome. Fertil Steril. 2004;81:19-25.
5. Sathyapalan T, Atkin SL. Recent advances in cardiovascular aspects of polycystic ovary syndrome. Eur J Endocrinol. 2012;166:575-83.
6. Velazquez EM, Mendoza S, Hamer T, Sosa F, Glueck CJ. Metformin therapy in polycystic ovary syndrome reduces hyperinsulinemia, insulin resistance, hyperandrogenemia, and systolic blood pressure, while facilitating normal menses and pregnancy. Metabolism. 1994;43:647-54.

Association of Subfertility with Endometriosis

Approximately 40–60% of women in the reproductive age suffer from the problem of subfertility in association with pelvic endometriosis. Often they remain asymptomatic. Laparoscopic pelvic evaluation is the **gold standard** to detect pelvic endometriosis even if they are without any symptoms.

Endometriosis is a progressive disease. Treatment of endometriosis is justified regardless of the symptoms because in 30–60% of women, it progresses within a year.

However, association of subfertility and minimal or mild endometriosis is not well-established. Management of infertile women with minimal to mild endometriosis is therefore controversial.

Current evidence suggests that **medical treatment** has no benefit over no treatment in terms of crude pregnancy rate.

Association between endometriosis and subfertility is established especially in women with moderate to advanced stage disease.

COMMON CAUSES OF SUBFERTILITY IN A WOMAN WITH PELVIC ENDOMETRIOSIS

- Alteration of pelvic anatomy due to adhesion formation
- Anovulation or oligoovulation
- Failure of ovum pick-up due to distorted anatomy
- Impaired fertilization (increased macrophages to cause phagocytosis, growth factors, cytokines)
- Poor oocyte quality
- Luteal phase defect
- Reduced endometrial receptivity
- Peritoneal fluid inflammatory mediators
- Implantation failure

TABLE 10.1: Common causes of subfertility related to pelvic pathology.

Minimal or mild endometriosis and subfertility	Infertility in severe endometriosis
The precise association is not clearly understood: ■ Peritoneal factors (macrophages, lymphocytes, cytokines, growth factors) to cause damage to sperm ■ Raised levels of peritoneal prostaglandins inhibit ovulation, increases uterine contractility ■ Impaired follicular development ■ Pelvic pain and dyspareunia	■ Pelvic pain ■ Dyspareunia ■ Adhesion covering the tubes and ovaries ■ Ovarian endometriosis causing anovulation and destruction of ovarian tissues

Ovarian Surgery and IVF Outcomes

Ovarian surgery (cystectomy and cyst aspiration) for endometriomas prior to IVF treatment is not routinely recommended as there is no improvement in outcomes. Management approach must be balanced considering the risk of reducing ovarian reserve and worsening the pelvic anatomy with ovarian surgery. Ovarian reserve assessment should be done before any ovarian surgery.

Surgical procedures and fertility outcomes.
- Open surgery
  - ♦ Cystectomy
  - ♦ Cyst aspiration
- Laparoscopic surgery
  - ♦ Bipolar electrosurgery
  - ♦ Plasma or Laser surgery
- Comparative studies have shown laser ablation or plasma energy is superior to bipolar coagulation. Hemostatic sealants are favored to bipolar surgery.

Indications for assessment of ovarian reserve before ovarian surgery.
- Women requiring repeat surgery on the same or the contralateral ovary
- Cases with advanced endometriosis or bilateral endometriomas
- Women's age ≥35 years

Indications of ovarian surgery in women with endometriomas prior to IVF.
- Worsening pain and failed medical therapy
- Unilateral endometrioma
- Rapidly progressing endometriosis
- Women with adequate ovarian reserve
- No previous surgery
- Suspicion of malignancy (USG features)

Factors for Future Fertility Following Ovarian Cystectomy

1. Nature of the cyst
2. Size and number of the cyst
3. Unilateral or Bilateral
4. Risk of recurrence

The follicular density in the endometriotic cyst is much less compared to a dermoid or serous cyst. The ovarian cortex is stretched out but not damaged in a case with the dermoid cyst. Therefore, the results of IVF treatment in patients with dermoid cyst, showed no difference in the number of eggs collected. On the contrary, surgery for endometriomas and their effects on fertility is poor. Endometriomas (endometriotic cysts) are reported in 17–44% of women with endometriosis. It is the marker of more severe and deeper disease. Nearly 28% of endometriomas are bilateral. The risk of recurrence of endometriomas in the same or the contralateral ovary following surgery is 12–13% after 2–5 years. Most recurrence occurs in the same ovary due to the presence of residual loci. Causes of impaired fertility in women with endometriomas are multifactorial.

Causes of impaired fertility due to endometriomas (endometriotic cysts).
- Persistent chronic inflammatory state (presence of raised levels of IL-2, 6, 8, TNF-α, VEGF) affecting the quality of the oocytes
- Impaired ovarian function, defective folliculogenesis
- Reduced fertilization
- Poor embryo quality
- Failure of implantation, increased rate of miscarriage
- Poor ovarian reserve secondary to fibrosis, (increased tissue oxidative stress)
- Failure of oocytes for in vitro maturation
- There is reduced cytoplasmic mitochondrial content
- Lower mean number of oocyte retrieval and higher cycle cancellation rates
- Reduced ovarian reserve, as confirmed with lower AMH levels and antral follicle count (AFC)
- There is destruction of ovarian cortical tissue due to invasion of endometriosis
- Low follicular density in the ovarian cortex
- Tubal damage, anatomical distortion or tubal occlusion due to adhesion formation.

Management of Women with Minimal or Mild Endometriosis

Women with minimal to mild pelvic endometriosis have been found to have more chance of spontaneous conception compared to women with unexplained infertility. The monthly fecundity rate is 5–10%. An expectant management approach is appropriate in these couples for up to 2 years. Undue delay should be avoided with expectant management especially when the woman is over 35 years of age and other factors for infertility are there.

Medical Management

Medical management to control pelvic endometriosis is not good for the women who try to conceive. Drugs commonly used to control pain are gonadotropin-releasing hormone (GnRH) analogs, combined oral contraceptives (COCs) and nonsteroidal anti-inflammatory drugs (NSAIDs). These drugs inhibit ovulation. These drugs usually delay conception and are not to be prescribed.

Surgical Management

Laparoscopic surgical management (excision of endometriotic deposits, ovarian cystectomy for endometriomas, deep rectovaginal septum endometriosis, restoration of normal pelvic anatomy and adhesiolysis) has got some advantages over medical management to improve pregnancy rate (44%). However, **role of surgery in minimal to mild endometriosis is yet to be established**.

Laparoscopic ablation or excision of endometriotic lesions may be done with improved outcome. Laparoscopic procedure has been done with less morbidity and is preferred compared to laparotomy. Moreover, laparoscopic procedure gives better visualization and minimal tissue damage. However, surgical intervention carries some tissue damage and complications also. There is doubt about the benefits of surgical management especially in cases with mild-to-moderate endometriosis with infertility.

Endometriosis is a progressive disease in about 50% of cases. Surgical intervention is a sensible option to arrest the progress of the disease and to reach the advance stage. It is not yet possible to predict which women will experience progression of the disease and which may go for spontaneous regression.

Superovulation

Superovulation may be done using gonadotropins to increase pregnancy rate. The benefits are—to get more than one oocyte, improved endometrium, improving the timing of coitus or insemination. All these may improve the success rate of pregnancy. Overall pregnancy rate 10–15% per cycle of treatment of a woman with <40 years age with minimal-to-mild endometriosis.

***Intrauterine insemination (husband)*, along with controlled ovarian stimulation (superovulation)** is found to improve pregnancy rate in women with mild to moderate disease.

IVF is an effective method to achieve pregnancy, irrespective of the stage of the disease. IVF may be considered following surgical treatment of endometriosis.

Place of In Vitro Fertilization in Cases with Minimal or Mild Endometriosis

Women with minimal or mild endometriosis and unable to conceive in a period of 2 years duration or more may be considered for in vitro fertilization (IVF). It is important that chance of conception and live birth rate decline sharply as the age of the woman increases. Overall, live birth rate for a woman with age <34 years is over 25–30% following IVF, whereas it goes down to about 10% at the age of 40 years.

Management of Moderate to Severe Endometriosis

Place of Expectant Management

There is significant pelvic structural and anatomical distortion in such a woman. There are several reasons for infertility for the women with advanced stage. The prospect of spontaneous pregnancy for such a woman with moderate-to-severe endometriosis is significantly low. Monthly fecundity is approximately 3% or less. Rate of expectant management is limited.

Surgical Management

The principles of surgery is to:
- Excise or ablate or destroy all visible endometriosis adhesions, and
- To restore the pelvic anatomy as much as possible.

Endometriomas (chocolate cysts of the ovary) can be either ablated, drained or excised. There remains the risk of ovarian tissue damage due to the process of excision or electrosurgery. Ovarian tissue excision or ablation may reduce the ovarian reserve. Pelvic endometriosis has the risk of recurrence. On the other hand, damage to ovarian reserve may cause failure of ovarian response during treatment with IVF procedure. Laparoscopic surgery unless done by a skilled person may cause complications of thermal damage to the bowel, bladder and the ureter.

Large endometrioma (≥5 cm in diameter) needs to be drained and peeled off the cyst lining to prevent recurrence.

In Vitro Fertilization

In vitro fertilization appears to be the optimum option for a woman with advanced endometriosis where other treatments option have failed. In case following unsuccessful surgery for infertility, IVF is preferable to reoperation. Downregulation with GnRH analog for at least 3–4 months before IVF treatment cycle can improve the live birth rate. It is recommended to perform surgical treatment (endometrioma) of moderate-to-severe grade of endometriosis before IVF. However, it is important to note that destruction of ovarian cortex reduces ovarian reserve and reduces the prospect of fertility.

However, it is yet uncertain whether the surgery or the disease process or the patient characteristics (genetic inheritance) itself is the cause of subfertility.

Suggested Reading

1. Baracat CMF, Abdalla-Ribeiro HSA, Araujo RSDC, Bernando WM, Ribeiro PA. The Impact on Ovarian Reserve of Different Hemostasis Methods in Laparoscopic Cystectomy: A Systematic Review and Meta-analysis. Rev Bras Ginecol Obstet. 2019;41:400-8.
2. Chen Y, Pei H, Chang Y, Chen M, Wang H, Xie H, et al. The impact of endometrioma and laparoscopic cystectomy on ovarian reserve and the exploration of related factors assessed by serum anti-Mullerian hormone a prospective cohort study. J ovarian Res. 2014;7:108.
3. Dunselman GA, Vermeulen N, Becker C, et al. ESHRE guideline management of women with endometriosis. Hum Reprod. 2014;29(3):400.
4. Dutta DC, Konar H. Endometriosis and adenomyosis. In: Konar H (ed). Textbook of Gynecology, 8th edition. New Delhi, India: Jaypee Brothers Medical Publishers; 2020. p. 257.
5. Harb HM, Gallos ID, Chu J, Harb M, Coomarasamy A. The effect of endometriosis on in vitro fertilisation outcome: a systematic review and meta-analysis. BJOG. 2013;120:1308-20.
6. Jacobson TZ, Duffy JM, Barlow D, Farquhar C, Koninckx PR, Olive D. Laparoscopic surgery for subfertility associated with endometriosis. Cochrane Database Syst Rev. 2010;1:CD001398.
7. Kennedy S, Bergqvist A, Chapron C, D'Hooghe T, Dunselman G, Greb R, et al. ESHRE guideline for the diagnosis and treatment of endometriosis. Hum Reprod. 2005;20(10):2698-704.
8. Muzii L, Di Tucci C, Di Feliciantonio M, Marchetti C, Perniola G, Panici PB. The effect of surgery for endometrioma on ovarian reserve evaluated by antral follicle count: a systematic review and meta-analysis. Hum Reprod. 2014;29:2190-8.
9. Posabella A, Galetti K, Engelberger S, Giovannacci L, Gyr T, Rosso R. A huge mucinous cystadenoma of ovarian: a rare case report and review of the literature. Rare Tumors. 2014;6:5225.
10. Sanchez AM, Vanni VS, Bartiromo L, Papaleo E, Zilberberg E, Candiani M, et al. Is the oocyte quality affected by endometrosis? A review of the literature. J Ovarian Res. 2017;10:43.
11. Scottish Intercollegiate Guidelines Network. Management of epithelial ovarian cancer. SIGN publication no. 135. Edinburgh: SIGN; 2013.
12. The effect of surgery for endometriomas on fertility: Scientific impact paper no. 55. BJOG. 2018;125(6):e19-28.
13. Timmerman D, Valentin L, Bourne TH, Collins WP, Verrelst H, Vergote I; International Ovarian Tumor Analysis (IOTA) Group. Terms, definitions and measurements to describe the sonographic features of adnexal tumors: a consensus opinion from the International Ovarian Tumor Analysis (IOTA) Group. Ultrasound Obstet Gynecol. 2000;16(5):500-5.
14. Uncu G, Kasapoglu I, Ozerkan K, Seyhan A, Oral Yilmaztepe A. Ata B. Prospective assessment of the impact of endometriomas and their removal on ovarian reserve and determinants of the rate of decline in ovarian reserve. Hum Reprod. 2013:28:2140-5.

Management of Pain in Endometriosis

CAUSES OF PAIN IN ENDOMETRIOSIS

Ectopic endometrium lies outside the uterine cavity whereas eutopic endometrium lines uterine cavity. Ectopic endometrium differs from eutopic endometrium in molecular levels of expression. ***The growth of ectopic endometrium is characterized by the following features:***
- Estrogen-dependent
- State of chronic inflammation
- Progesterone resistance
- Local invasion
- Neurovascular proliferation
- Cells are resistance to apoptosis
- Expression of aromatase and 17β-hydroxysteroid dehydrogenase type-1 enzymes.

These enzymes convert peripheral androgens (androstenedione) to estrone and estradiol. The enzymatic effects create an estrogenic environment that stimulates the proliferation of ectopic endometrial tissues.

Eutopic endometrium do not secrete aromatase enzymes. The inflammatory mediators involved in endometrosis are: Prostaglandin E2, cytokines, TNF-α, VEGF, matrix metalloproteinase (MMP-3), macrophages, interleukins (IL-1, IL-6, IL-8).

Endometriosis has a polygenic and multifactorial pattern of inheritance. Endometriosis may remain static but often progressive in nature. Rarely it may regress.

Sign and Symptoms of Endometriosis

Frequently associated symptoms are:
- Pelvic pain
- Dysmenorrhea
- Dyspareunia
- Dyschezia (painful or defecation).

Deep infiltrating endometriosis (DIE) involving bowel, bladder and rectovaginal septum is often associated with pelvic adhesions and pain.

Diagnosis

Diagnosis of endometriosis is often made late. About 25% of women with endometriosis remain asymptomatic. Onset of symptoms to definitive diagnosis of endometriosis is often delayed with a mean latency of 6–7 years throughout the world. Common conditions that create the diagnostic errors are—chronic pelvic inflammatory disease, inflammatory bowel disease or interstitial cystitis.

Characteristic type of pain in endometriosis may be helpful to suspect the disease. Woman is not free of pain even in the intermenstrual period. Crescendo type of pain to start with and reaching the peak and plateau, and then decrescendo is observed.

Vaginal examination alone may be insufficient to make the diagnosis. Presence of nodules in the pouch of Douglas in cases with DIE may be felt. Vaginal speculum examination may reveal the dark blue nodules in the posterior fornix of the vagina. These nodules are tender and increase in size and often bleeds during menstruation.

Recently the noninvasive imaging modalities like ultrasonography (USG) and magnetic resonance imaging (MRI) are helpful in the diagnosis. MRI is superior to USG and CT especially for a deep infiltrating endometriosis.

When endometriosis is suspected, the patient may have the benefit of empirical therapy (hormones) for relief of pain. This may lead to amonorrhea also. Otherwise *"see and treat"* policy of confirmation with laparoscopy and simultaneous therapy could be the alternative. Diagnosis of endometriosis may remain presumed or probable till confirmation is done by laparoscopy or laparotomy. Details of therapy either medial or surgical or a combination of both depend on the extent and spread of the disease (staging) and her primary objective of therapy.

Determination of Therapeutic Options

- Age of the patient
- Size and extent of lesions
- Severity of symptoms
- Location of disease
- Desire for fertility
- Results of previous therapy
- **Expectant management** cases with minimial endometriosis may be followed up under observation only.
- **Medical management** is considered for woman with **pelvic pain** that may be mild, moderate or severe or due to other symptoms of **infertility**. Women with moderate-to-severe pain with or without infertility need confirmation

of diagnosis with laparoscopy. Women with infertility with probable or presumed clinical diagnosis of endometriosis should get the benefit of laparoscopy.

Commonly used Drugs

- Nonsteroidal anti-inflammatory drugs (NSAIDs) are widely used to relieve the endometriosis related pelvic pain.
- Both COX-1 and COX-2 enzymes promote synthesis of prostaglandins. NSAIDs commonly used are: Ibuprofen, naproxen mefenamic acid and ketoprofen. All these inhibit both COX-1 and COX-2 enzymes and the pain and inflammation associated with endometriosis.

The common adverse effects associated with the use of NSAIDs are inhibition of ovulation, gastric irritation, ulceration, and cardiovascular disease.

Hormonal Therapies

- **Combined Oral Contraceptives (COCs)** work by inhibiting the release of gonadotropins and suppress the cyclic increase in hormones. COCs decrease the menstrual flow at the same time causes decidualization of ectopic endometrial implants. They also work as contraceptive having other noncontraceptive benefits. COCs may be used cyclically or continuously without a break, with a phase of amenorrhea. COCs were found to be as effective as GnRH analogs for relief of dysmonorrhea and the chronic pelvic pain (CPP). Emperical use of COCs for the relief of pain in cases with clinical presumed diagnosis of endometriosis is recommended.
- **Progestins:** They are widely used in the management of endometriosis. Progestins cause decidualization of the ectopic endometrium by antagonizing estrogen. Latter on, it causes atrophic changes. The common preparations of progestins used to treat endometriosis are—oral progestin pills, e.g., medroxyprogesterone acetate, dydrogesterone, norethisterone including LNG-IUS, depot medroxy porogesterone acetate (DMPH), norethisterone acetate (NETA) and also levonorgestrel-releasing intrauterine system (LNG-IUS). Subcutaneous form of DMPA, depo-subQ provera 104, are also used and found to be effective. Prolonged DMPA use may cause loss of bone mineral density. However, it is reversible.
- **Dienogest** is 19-nortestosterone, a synthetic progesterone. It is used for the control endometriosis associated pain. Its effectiveness is equivalent to half of GnRH agonists. Currently, it is used in a dose 2 mg/day for the relief of endometriosis-related pain.
- **LNG-IUS** is effective in the improvement of endometriosis-related pain. However, it is ineffective in cases with bowel-related endometriosis. Use of progestin containing implant (etonogestrel) and LNG-IUS have shown comparable efficacy in terms of pain relief.

Progesterone-only pill has also been observed to be effective as it causes anovulation and amenorrhea.

GnRH Agonists

Commonly used GnRH agonists are leuprolide acetate (3.75 mg IM monthly), goserelin (3.6 mg SC monthly), triptorelin (3.75 mg IM monthly) and nafarelin (200 mg twice daily nasal spray). Gn-RH agonists results in medical hypophysectomy as it causes profound downregulation of the anterior pituitary after 1–3 weeks. Initially there is an upregulation (flare effect). There is pituitary desensitization and suppression of ovarian sterioidogenesis. This hypoestrogenic condition suppresses the endometriotic implants and creates a pseudomenopausal state throughout the course of treatment. Emperical therapy with GnRH agonists may be used with the presumed clinical diagnosis of endometriosis, in women with chronic pelvic pain (CPP). GnRH agonists improve pain satisfactorily in cases with laparoscopically confirmed endometriosis.

Side effects: GnRH agonists are relatively safe and have got less side effects when used for a limited period of 6 months or less. The hypoestrogenic symptoms are at times severe. The symptoms include—hot flush, insomnia, irritability mood swings, decreased libido, vaginal dryness and headaches. The major problem is decrease in bone mineral density (spine and hip bones). It should not be given to young girl <16 years of age because of its long-term effects on bone mineral density.

Add-back therapy: Estrogen is added to GnRH agonist therapy to counteract the side effects of hypoestrogenic state and bone loss. However, the replacement therapy is used to minimize the side-effects while still maintaining a hypoestrogenic state, sufficient to suppress the growth of endometrosis. The optimum level of estrogen is thought to be 30–40 pg/mL of estradiol. The commonly used regimens are low dose combined estrogen (conjugated equine estrogen 0.625 mg) and progesterone (MPA 2.5 mg) daily. Alternative regimen of transdermal estradiol 25 µg plus daily 5 mg of MPA orally. Traditional COCs may be used effectively also.

GnRH antagonists: It may be used as it suppresses the gonadotropin release. GnRH antagonists do not produce an initial flare of gonadotropin release. Its suppression effect is immediate. Cetrorelix 3 mg SC weekly for 8 weeks is found to be equally effective to GnRH agonists. Elagolix, a new nonapeptide, GnRH antagonists has been found with similar efficacy with DMPA.

Aromatase inhibitors (AI): AI block aromatase action and production of estradiol in both the ovaries, extraovarian sites including the ectopic sites of endometrial implants. Estradiol is produced locally in the ectopic endometriosis implant sites from the circulating androgens. As the AI creates an hypoestrogenic state, the growth of ectopic endometrium is arrested. Commonly used AI are—anastrozole and letrozole.

Side effects of AI are due to hypoestrogenic state and are similar to GnRH agonists. Ovarian cysts formation is a common side effect due to evaluated levels of LH. To minimize the side effects of AI may be combined with a progestin or CoCs.

Selective Progesterone Receptor Modulators (SPRMs)

Progesterone antagonists and SPRMs act binding on the receptor. Mifepristone (RU-486) is a commonly used progesterone antagonist. Mifepristone reduces endometriosis associated pain and growth of endometriosis.

Side effects: Endometrial hyperplasia—It is known as progesterone receptor modulator associated endometrial changes (PAEC). Ulipristal acetate has been used in endometriosis. Long-term endometrial safety for both eutopic and ectopic endometrial is still awaited.

Androgens: Danazol is an isoxazole derivative of 17α-ethynyl-estradiol testosterone. It is strictly antigonadotropin but acts as an androgen agonist. It causes anovulation. It reduces liver synthesis of SHBG; therefore, levels of free testosterone is increased. It creates a hypoestrogenic and hyperandrogenic state that induces endometrial atrophic changes. This increased levels of testosterone causes both eutopic and ectopic endometrial atrophy. Danazole is given orally at doses 200 mg three times a day. Higher doses may cause significant androgenic side effects. The common androgenic side effects are many (*See* Dutta's Textbook of Gynecology, 8th Edition, p. 451). Due to adverse effect, it is either not commonly used these days or used for a short duration.

Gestrinone: It has got antiprogestional antiestrogenic and androgonic effects. It reduces endometriosis related pain similar to that of danazol and GnRH agonist.

Gestrinone dose: It is used orally 3–10 mg weekly in divided doses.

Side effects: It lowers the level of HDL.

SURGICAL MANAGEMENT OF PAIN RELIEF IN CASES WITH ENDOMETRIOSIS

A. Commonly used surgical method is laparoscopy.
Laparoscopy is the primary method of diagnosis and treatments (*see-and-treat*). Laparoscopic surgery using laser is more precise and causes less damage to tissues.

Indications of laparoscopy	Advantages of MIS
■ To make a definitive diagnosis	■ Superior view of pelvic viscera
■ As a part of investigation for fertility	■ Less postoperative pain
■ Symptoms suggestive of moderate-to-severe endometriosis	■ Short-hospital stay
■ Ovarian endometriosis	■ Quick recovery
■ DIE with several symptoms	■ Less analgesia
	■ Better cosmesis

B. Surgical procedures for endometriosis are:

Surgical procedures with laparoscopy	
■ Excision	■ Ovarian cystectomy
■ Electrofulguration	■ Resection of rectovaginal nodules
■ Laser ablation of implants	
■ Drainage of endometriosis	■ Adhesiolysis

Objectives of Surgery

A. Remove all the visible endometriotic lesions

B. Restore the normal pelvic anatomy
The place of laparoscopic uterosacral nerve ablation (LUNA) has not been found to have any benefit.
Presacral neurectomy (PSN) combined with removal of endometrial tissue significantly improved the pain of endometriosis (dysmenorrhea, and other midline pain). Surgery for presacral neurectomy needs a high degree of skill as the adverse effects are more.

C. Endometrioma resection
Ovarian endometrioma is best treated laparoscopically by ovarian cystectomy compared to cyst aspiration and cyst wall ablation. Ovarian endometrioma excision reduces the ovarian reserve. The surgery increases the risk of adhesion formation. Both decreases future fertility.

SURGERY FOR DIE

DIE in the uterosacral ligaments, rectovaginal septum, bowel, bladder, ureters, pelvic side walls, are difficult to treat.

- **Medical management of DIE** with colorectal symptoms may prevent the progression of the disease. Often these need surgical treatment. These may need superficial shaving, segmental resection. However, the complication rates are high (13%). The recurrences following resection are not uncommon (5–25%). Ureteric involvement need to be treated surgically depending upon the severity of the disease. Surgery may be done (a) ureterolysis (stenting the ureters), (b) segmental resection and reanastomosis and (c) ureteric reimplantation into the bladder (ureteroneocystostomy).

- **Hysterectomy for endometriosis:** Hysterectomy with bilateral salpingo-oophorectomy is generally done for women with moderate-to-severe endometriosis with debilitating symptoms and those who have completed their families. This may be an indication for a woman with failed medical therapy. Conservation of ovaries during hysterectomy may cause higher risk (6.1 times) of persistence of pain and higher (8.1 times) risk of reoperation. Postoperative hormone replacement therapy needs combined estrogen and progesterone or tibolone (ESHRE). Ovarian conservation may be considered when the ovaries appear normal (ACOG-2014b).

- **Other measures for treatment of pain:** Acupuncture and Chinese herbal medicine for endometriosis have been tried but it needs further studies to establish.

- **Pain support groups and self-management:** Some women with endometriosis may be benefitted with counseling with a psychologist. Breaking the pain cycle and overcoming the stress and anxiety may be helpful.

CONCLUSION

The clinical presentation of endometriosis is highly variable and does not correlate with the stage of the disease. Emperical therapy with hormones may be tried initially. Features of presumed endometriosis or with DIE should be confirmed by laparoscopic procedure where ***see-and-treat*** could be done. Medical treatment is effective for a large number of women with symptoms of pain. Surgical treatment often improves fertility. Women with debilitating symptoms due to moderate-to-severe endometriosis may have benefit of surgery. Laparoscopic surgery is preferred compared to laparotomy.

Suggested Reading

1. Allen C, Hopewell S, Prentice A, Gregory D. Nonsteroidal anti-inflammatory drugs for pain in women with endometriosis. Cochrane Database Syst Rev. 2009;(2):CD004753.
2. Brown J, Pan A, Hart RJ. Gonadotrophin-releasing hormone analogues for pain associated with endometriosis. Cochrane Database Syst Rev. 2010;(12):CD008475.
3. Busacca M, Riparini J, Somigliana E, Oggioni G, Izzo S, Vignali M, et al. Postsurgical ovarian failure after laparoscopic excision of bilateral endometriomas. Am J Obstet Gynecol. 2006;195:421–5.
4. Dunselman GA, Vermeulen N, Becker C, Calhaz-Jorge C, D'Hooghe T, De Bie B, et al. ESHRE guideline: management of women with endometriosis. Hum Reprod. 2014;29:400–12.
5. Ferreira RA, Vieira CS, Rosa ESJC, Rosa-e-Silva AC, Nogueira AA, Ferriani RA. Effects of the levonorgestrel-releasing intrauterine system on cardiovascular risk markers in patients with endometriosis: A comparative study with the GnRH analogue. Contraception. 2010;81:117–22.
6. Flower A, Liu JP, Lewith G, Little P, Li Q. Chinese herbal medicine for endometriosis. Cochrane Database Syst Rev. 2012;(4):CD006568.
7. Harada T, Momoeda M, Taketani Y, Hoshiai H, Terakawa N. Low-dose oral contraceptive pill for dysmenorrhea associated with endometriosis: A placebo-controlled, double-blind, randomized trial. Fertil Steril. 2008;90:1583–8.
8. Hart RJ, Hickey M, Maouris P, Buckett W. Excisional surgery versus ablative surgery for ovarian endometriomata. Cochrane Database Syst Rev. 2008;(2):CD004992.
9. Healey M, Ang WC, Cheng C. Surgical treatment of endometriosis: A prospective randomized double-blinded trial comparing excision and ablation. Fertil Steril. 2010;94:2536–40.
10. Royal College of Obstetricians and Gynaecologists. The Investigation and Management of Endometriosis. Green-top Guideline No. 24. London: RCOG; 2006.

Chapter 12: Adenomyosis Uterus

Adenomyosis uteri are defined as the presence and proliferation of endometrium in the myometrium. Histologically, uterine adenomyosis is characterized by presence of non-neoplastic endometrial glands and stroma within the myometrial fibers which are hypertrophic and hyperplastic.

In the uterus, there is no submucosa between the layers of myometrium and endometrium. As a result, endometrial glands and stroma lie in direct contact of the myometrium. When the endometrial glands extend > 2.5 mm below the endometrial-myometrial interface, it is considered as adenomyosis of the uterus.

Adenomyosis uteri can involve the whole muscle thickness of the uterus extending up to the level of serosa. Adenomyosis uteri could be either focal or diffuse. In the diffuse variety of the adenomyosis, the uterus becomes diffusely enlarged. It appears more globular. On cut section of the uterus, focal areas are seen. These are due to deposition of brown hemosiderin pigment. These focal lesions may often resemble leiomyomas. As opposed to leiomyomas, adenomyosis has got no capsule. It cannot be enucleated.

The endometrial glands are in the basal layer of the endometrium predominantly. The endometrial glands and stroma of adenomyotic uteri show limited changes unlike that of the normally located endometrium.

Hyperplasia and the hypertrophy of the myometrial fibers are thought to be due to the local hyperestrogenic state. Hyperprolactinemia (drug-induced) has also been considered in the pathogenesis of adenomyosis. Endometrial glands and the stroma invade the endometrial-myometrial interface during the periods of endometrial regeneration or following menstruation or trauma (D/C). However, other etiological factors in the pathogenesis are—genetic and immunological.

Other Lesions Associated with Adenomyosis Uteri

a. Leiomyoma (common)
b. Pelvic endometriosis
c. Endometrial hyperplasia
d. Atypical endometrial hyperplasia and endometrial carcinoma

Exact prevalence of the disease is unknown. Based on MRI criteria, overall incidence was 11%.

Clinical Features and Diagnosis of Adenomyosis

- Adenomyosis is commonly seen in elderly (> 40 years) and parous women.
- Disruption of endometrial-myometrial interface is thought to be cause of adenomyosis.
- Associated with spontaneous abortion
- Sharp endometrial curettage often associated with invasion of endometrium within the deep myometrium.

Risks factors for adenomyosis	
■ Increased age	■ Preterm birth
■ Increased parity	■ Infertility
■ Medical termination of pregnancy	■ Endometriosis
■ Endometrial curettage postabortal/postpartum	■ Menorrhagia

Clinical Features of Adenomyosis

- **Infertility**: Due to abnormal uterine peristalsis and/or hyperperistalsis. This impairs sperm transport, fertilization and implantation.
- Other factors for infertility are—anovulation, endometrial hyperplasia
- Miscarriage
- Menorrhagia (40–50%)
- Dysmenorrhea (10–30%)
- Metrorrhagia (10–20%)
- Dyspareunia

Ultrasonographic (TVS) diagnostic criteria of adenomyosis	
■ Enlargement of the uterus—diffuse myohyperplasia	■ Myometrium heterogeneity
■ Asymmetric enlargement—either of the anterior or the posterior wall	■ Hyperechoic nodular areas
■ Absence of capsule or fibroids	■ Cystic spaces within the myometrium

MRI diagnostic criteria of adenomyosis
■ Focal or diffuse thickening of the junctional zone (JZ) ■ Thickness of JZ ≥ 12 mm ■ Poor identification of JZ border ■ Areas of high signal intensity (ectopic endometrium) foci within an area of low-signal intensity (smooth muscle hyperplasia) could be seen ■ MRI is superior to TVS in the diagnosis of adenomyosis and to differentiate it from other conditions such as leiomyomas, endometrial polyps and other pathologies

Medical Management of Adenomyosis

- **Medical management** has been tried for symptomatic reliefs using mefenamic acid, tranexamic acid for control of menorrhagia and pain associated with adenomyosis.
- **Hormonal treatment** has been tried using: Progestins, combined oral contraceptive pill (COCs), and GnRH analogs. The relief of symptoms often remains unpredictable and usually limited to the duration of treatment.
- **Danazole-containing IUCD** has been used with improved control of dysmenorrhea. Pregnancies have been reported following discontinuation of the treatment. Serum levels of danazol were undetectable.
- **LNG-IUS** have been found to be effective in the control of menorrhagia (>90%) and improvement of anemia. The other beneficial effects were reduction in uterine size and improvement of dysmenorrhea.
- **Mifepristone** (RU-486) has been used for the treatment of endometriosis.
- **Aromatase inhibitor** (anastrozole) has been tried but with limited benefits.

Surgical Management of Adenomyosis

A laparoscopic myometrial electrocoagulation (monopolar or bipolar) has been tried at different sites to induce coagulation of endometriotic foci. It is difficult, at the same time, less precise method. It may be used for women > 40 years of age who have completed their families and who wish to avoid hysterectomy.

Complications: Uncontrolled bleeding, adhesion formation, may need emergency hysterectomy.

Adenomyomectomy

Localized excision of myometrium with areas of endometriotic foci can be done with prior assessment of exact location. This may be an option for women intending to preserve their fertility.

Complications: Obstetric complications of adenomyomectomy are—reduced expansive capacity of the uterus, reduced bulk of myometrium and uterine rupture.

Uterine artery embolization has been done for the relief of symptoms and to improve the quality of life.

Uterine artery ligation using laparoscopic method has been tried and found to be effective with better symptomatic improvement.

Endometrial resection or ablation is an alternative for women with symptoms of menorrhagia. Women desiring pregnancy or women with deep-seated adenomyosis should be excluded from this method.

Hysterectomy is the only method of treatment for women not intending to have a baby.

Suggested Reading

1. Hauth EA, Jaeger HJ, Libera H, Lange S, Forsting M. MR imaging of the uterus and cervix in healthy women: determination of normal values. Eur Radiol. 2007;17:734–42.
2. Kunz G, Beil D, Huppert P, Noe M, Kissler S, Leyendecker G. Adenomyosis in endometriosis—prevalence and impact on fertility. Evidence from magnetic resonance imaging. Hum Reprod. 2005;20:2309–16.
3. Siskin GP, Tublin ME, Stainken BF, Dowling K, Dolen EG. Uterine artery embolization for the treatment of adenomyosis: clinical response and evaluation with MR imaging. Am J Roentgenol. 2001;177:297–302.
4. Wang CJ, Yen CF, Lee CL, Soong YK. Laparoscopic uterine artery ligation for treatment of symptomatic adenomyosis. J Am Assoc Gynecol Laparosc. 2002;9:293–6.

Chapter 13: High Intensity Focused Ultrasound in the Management of Leiomyomas and Adenomyosis

Currently, the management protocol using magnetic resonance imaging-guided (MRg)/ultrasound-guided (USg) high intensity focused ultrasound (HIFU) for women with symptomatic fibroids and adenomyosis is considered to be superior to many other noninvasive or invasive procedures.

Since the establishment (July 2013) of International Society for Minimally Invasive and Noninvasive Medicine (ISMINIM), more than 13 countries in the world are making continued progress in the field of noninvasive treatment. Earlier study reports raised the concern as regard to the effect of HIFU on ovarian reserve. Principally the technique focuses ultrasound energy to the target tissue necrosis during the treatment period. The procedure is done with conscious sedation. Ablation of an average size myoma takes around 60–90 minutes. Once the HIFU treatment is conducted with precise imaging guidance only the leiomyoma is ablated without affecting the smooth muscles of the uterus. After treatment, the fibroid is absorbed. The normal uterine shape and the cavity is restored gradually. It is stated that the myometrium maintains uterine wall integrity and tension during pregnancy and labor.

Moreover, there is no adverse effect on the functions of ovary and endometrium. With this mechanism there is no extra risk for the patient to conceive soon after the HIFU treatment. Besides this has got many other advantages like it is a noninvasive method with rapid necessary time and quick return to daily activities and it preserves the uterus. However, some patients may need repeat treatment or some other alternative method of treatment as the symptoms may remain either uncontrolled or poorly controlled.

As with any method of treatment, not all women with fibroids or adenomyosis could be benefitted with this treatment.

Common contraindications for MRg/USg HIFU
- Abdominal wall scars
- Uterine size >24 weeks and woman desiring future pregnancy
- Any contraindications to MRI itself is an independent factor
- Leiomyoma that is much vascular responds poorly to this treatment

Long-term data regarding the duration of symptomatic relief following treatment are awaited. Initial study reports suggest that MRg/USg HIFU is safe and effective. It can be used as an alternative to hysterectomy for women not responding to medical therapy.

Treatment with HIFU focuses with symptomatic fibroid and adenomyosis has been approved by FDA (2008).

Concerns were expressed as regard to the effect of HIFU on ovarian reserve when evaluated with the levels of serum anti-Mullerian hormone (AMH) before and after the treatment.

Serum AMH levels are found to correlate strongly with the number of antral follicles in the ovary. With this observation, the levels of AMH is taken as an indicator of ovarian reserve. Levels of AMH as a biomarker for ovarian reserve were evaluated following treatment with HIFU. The main interest in measuring AMH before any assisted reproductive cycle (ART) is to assess: (a) ovarian follicular pool reserve, (b) ovarian responsiveness and (c) prediction of any excess ovarian response to ovarian hyperstimulation syndrome (OHSS).

More published reports are now available to evaluate the changes in AMH levels after HIFU treatment in cases with symptomatic fibroid or adenomyosis (Lee JS et al.).

Overall used median treatment time 140.5 minutes, median ablation (sonication) time 24 minutes, median energy delivered was 400 W. This was correlated with serum AMH levels before and 6 months after HIFU. There was no significant difference in AMH levels between two time points ($p > 0.05$). Neither any woman becomes amenorrhoeic nor anyone presented with symptoms of menopause. The study concluded, HIFU is a safe and effective treatment of a woman with symptomatic fibroids and adenomyosis and this does not affect ovarian function or reserve.

Subsequent studies (Lee et al.) concluded HIFU treatment for woman with symptomatic fibroid or adenomyosis was effective and did not affect the ovarian reserve. It is observed that initial studies included women with age < 40 years hence the result was affected adversely. The clinical use of HIFU as the noninvasive treatment of symptomatic fibroids and adenomyosis is considered a priority in many countries.

Uterine fibroids may be the cause of subfertility in about 10–15% of women.

Important factors for infertility due to fibroids

- Anatomical distortion of uterus along with uterine cavity
- Association of anovulation due to high estrogen levels
- Myometrial contractions which is dysrrhythmic
- Poor receptivity of the endometrium
- Failure of implantation
- Increased miscarriage
- Blockage of the cervical canal or uterine ostium (fallopian tube) by the fibroid

Features of high intensity focused ultrasound (HIFU) in the management of uterine fibroids and adenomyosis

- Selective ablation of myoma is done.
- It does not affect the normal smooth muscle fibers of uterus.
- Myometrial tissue texture and tension are maintained. No adverse effects during the course of subsequent pregnancy.
- Reduction on volume of fibroid up to 60% is obtained by 6 months follow-up period.
- The waiting period for pregnancy following HIFU is significantly less compared to myomectomy (1 year).
- Myoma shrinks gradually (60%) by 3–6 months time. There is anatomical restoration of uterine shape, size and endometrial cavity. With reduction of paracrine action, there is improvement of high levels of estrogenic environment.
- There is no adhesion formation as opposed to myomectomy.
- There is no reduction in blood flow to the ovaries and endometrium as in UAE.
- Miscarriage rate is low.

Limitations of other alternative methods compared to HIFU

Limitations of myomectomy	Limitations of UAE
a. Increased operative blood loss	a. Reduces blood supply to myoma and the myometrium to reduce size
b. Complications of surgery—infections, adhesions that mainly reduces pregnancy rate	b. Reduce blood supply to ovaries and endometrium to cause infertility
c. Risk of uterine rupture (0.5–1.2%) during 3rd trimester or during labor	c. Increased miscarriage rate
d. Long-waiting period for conception (1 year) following surgery	d. Abnormal placentation
e. HIFU treatment for symptomatic fibroids and adenomyosis is approved by FDA (2008)	e. ACOG does not recommend UAE for women desiring pregnancy

HIFU is a safe and noninvasive procedure for the treatment of symptomatic uterine fibroids which are not responding to medical therapy. It reduces the volume of the fibroid by 60% or more.

Several studies have shown that serum AMH levels were temporarily reduced after myomectomy, and it returned to the previous levels within a short period of time. Most of the studies suggest that HIFU ablation is an effective mode of therapy for uterine fibroids and it does not affect the ovarian reserve.

Report of pregnancy following treatment with HIFU has been currently observed and found to be encouraging. Eighty pregnancies have been reported in 78 patients following treatment with HIFU.

However, it is essential that pregnancy and labor management must be done with intensive monitoring till sufficient data are available with satisfactory outcome measures.

Suggested Reading

1. Keltz J, Levie M, Chudnoff S. Pregnancy outcomes following direct uterine fibroid thermal ablation: A review of the literature. J Minim Invasive Gynecol. 2017;24:538–45.
2. Lee JS, Hong GY, Lee KH, Kim TE. Changes in anti-mullerian hormone levels as a biomarker for ovarian reserve after ultrasound guided high-intensity focused ultrasound treatment of adenomyosis and uterine fibroid. BJOG. 2017;124(S3):18–22.
3. Lee JS, Hong GY, Park BJ, Kim TE. Ultrasound-guided high-intensity focused ultrasound treatment for uterine fibroid adenomyosis: A single center experience from the Republic of Korea. Ultrason Sonochem. 2015;27:682–7.
4. Zou M, Chen L, Wu C, Hu C, Xiong Y. Pregnancy outcomes in patients with uterine fibroids treated with ultrasound-guided highintensity focused ultrasound. BJOG. 2017;124(S3):30–5.
5. Wang W, Wang Y, Tang J. Safety and efficacy of high intensity focused ultrasound ablation therapy for adenomyosis. Acad Radiol. 2009;16:1416–23.
6. Wang W, Wang Y, Wang T, Wang J, Wang L, Tang J. Safety and efficacy of US-guided high-intensity focused ultrasound for treatment of submucosal fibroids. Eur Radiol. 2012;22:2553–8.
7. Zhang X, Li K, Xie B, He M, He J, Zhang L. Effective ablation therapy of adenomyosis with ultrasound-guided high-intensity focused ultrasound. Int J Gynaecol Obstet. 2014;124:207–11.

Chapter 14: Menopause and the Management Issues

INTRODUCTION

Menopause is the permanent cessation of the menstruation due to loss of ovarian follicular activity. As such a woman is declared to have attained menopause only retrospectively. There are significant changes in the reproductive endocrinolgy during the menopause transition and menopause. Menopausal symptoms are many. At times, symptoms are so severe to cause incapacitation of the day-to-day work. Many modes of therapy are available for the management of menopause. Hormone therapy (HT) is indicated to overcome the short-term and the long-term consequences of estrogen deficiency (Table 14.1).

TABLE 14.1: Women's health condition and selection of the type of HT and mode of therapy.

Women's condition	Hormone therapy
Postmenopaual women (intact uterus)	Continuous estrogen/cyclical progestogen
Hysterectomized women	Estrogen only
Perimenopausal women (intact uterus)	Mirena (± systemic estrogen)
Early (premature) menopause	Low-dose estrogen to start, needs dose adjustment
Women potential malabsorption	Non-oral route
Postmenopausal women, low libido	Tibolone
Non-responders to standard treatment	Subcutaneous implants of estrogen (E2)
Young women with surgical menopause	Subcutaneous implants of estrogen (E2)

AVAILABLE PREPARATIONS AND ROUTES OF ESTROGEN THERAPY

- **Oral**: Estradiol can be delivered orally (micronized estradiol, estradiol valerate, estrone, estriol or conjugated equine estrogen).
- **Transdermal** (17-β-estradiol) to bypass the first pass hepatic metabolism. Risks are less compared to oral route.
- **Subdermal implants:** Inserted subcutaneously in the anterior abdominal wall using local anesthesia.
- 17-β-estradiol implants are commonly used in doses of 25 mg or 50 mg for a period of 6 months.
- **Topical vaginal administration** of estrogen is used for localized symptoms. It is used in the form of a cream or gel.
- **Progestogens** are mostly administered orally. Various progestogens are used in combination with estradiol, either in a sequential cyclical regimen or as continuous combined therapy.
- **The levonorgestrel-releasing intrauterine system (Mirena)** is used either alone or with oral estrogen.
- **Tibolone** (19-nortestosterone derivative) is an oral synthetic steroid with estrogenic, androgenic and progestogenic actions. This may be used as hormone replacement therapy (HRT) in postmenopausal women.

Vasomotor symptoms (hot flushes, night sweat and sleep disturbances) are common. These may affect about 80% of women. This usually subsides by 2–3 years. However, in some women (10%), this may continue for few years. Menopausal symptoms adversely affect quality of life. HRT is the most effective treatment (Table 14.2). Presently, the risk–benefit ratio for the use of HRT has been much debated.

TABLE 14.2: Benefits of estrogen therapy.

- Improves vasomotor symptoms (80%)
- Improves urogenital atrophy
- Increases bone mineral density (2–5%)
- Decreases the risk of vertebral and hip fractures (25–50%)
- Reduces atherosclerosis due to its antioxidant property
- Increases HDL-cholesterol
- Decreases LDL-cholesterol and total cholesterol
- Promotes coronary artery vasodilatation with release of nitric oxide (NO)
- Prevents platelet aggregation (thrombus formation)
- Reduction in colorectal cancers (20%)
- Decreases lipoprotein-A and inhibits LDL-cholesterol oxidation

(HDL: high-density lipoprotein; LDL: low-density lipoprotein)

Studies: The important studies in this respect are mentioned below.

The Heart and Estrogen/Progestin Replacement Study (HERS)

The first study was the Heart and Estrogen/Progestin Replacement Study (HERS) designed to identify if HRT prevented recurrence of coronary heart disease (CHD) in women with established CHD.

Postmenopausal women (with an average age of 66.7 years) were randomized to conjugated equine estrogens (CEE)/medroxyprogesterone acetate. Therapy did not show benefit.

The treatment did increase the risk of venous thromboembolism (VTE) (more pronounced in the first year) and gallbladder disease. The oral route of delivery, the dose given and the type of HRT could, together have promoted the thrombotic effect seen in these older women.

A follow-up study of this cohort, the HERS II in 2002 concluded that this benefit did not persist and stated that HRT should not be used for secondary prevention in women with established heart disease.

The Women's Health Initiative Study

It was an RCT planned to evaluate the effect of HRT on healthy postmenopausal women with special interest to cardiovascular outcome. The women belonged to the age range of 50–79 years. Women with hysterectomy were randomized to CEE only or placebo. The women with intact uterus were randomized to CEE and medroxyprogesterone or placebo.

In 2003, the study was closed. Increase in breast cancer, heart disease, stroke, and VTE, were reported. While a reduction in fracture rate, bowel cancer, and diabetes was the advantage observed. These adverse effects were not observed in the CEE arm.

The Million Women Study

Women aged 50–60 years in the UK attending the NHS breast screening program were invited and subsequently followed by completion of a questionnaire. A significant increased risk of breast cancer was seen in the women on combine HRT (estrogen and progestogens) and less so with estrogen-only and tibolone.

It was concluded that this study did not establish causality and that the size (one million women) alone does not guarantee that the findings are reliable.

Summary of these Studies

The above studies, while extensive, were for the most part focused on cardiovascular risk and failed to accurately assess the effect of HRT in the symptomatic younger postmenopausal women. They have not, therefore, addressed the benefits of HRT given at 'the window' of opportunity before aging has advanced and collagen has been lost.

The absolute increase in breast cancer risk is six extra cases per 1000 women for 5 years of estrogen and progestogens, and reverts back to the population risk 5 years after stopping.

Recommendations

- Counseling the woman with evidence on the use of hormone therapy.
- Special health conditions of the woman need to be considered.
- Indications of HRT are to be fulfilled.
- Contraindications of HRT are to be judged carefully.

TABLE 14.3: Main indications of HRT.
- Relief of vasomotor symptoms
- Relief of other menopausal symptoms
- Premature menopause
- Cases with ovarian failure
- Cases with surgical menopause
- Risk factors for osteoporosis
- To maintain the quality of life

TABLE 14.4: Important considerations for therapy.
- History of hysterectomy
- Selection of the type of hormone therapy
- Duration of therapy
- Monitoring the side effects
- Adjustment of the dose
- Consideration of change of therapy or stoppage of therapy
- Annual review to assess the risks and the benefits of therapy

Overall, a period of 3 years of therapy may be maintained

TABLE 14.5: Medical and other health conditions where HRT may be prescribed following assessment and with follow-up.
- Asthma
- Past history of benign breast disease
- Diabetes
- Controlled blood pressure
- Hyperlipidemia
- Multiple sclerosis
- Obesity
- Renal failure
- Sickle cell anemia
- Thyroid disease
- Osteoporosis prevention in young women
- Women with premature ovarian failure

TABLE 14.6: Contraindications to HRT.
- Estrogen-dependent neoplasm in the body
- Existing cardiac disease
- Active liver disease
- Known breast cancer
- Previous ovarian/endometrial cancer
- Undiagnosed genital tract bleeding
- History of venous thromboembolism or active DVT

The woman with intact uterus should be given combined estrogen and progesterone to get the benefits of hormone therapy.

TABLE 14.7: Indications of transdermal route therapy of HT.
- Personal preference
- Migraine
- Diabetes
- Controlled hypertension
- Existing gallbladder disease
- Hyperlipidemia
- Obesity
- Smoking
- Previous venous thromboembolism
- Varicose veins

Non-hormonal treatments for menopausal symptoms are there. SERMs (raloxifene), colinidine, gabapentin, increase in exercise, reducing coffee/alcohol intake are helpful.

CONCLUSION

Symptomatic women are benefitted with the use of HRT. Counseling the woman is important. Selection of the type of HT must be carefully made excluding the contraindications. Short-term therapy is recommended with the low dose so as to control the symptoms. Non-hormonal treatment options are to be discussed including the lifestyle modification.

Suggested Reading

1. Burger HG, MacLennan AH, Huang KE, Castelo-Branco C. Evidence-based assessment of the impact of the WHI on women's health. Climacteric. 2012;15:281–7.
2. Chlebowski RT, Hendrix SL, Langer RD, Stefanick ML, Gass M, Lane D, et al. WHI investigators. Influence of estrogen plus progestin on breast cancer and mammography in healthy postmenopausal women: the Women's Health Initiative Randomized Trial. JAMA. 2003;289:3243–53.
3. Crawford SL. The roles of biologic and nonbiologic factors in cultural differences in vasomotor symptoms measured by surveys. Menopause. 2007;14:725–33.
4. Gold EB, Bromberger J, Crawford S, Samuels S, Greendale GA, Harlow SD, et al. Factors associated with age at natural menopause in a multiethnic sample of midlife women. Am J Epidemiol. 2001;153:865–74.
5. Grady D, Herrington D, Bittner V, Blumenthal R, Davidson M, Hlathy M, et al. Cardiovascular disease outcome during 6.8 years of hormone therapy Heart and Estrogen/progestin Replacement Study follow-up (Hers II). JAMA. 2002;2888:49–57.
6. Hulley S, Grady D, Bush T, Furberg C, Herrington D, Riggs B, et al. Randomized trial of estrogen plus progestin for secondary prevention of coronary heart disease in postmenopausal women. Heart and Estrogen/progestin Replacement Study (HERS) Research Group. JAMA. 1998;280(7):605–13.
7. Million Women Study Collaborators. Breast Cancer and HRT in the Million Women Study. Lancet. 2003:362:419–27.
8. Panay N. Commentary Regarding Recent Million Women Study critique and subsequent publicity. Menopause Int. 2012;18:33–5.
9. Shapiro S, Farmer RD, Mueck AO, Seaman H, Stevenson JC. Does hormone replacement therapy cause breast cancer? An application of causal principles to three studies. Part 2. The Women's Health Initiative: estrogen plus progestogen. J Fam Plann Reprod Health Care. 2011;37:165–72.
10. Shapiro S, Farmer RD, Mueck AO, Seaman H, Stevenson JC. Does hormone replacement therapy cause breast cancer? An application of causal principle to three studies. Part 4. The Million Women Study: J Fam Plann Reprod Health Care. 2012;38:102–9.
11. Shapiro S, Farmer RD, Seaman H, Stevenson JC, Mueck AO. Does hormone replacement therapy cause breast cancer? An application of causal principles to three studies. Part 1. The Collaborative Reanalysis. J Fam Plann Reprod Health Care. 2011;37:103–9.
12. Shapiro S, Farmer RDT, Mueck AO, Seaman H, Stevenson JC. Does hormone replacement therapy cause breast cancer? An application of causal principle to three studies. Part 3. The Women's Health Initiative: unopposed estrogen. J Fam Plann Reprod Health Care. 2011;37:225–30.
13. West Midlands Menopause Society. HRT Guidance. [online] Available from: http://www.menopausesociety.co.uk/hrt_guidance.

15 Chapter — Abnormal Uterine Bleeding

Any menstrual flow outside of normal volume, duration, regularity or frequency is considered as abnormal uterine bleeding (AUB). Significant number of women (70%) in a gynecology clinic are seen due to AUB. In order to avoid the confusion of different terminology used, FIGO introduce this universally accepted nomenclature. The acronym 'PALM-COEIN' is used (see below) to described AUB. AUB in an individual may be due to one or more than one causes. The nomenclature used terms such as menorrhagia, metrorrhagia or polymenorrhea are often inconsistent and confusing. This also makes investigation and management approach difficult. To avoid these difficulties newer classification system has been introduced by FIGO and approved by ACOG.

CLASSIFICATION OF AUB (FIGO 2011): PALM-COEIN

Structural causes: PALM		Nonstructural causes: COEIN	
Polyp	AUB-**P**	**C**oagulopathy	AUB-**C**
Adenomyosis	AUB-**A**	**O**vulatory dysfunction	AUB-**O**
Leiomyoma (Fig. 15.1)	AUB-**L**	**E**ndometrial	AUB-**E**
Malignancy and hyperplasia	AUB-**M**	**I**atrogenic	AUB-**I**
		Not yet identified	AUB-**N**

Subclassification of Leiomyoma (AUB-L) (Figs. 15.1 and 15.2)

Submucosal (SM)	0	Pedunculated intracavitary
	1	< 50% intramural
	2	≥ 50% intramural
Others (O)	3	100% intramural; contacts endometrium
	4	Intramural
	5	Subserosal ≥ 50% intramural
	6	Subserosal < 50% intramural
	7	Subserosal pedunculated
	8	Others (cervical, parasitic)
Hybrid (both endometrium and serosa)	2–4	Two numbers are listed separated by a hyphen. The **first** number refers to the relationship with endometrium and the **second** refers to that of serosa. Example: 2–4 = submucosal (≥ 50% intramural) and intramural.

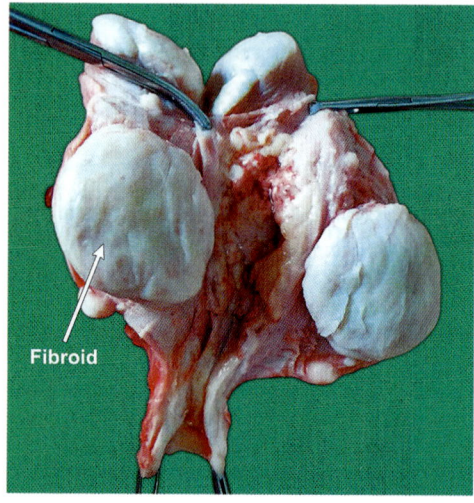

Fig. 15.1: AUB due to fibroid (leiomyoma) uterus (AUB-L).

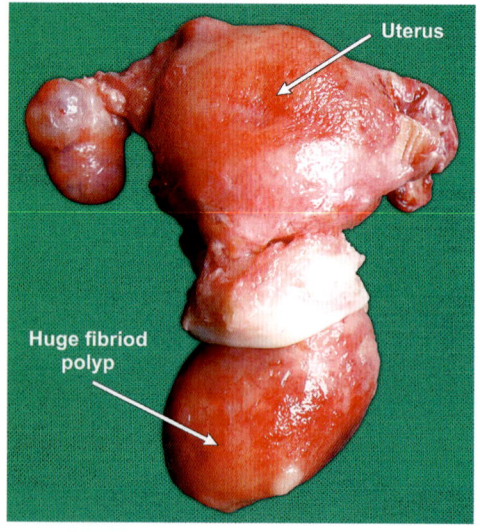

Fig. 15.2: AUB due to polyp (AUB-P).

Therefore, AUB includes a wide range of abnormalities (pelvic or systemic) that need to be investigated for diagnosis.

According to the new FIGO classification system of AUB, the 'PALM-COEIN' terminology used for expressing the pathology is as follows—AUB due to Polyp = AUB–**P** (Fig. 15.3).

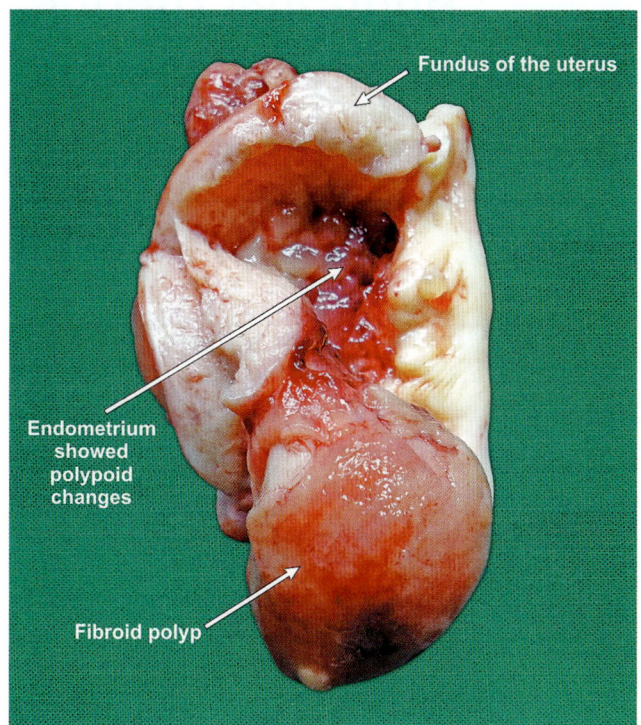

Fig. 15.3: Uterus is cut opened to show—a huge polyp protruding out of the cervical external os. Endometrium showed polypoid changes.

Similarly for the others: (1) AUB-*A* (adenomyosis), (2) AUB-*L* (leiomyoma), (3) AUB-*M* (malignancy and hyperplasia), (4) AUB-*C* (coagulopathy), (5) AUB-*O* (ovulatory dysfunction), (6) AUB-*E* (endometrial), (7) AUB-*I* (iatrogenic) and (8) AUB-*N* (not yet classified).

Women with AUB may have one or more factors that may be responsible for the bleeding. The investigations should be comprehensive depending upon the available resources. However, it should be kept in mind that a mere presence of any abnormality may not be the contributory factor for AUB. Presence of a small subserous fibroid may not be the cause for AUB.

Notation

All the cases of AUB are evaluated in terms of presence or absence of each criterion. It is expressed as '*O*' if the criterion is absent; '*I*' if present and '*N*' if not yet assessed.

Once the investigations have been completed and the causes have been evaluated, the categorization of pathology and notation is done in a fashion for simpler understanding. For example, if a woman with AUB was found to have leiomyoma (type-1) and endometrial hyperplasia and no other abnormalities, the pathology would be categorized and notified as AUB $P_0A_0L_{1(SM)}M_0 - C_0O_0E_1I_0N_0$.

This notation may also be done in a simple form of categorization—AUB $(L_{(SM)}E_1)$.

Example

$P_1 \quad A_0 \quad L_0 \quad M_0 - C_0 \quad O_0 \quad E_0 \quad I_0 \quad N_0$

In this case, endometrial polyp is the only cause of AUB and the rest are absent.

Diagnosis of Chronic AUB

It is made when a woman has suffered for a period of 3 months or more. In such a case, the following procedures are to be followed:
- **Structured history:** It is designed to determine: (a) Ovulatory function, (b) Fertility status, (c) Medical disorders, (d) Medications and (e) Thyroid function.
- **Physical examination:** Systemic and pelvic examination.
- **Investigations**
  - (i) Complete blood count (CBC), (ii) Hormone profile (thyroid function), (iii) Pap smear.
  - *Uterine evaluation*
    - Transvaginal sonography (TVS) → for any structural abnormality
    - Outpatient endometrial biopsy for women > 40 years age ⎤ To detect endometrial hyperplasia/atypia/carcinoma
    - Saline infusion sonography (SIS) is superior to TVS in detecting cavitary abnormalities ⎦
  - *Hysteroscopy and biopsy:* Hysteroscopy is highly accurate in diagnosing endometrial cancer
  - *Magnetic resonance imaging (MRI):* When needed (second-line test in cases like adenomyosis).

Differential Diagnosis of AUB (Age-based)

- **13–19 years**
  - *Anovulatory bleeding* due to dysregulation of hypothalamic-pituitary-ovarian axis.
  - *Coagulopathy* (laboratory tests needed are: CBC with platelets, PT and PTT).
  - *Irregular intake* of hormonal contraceptives (sexually active adolescents).
- **20–40 years**
  - Pregnancy complications
  - Uterine structural lesions (leiomyoma)
  - Anovulatory bleeding (PCOS)
  - Hormonal contraceptions
  - Endometrial hyperplasia.
- **41 years to menopause**
  - Anovulatory bleeding (declining ovarian function)
  - Cervical carcinoma (in developing countries)
  - Endometrial hyperplasia or carcinoma
  - Leiomyomas.
- **Management options:** Based on individual patient (*See* Ch 4, 16, 57).

Suggested Reading

1. Committee on Practice Bulletins—Gynecology. Practice Bulletin no. 128: Diagnosis of abnormal uterine bleeding in reproductive–aged women. Obstet Gynecol. 2012;120(1):197-206.
2. Munro MG, Critchley HO, Broder MS, et al. FIGO classification system (PALM-COEIN) for causes of abnormal uterine bleeding in nongravid women of reproductive age. Int J Gynecol Obstet. 2011;113(1):3-13.

Chapter 16: Abnormal Uterine Bleeding: Investigations and Management Issues

Q.1 What are the common causes of abnormal uterine bleeding (AUB)?

Ans. Neoplasm (fibroid, polyps, cancers), hormonal therapy, trauma, infection, coagulopathies and pregnancy complications (*See* Ch 15) are the common causes of AUB.

Q.2 What is the prevalence of AUB?

Ans. Overall prevalence in the women of reproductive age is 10–30%. It is as high as 50% in the premenopausal age group.

Q.3 How to assess the severity of AUB?

Ans. There are several methods in practice to assess the severity of uterine bleeding.
- Estimation of blood hemoglobin (usually <12 g/dL). However, a normal level does not rule out HMB
- Hematocrit level
- Estimation of hematin (spectrophotometrically) not commonly done
- Pictorial blood assessment chart (PBAC): By assessment of pads soaked—lightly, moderately or completely
- Measurement of clots (> 1 cm in diameter). Small clots are scored 1 and large clots scored 5 (Fig. 16.1).
- **Pad changing with time (frequency):** Pad changing more frequently than every 3 hours has got positive correlation for HMB.
- **Scoring system:** Scoring system has been introduced with scores 1, 5, 20 points—1 is for each lightly stained pad, 5 for moderately and 20 for completely soaked pad.
  ♦ Total score >100 points suggests menorrhagia.

Q.4 How saline infusion sonography (SIS) is correlated with transvaginal sonography (TVS)?

Ans. Saline infusion sonography is more helpful to detect the uterine intracavity pathology like polyps, submucous fibroid and blood clots. With these advantages SIS is found superior to TVS.

Q.5 What are the contraindications of SIS?

Ans.
- Pregnancy
- Pelvic inflammatory diseases
- Unexplained abdominal tenderness.

Fig. 16.1: Pictorial blood assessment chart (PBAC) and the scoring system. Total score is made joining each point. Score total more than 100 suggests menorrhagia.

Q.6 What are the disadvantages of SIS?

Ans. Performance of SIS is cycle dependent. Thickened endometrium in the second half of the cycle may cause difficulty in diagnosis. The risk of false-positive diagnosis is more. SIS is good for the detection of focal lesion. Difficulty is there when the lesion is diffuse. Moreover difficulties are faced in cases where there is cervical stenosis and in postmenopausal women.

Q.7 How do you correlate AUB with different clinical scenarios?

Ans. The different clinical situations manifested with AUB are:
- Obesity
- Polycystic ovary syndrome (PCOS)
- Thyroid dysfunction
- Infections (chlamydia)
- Coagulopathies [idiopathic thrombocytopenic purpura (ITP), thrombocytopenia, leukemia, Von Willebrand disease]
- Uterine arteriovenous malformation
- Cervical ectopy
- Cervical pathology
- Enlarged uterus:
  ♦ Fibroid
  ♦ Adenomyosis
- Endometrial carcinoma

- Uterine sarcoma
- Adnexal pathology
    - Tubo-ovarian mass
    - Fallopian tube cancer

Q.8 What are the causes of uterine arteriovenous (AV) malformations?

Ans. Exact cause is not well understood. Common observations are: trauma (difficult cesarean delivery), cancer [cancer cervix, endometrium or gestational trophoblastic neoplasia (GTN)] or congenital.

Q.9 How do the women with AV malformations present?

Ans. Women may present with irregular or intermittent bleeding. Bleeding may at times be heavy and life-threatening.

Q.10 How the diagnosis of AV malformations could be made?

Ans. *Exclusion* of other causes for AUB is essential: (a) TVS may show hypoechoic tubular structure, and with, (b) color Doppler study: reverse blood flow is observed. However (c) contrast-enhanced computed tomography (CECT), (d) magnetic resonance imaging (MRI) may be used when needed, (e) angiography is considered as the gold standard for the diagnosis.

Q.11 How AV malformation could be treated?

Ans.
- Hysterectomy may be considered for women who have completed their family.
- Uterine artery embolization is an option where facilities are available (*See* Ch 57).

Q.12 What is procedure of UAE?

Ans. *See* Ch 57.

Q.13 What are the contraindications of UAE?

Ans.
- Pregnancy
- Acute pelvic infection
- Endometrial hyperplasia
- Genital tract cancer
- Postmenopausal women
- Women desiring to presence fertility
- Intrauterine contraceptive device (IUCD) in place
- Larger or distorted endometrial cavity.

Q.14 What are the complications of UAE?

Ans.
- Nausea, vomiting
- Malaise, fever
- Infection
- Ovarian failure (rare).

Q.15 Outline your approach for management of a woman with AUB.

Ans. Details of history-taking and physical examination are done:
- Pregnancy is to be excluded [serum, beta-human chorionic gonadotropin (β-hCG), ultrasonography (USG)]
- *Hematological parameters:*
    - Complete blood count (CBC), platelets, thyroid-stimulating hormone (TSH), prolactin
    - Coagulation studies [partial thromboplastin time (PTT), prothrombin time (PT)]
- *Infections:* Chlamydia, others sexually transmitted infections (STIs)
- Cervical cytology (Pap smear)
- Ultrasonography (Flowchart 16.1).
- *Endometrial thickness on TVS*
    - Thickness 3.4 ± 1.2 mm mostly (postmenopausal atrophic endometrium)
    - Thickness 9.7 ± 2.5 mm (commonly endometrial hyperplasia)
    - Thickness 18.2 ± 6.2 mm (endometrial cancer).

Endometrial thickness > 4 mm requires additional evaluation with SIS, hysteroscopy, EB [American Congress of Obstetricians and Gynecologists (ACOG) 2009].

SIS is simple, minimally invasive sonographic procedure to evaluate endometrium, myometrium and the endometrial cavity.

Flowchart 16.1: Evaluation of uterine cavity, myometrium and endometrium through transvaginal sonography.

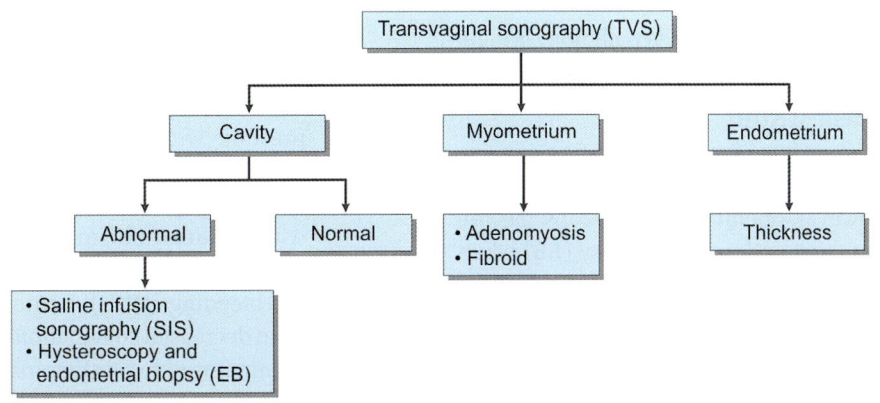

Q.16 What are the iatrogenic causes of AUB?
Ans.
- IUCD (CuT380 A)
- Mirena
- Combined oral contraceptive (COC) (breakthrough bleeding)
- Progestin-only pill (POP)
- Hormone replacement therapy (HRT) (discontinuation)
- Tamoxifen.

Q.17 How does IUCD cause AUB?
Ans. Initiation of subclinical inflammatory changes in the endometrium. There is release of prostaglandins, thromboxanes, and increase in local leukocyte population. All these results in increased endometrial vascularity, thrombosis and infarction.

Q.18 How tamoxifen is associated with AUB?
Ans. Tamoxifen is a selective estrogen receptor modulator. It is commonly used in the management of breast carcinoma following surgery. Tamoxifen is an estrogen receptor antagonist in the breast tissue as well as an agonist in the endometrium. Prolonged use results in endometrial hyperplasia and carcinoma. Women with tamoxifen therapy need to be screened for endometrial abnormalities.

Q.19 What are the advantages of USG in the management of AUB?
Ans. Ultrasonography is considered as the first-line tool in the management of AUB. USG either transabdominal sonography (TAS) or TVS can detect any anatomical abnormality located in the myometrium or endometrium or with other pathologies like fibroid uterus, adenomyosis or submucous polyps. However, limitations are: high false-negative rate due to focal uterine cavity pathology. In such a situation, hysteroscopy or SIS is performed.

Q.20 What are the limitations of pipelle endometrial sampling?
Ans.
- Collected sample may be inadequate.
- False-negative rate for detection of endometrial cancer is 0.91%.
- False-negative rate due to local pathology is high.

Q.21 How do you evaluate the place of TVS versus SIS in the management of AUB?
Ans. Both the procedure have similar diagnostic accuracy. But limitations for the both are due to lack of histological diagnosis. However, operative hysteroscopy has the advantage of taking endometrial biopsy (EB) when desired.

Q.22 What are the advantages of hysteroscopy?
Ans. Hysteroscopy (3–5 mm diameter) may be considered as a primary tool in the diagnosis of uterine polyps, submucous fibroid. Operative hysteroscopy may be helpful as biopsy could be done simultaneously when endometrial carcinoma is suspected.

Q.23 What are the limitations of hysteroscopy?
Ans. It is an invasive procedure and is expensive. Difficulties may be faced due to cervical stenosis and in postmenopausal women. Complications may occur due to uterine perforation, spread of infection in the peritoneal cavity or peritoneal spillage of cancer cells in a case with endometrial carcinoma.

Q.24 What are the different structural abnormalities?
Ans.
- Endometrial polyps
- Cervical ectopy
- Adenomyosis
- Infections—chlamydia, other STIs
- Leiomyoma
- Hypertrophic myometrium
- Arteriovenous malformation (fistulous communications).

Q.25 What are the different systemic diseases that may cause AUB?
Ans.
- Severe renal dysfunction
- Liver disease
- Thyroid dysfunctions
    - Hypothyroidism
    - Hyperthyroidism (5%)
- Coagulopathy.

Q.26 What are the underlying basic pathology of AUB where the woman suffers with such a systemic disease?
Ans.
A. *Renal dysfunction* is accompanied by endocrine disturbances. This causes hypoestrogenism and this ultimately leads to amenorrhea and infertility.
B. *Liver disease*: There is often association of hypothalamic-pituitary ovarian dysfunction as in a case with renal dysfunction. Liver dysfunction is associated with high level of serum estradiol. This causes low levels of serum follicle-stimulating hormone (FSH) and luteinizing hormone (LH). Hemostatic dysfunction have also been observed in such cases.
C. *Thyroid dysfunction*: Hyperthyroidism often presents with amenorrhea or hypomenorrhea and menorrhagia in about 5% of cases. Hypothyroidism presents with menorrhagia. Women with hypothyroidism suffers from anovulation, amenorrhea and anovulatory dysfunctional uterine bleeding (DUB). Some woman also suffers from decreased coagulation factors to cause AUB. Treatment of hyperthyroidism corrects the AUB abnormalities.

D. ***Coagulopathy:*** AUB in women with coagulopathy is due to:
- Deficient platelet number (thrombocytopenia)
- Dysfunction of platelets (thrombasthenia)
- Defects in platelet plug stabilization
- Deficient clotting factors (factors VIII, IX disorder)
- Disorder of Von Willebrand factor (VWF).

Q.27 What are the different options for operative management of AUB?

Ans. Selection of cases is important. The management options are:
- Dilatation and curettage: Intractable cases when medical management has failed (ACOG). Endometrium can be tested for histological diagnosis.
- Endometrial ablation or resection
  Indications are:
  - Women with failed medical treatment
  - Women not desirous to preserve menstrual or reproductive function
  - Women with normal uterine size (< 10 weeks pregnant size)
  - Fibroid uterus but fibroids < 3 cm in diameter
  - Where longer surgical time is to be avoided.
- Myomectomy (*See* Ch 4)
- Uterine artery embolization
- Hysterectomy.

Q.28 What is the overall success rate of endometrial ablation or resection?

Ans. Overall success rate is 70–80%. About 30–40% women become amenorrheic and another 50% get significant decrease in blood loss. But 10% women need repeat procedures or hysterectomy.

Q.29 How one should organize the investigations for the management of a case with AUB?

Ans. There is no such clear sequence of events. However, investigations should preferably be simple, less invasive with less discomfort and with much information. Considering all these TVS appears the logical first step. It can differentiate the pathologies that are focal, diffuse or located in the endometrial cavity, endometrium itself or in the myometrium.

Once anatomical localization is made, subsequent investigations are carried out as follows:
- Endometrial hyperplasia → EB (Pipelle)
- Focal lesion:
  - Hysteroscopy ⎫
  - SIS ⎭ → Biopsy

> Endometrial thickness: 3.4 ± 1.2 mm → Atropic endometrium (postmenopausal)
> 9.7 ± 2.5 mm → Hyperplasia
> 18.2 ± 6.2 mm → Endometrial cancer

Q.30 Describe the management options cases with hormonal abnormality (DUB)?

Ans.
- ***Acute bleeding:*** Premarin 25 mg IV 4 hourly 3 doses.
  → Then tablet 2.5 mg 6 hourly till bleeding stops.
- ***Chronic cases:*** Inhibitor of cyclooxygenase (COX-1 and COX-2).
  Reduces blood loss by 90%.
- ***Progestogens***
  - Medroxyprogesterone acetate
  - Norethisterone
- ***Levonorgestrel-intrauterine system (LNG-IUS)*** reduces blood loss by 70–90%.
- ***Danazol/gestrinone:*** 17α-isoxazole derivative of testosterone. Reduces serum estradiol levels and increases androgen levels. There is amenorrhea. It is the second-line drug of choice.
- ***Tranexamic acid:*** It is an antifibrinolytic agent. It is contraindicated in patients with risks of thrombosis.
- ***Ethamsylate:*** It is used as a hemostatic. It is not so effective.

Surgery

- Dilatation and curettage; cases with severe bleeding and refractory to medical management
- Uterine artery embolization in selective cases (*See* Clinics in Obstetrics, Ch 1, Case 12 and Ch 57 of this book)
- Endometrial ablation/resection
- Hysterectomy in a selected case.

Suggested Reading

1. Granberg S, Wikland M, Karlsson B, et al. Endometrial thickness as measured by endovaginal ultrasonography for identifying endometrial abnormality. Am J Obstet Gynecol. 1991;164(1 Pt 1): 47-52.

Chapter 17: Management of Adnexal Mass in Peri- and Post-menopausal Women

ADNEXAL MASS IN PERI- AND POST-MENOPAUSAL WOMEN

Case Summary

Mrs AR, 48-year-old (menopause transition) parous lady, was admitted with pelvic pain and heaviness. Clinical examination was unremarkable. Pelvic examination did not reveal any abnormality. USG (TVS) revealed a cyst in left adnexa measuring 7.5 cm × 8.0 cm. The cyst had homogenous internal echoes. The wall was thick. There was no nodularity, septations, no significant vascularity. Uterus was studded with multiple myomas. Serum CA-125 revealed 69 IU/mL, RMI <250. Considering the low-risk for malignancy, laparotomy was done. Pelvic adhesions were present. Exploration of the whole abdomen did not reveal any abnormality suggestive of malignancy. Total abdominal hysterectomy and bilateral salpingo-oophorectomy (TAH-BSO) were done. Her recovery was uneventful. Histopathology confirmed chocolate cyst of the ovary (Fig. 17.1).

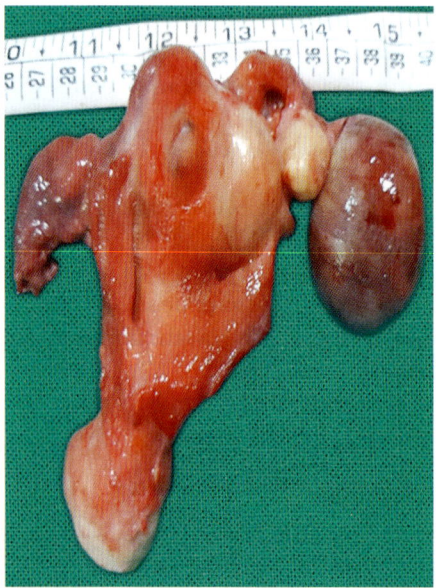

Fig. 17.1: Chocolate cyst of the left ovary, with multiple fibroids of uterus.

Q.1 What constitutes an adnexal mass and what is its importance?

Ans. Adnexal mass may arise from: Ovary, fallopian tube or from the surrounding tissues (Figs. 17.2A and B).
- Detection is often late
- Incidental observation on vaginal examination
- Otherwise mostly on pelvic imaging
- At times it is associated with acute/intermittent pelvic or lower abdominal pain
- *Diagnostic evaluation is needed to exclude malignancy*
- **Management depends on:** Age of the women, need of child-bearing and nature of *Pathology*.

Differential Diagnosis for an Adnexal Mass

Gynecological (ovary and others)

- **Benign**
  - Functional cysts (ovary)
  - Chocolate cyst
  - Teratomas (dermoids)
  - Epithelial tumors
  - Tubo-ovarian mass
  - Hydrosalpinx
  - Mullerian anomalies
  - Ectopic pregnancy
- **Malignant**
  - Epithelial carcinoma
  - Metastatic cancers
  - Germ cell tumor
  - Sex cord stromal tumor
- **Others**
  - Myomas

Adnexal Mass: Non-gynecologic

- **Benign**
  - Appendiceal mass
  - Urethral diverticulum
  - Pelvic kidney
  - Bladder diverticulum
- **Malignant**
  - GI cancers
  - Retroperitoneal sarcomas
  - Metastatic cancer

EVALUATION OF THE WOMEN

- Physical examination
  - Imaging studies
  - Serum markers
- Medical and family history
  - Breast and ovarian cancers
  - Acute or chronic dysmenorrhea
- Presence of bloating, pain and early satiety:
  - Suggests malignancy.

PHYSICAL EXAMINATION (PE)

Comprehensive PE is needed. It includes:
- Examination of regional lymph nodes
- Pelvic examination (under GA)
- Limitations of PE are: BMI > 30
  - **Presence of a mass:** Irregular, tender, firm, fixed nodular, bilateral or with ascites—suggests malignancy
  - **Others:** Endometriosis, PID, TO abscess, or leiomyomas.

CHAPTER 17: Management of Adnexal Mass in Peri- and Post-menopausal Women

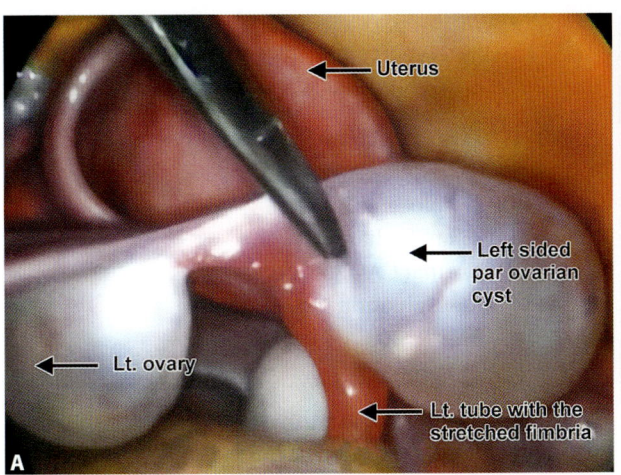 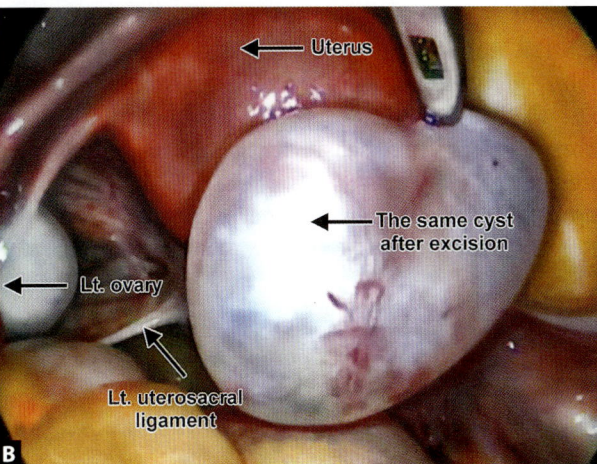

Figs. 17.2A and B: (A) Laparoscopic view of an adnexal mass (parovarian cyst) arising on the left side. The ovarian fimbria is stretched over the cyst; (B) Laparoscopic view of the same cyst after excision.

IMAGING

- TVS is the recommended imaging
- *No other alternative imaging is superior for routine use.*

Characteristic Features on TVS Imaging

Simple cyst	Complex cyst
■ Round or oval shape	■ Complete septations
■ Wall: Thin or imperceptible	■ Multilocular
■ Posterior acoustic enhancement present	■ Solid nodules
■ Anechoic fluid	■ Papillary projections
■ Absence of septations or nodules	■ Shape: Irregular

Imaging Studies

Complex ovarian cyst	
■ Multilocular cyst	■ ≥10 cm diameter
■ Solid nodules	■ Papillary projections
Risk of malignancy: 8 to 39%	

Imaging Studies USG

- *Abdominal sonography for a large mass encroaching beyond the field of view of TVS*
- *TVS may help for benign and malignant mass (sensitivity 89%, specificity 73%)*
- *Spectral and pulse Doppler indices (R1, P1) can differentiate benign from malignant mass*
- *3-D USG may be useful.*

MANAGEMENT OF AN ADNEXAL MASS

Case Summary

Miss C George, 31-year-old, joined the UK Familial Ovarian Cancer Screening Programme. Parameters included: Age, serum CA 125, USG for ovarian volume and the Doppler study for vascularity (indices). Follow-up study revealed all normal except marginal increase in volume with clear and distinct increase and alterations in vascularity. Repeat screening at 6 weeks interval revealed the same.

Decision for laparoscopy was made and it revealed several (> 5) papillary projections on the surface. Biopsy confirmed papillary serous cyst adenocarcinoma (anaplastic type). Provisional diagnosis: Familial Ovarian Cancer.

Place of Other Imaging Studies

- CT, MRI, PET are not recommended for initial evaluation
- MRI is superior for malignant masses (sensitivity 78%, specificity 87%)
- CT can detect ascites, metastases, enlarged lymph nodes and also peritoneal implants
- PET-CT is not recommended
- **RMI 1** = U × M × CA-125
  Score >200 (sensitivity 78%, specificity 87%) or score >250 with higher specificity (90%)
- **ROMA**: CA-125, HE4

Cut-off value 2.27; sensitivity 89%, specificity 75%

IOTA Group: Ultrasound Rules

B-rules	M-rules
■ Unilocular cysts	■ Irregular solid tumor
■ Presence of solid components where the largest solid component <7	■ Ascites
	■ At least four papillary structures
■ Presence of acoustic shadowing	■ Irregular multilocular solid tumor with largest diameter ≥100 mm
■ Smooth multilocular tumor with largest diameter <100 mm	■ Prominent blood flow on color Doppler
■ No blood flow on color Doppler	

IOTA Group: USG Rules and OVA1

- **IOTA:** USG features and logistic regression model (LGM-2); includes 6 variables (age and 5 USG findings for B-rules and M-rules) (B = Benign, M = Malignant).
  It is not recommended for routine use

- **OVA1**: It is a quantitative assay using 5 serum proteins: [CA-125, transthyretin, (prealbumin), apolipoprotein A1, beta-2 microglobulin and transferrin]: Numerical score 0.0—10.0; value >4.4 risk of malignancy in postmenopausal women. OVA1—high sensitivity, specificity and positive predictive value.
- **Serum biomarkers in ovarian germ cell tumors**

	β-hCG	AFP	LDH	CA-125
Dysgerminoma	+	−	+	−
Endodermal sinus tumor	−	+	−	−
Choriocarcinoma	+	−	−	−
Immature teratoma	−	+	+	+
Embryonal carcinoma	+	+	−	−

(AFP: alpha fetoprotein; CA: cancer antigen; LDH: lactate dehydrogenase)

- **Serum biomarker and multimodal test results considered abnormal in women with adnexal masses**

Test	Premenopausal	Postmenopausal
CA-125	±	>35 U/mL
MIA	≥ 5.0	≥ 4.4
ROMA	≥ 1.31	≥ 2.77
RMI	> 200	> 200

(CA: cancer antigen; MIA: multivariate index assay; ROMA: risk of ovarian malignancy algorithm; RMI, risk of malignancy index); ± Specificity and positive predictive vlalue of CA-125 are higher in post-menopausal women.

- **Recommendations on consensus with *expert opinion***
    - Serum biomarker panels are preferred as alternative to CA-125 alone
- **Serum CA-125 (biomarker)**
    - Specificity and PPV are higher in postmenopausal women
    - Serum biomarker panel testing is preferred (RM1, ROMA, OVI).

MANAGEMENT OF AN ADNEXAL MASS (OVARIAN CYST)

Q.2 What is the place of management with observation only?

Ans.
- The mass morphology on USG suggests a benign disease
- Compelling reason to avoid surgical intervention (multiple co-morbidities of the patient)
- CA-125 level normal
- Simple cysts are almost always benign
- Unilocular cysts ≤10 cm; when followed up by serial USG it was observed that resolution occurred in >66% cases.

Q.3 What is the place of conservative management?

Ans.
- Ovarian cyst—asymptomatic
- Simple—unilocular
- <5 cm in diameter
- Normal CA-125 values
- Re-evaluation in 4–6 months
- RMI 1 <200.

Q.4 What is the management of adnexal masses in perimenopausal women?

Ans.
- Simple cyst ≤10 cm diameter (TVS)—asymptomatic
- Suspected endometrioma
- Repeat imaging is needed on follow-up.

Q.5 What is the place of aspiration of an adnexal mass?

Ans.
- Generally it is contraindicated
- It is done in a case with tubo-ovarian abscess following antibiotic therapy
- Detection of malignancy following aspiration is low (sensitivity 50 to 70%)
- It induces spillage and seeding of cancer cells
- Even for a benign simple cyst, aspiration is not therapeutic as risk of recurrence is high (44%)
- Exception may be in an advanced case and the patient is unfit for surgery
- Aspiration may allow neoadjuvant chemotherapy.

Q.6 What are the high-risk (postmenopausal) women?

Ans.
- Raised CA-125 level
- USG findings—ascites, nodular fixed mass, metastasis
- Elevated score on—multivariate LR-2 (RM1, ROMA or IOTA).

Q.7 What are the different types of surgical intervention (presumed to be a benign adnexal mass)?

Ans.
- Minimally invasive surgery is preferred
- Fertility preservation rarely needed in such an age group
- Ovarian cystectomy/ovariotomy/Salpingo-oophorectomy (uni/bilateral), TAH + BSO may be done
- Conversion to laparotomy (0–1.5%) when there is suspicion of malignancy
- Robotic assisted surgery is an option
- Retrieval bag for the specimen should be used
- Full staging laparatomy is the option with the evidence of malignancy.

Q.8 When to make referral to a gynecological oncologist?

Ans. The indications are:
- Elevated level of CA-125
- USG suggestive of malignancy (ascites, nodular fixed mass)
- Evidence of abdominal or distant metastasis
- Raised score for RM1, ROMA or IOTA.

Q.9 Who should manage the woman?

Ans. It depends on the risk of malignancy:
- Low-risk of malignancy (RMI 1 <200): General gynecologist
- High-risk women: Gynecological oncologist

Actual surgery: Staging laparotomy includes:
- Exploration of the whole abdomen and to make clear documentation
- Malignant cell cytology from the ascites or washings
- TAH + BSO + omentectomy + biopsy of suspicious areas
- Selective pelvic and para-aortic lymphadenectomy
- In an advanced case, surgery may be delayed following administration of neoadjuvant chemotherapy.

Suggested Reading

1. Kaijser J, Sayasneh A, Van Hoorde K, Ghaem-Maghami S, Bourne T, Timmerman D, et al. Presurgical diagnosis of adnexal tumours using mathematical models and scoring systems: a systematic review and meta-analysis. Hum reprod update. 2014;20:449-62.
2. National institute for health and care excellence. Ovarian cancer; The recognition and initial management of ovarian cancer, NICE clinical guideline 122. Manchester NICE; 2021.
3. Scottish Intercollegiate Guideline Network. Management of epitbelial ovarian cancer. SIGN publication no 135. Edinburgh: SIGN; 2013.
4. Van calster B, Timmerman D, Valentin L, McIndoe A, Ghaem-Maghami S, Testa AC, et al. Triaging women with ovarian masses for surgery: observational diagnostic study to compare RCOG guidelines with an International Ovarian Tumour Analysis (I OTA) group protocol BJOG. 2012;119:662-71.

Chapter 18: Use of Selective Progesterone Receptor Modulators in Gynecology

Progesterone receptors (PRs) exist in multiple isoforms. PR isoforms are not interchangeable. **Mifepristone** is an antagonist for the receptors of progesterone (PR) as well as the glucocorticoid receptor (GR). More compounds are developed that they have both the properties of agonist and antagonist on PR. These compounds are classified as selective progesterone receptor modulators (SPRMs). It has been subsequently observed that some SPRMs have antagonistic effect on breast tissues. SPRMs do not influence the effect of estrogen on breast and endometrial tissues. Of the several SPRMs, **mifepristone** is commonly used.

Progesterone receptors are present in endometrium, myometrium and in mammary glands. Once progesterone binds the cell receptor (PR), dimerization occurs to form progesterone receptor complex. This complex enters the nucleus and initiates gene transcription. The main principles of action are:
- **PR agonist**: Initiates transcription via co-activators
- **PR antagonists**: Inhibits transcription via co-suppressors

There are two isoforms of the PR:
1. Human progesterone receptor A (hPR-A), and
2. Human progesterone receptor B (hPR-B)

The action of SPRMs is not clearly understood. SPRMs bind to both the isoforms and exert a mixed agonist and antagonist effect. The final action is mediated by the resultant effect of co-activators and co-suppressors.

Activation of progesterone receptors.
- PR-A: Blocks endometrial proliferation induced by E2
- PR-B: Promotes proliferation and differentiation of breast tissues

Ultimate effects depend on:
- Types of SPRM
- Ratio of PR isoform
- Tissue concentration of:
  - Co-activators
  - Co-suppressor

Mechanism of Action of Progesterone and SPRMs

- **Ulipristal acetate (UA)** downregulates the expression of vascular endothelial growth factor (VEGF). This reduces tissue neovascularization, cell proliferation. These ultimately lead to cell apoptosis. Asoprisnil also induces cellular apoptosis.
- UA increases the expression of matrix metalloproteinases. Thereby it reduces collagen deposition in fibroids.
- Asoprisnil and UA have been shown to modulate the ratio of PR isoforms (PR-A and PR-B) in the cultured leiomyoma cells. They reduced expression of growth factors, angiogenic factors and their receptors in these cells.
- Mifepristone and asoprisnil have also been observed to decrease the uterine artery blood flow.

Amenorrhea and SPRMs: SPRMs often induce amenorrhea. Period of amenorrhea varies as with type of SPRMs. Ulipristal has been observed to have higher amenorrhea rate.

Use of SPRMs in Gynecology

Commonly used SPRMs: Mifepristone, asoprisnil and ulipristal acetate and their effects on ovulation and endometrium.
- Inhibition of ovulation as there is no LH surge
- Endometrial suppression (counteracts estrogen-induced endometrial proliferation)
- Failure of implantation
- Induction of amenorrhea
- Prevention of pregnancy

Contraception: Ulipristal acetate and mifepristone have been found effective as a **contraception** when used up to 120 hours after unprotected sexual intercourse. Both mifepristone (20–30 mg) and ulipristal acetate (30 mg single dose) are found superior to levonorgestrel as an **emergency contraception**.

Mechanism of action of UA is to delay ovulation or inhibit ovulation. UA alters endometrial receptivity, exerting an anti-implantation effect. UA also alters tubal motility and sperm function. Amenorrhea that occurs with SPRMs is associated with low serum levels of estradiol.

Amongst all SPRMs, mifepristone has the pure antagonist activities. It is used for medical termination of pregnancy

Endometriosis and SPRMs

Common symptoms in endometriosis are: Dysmenorrhea, dyspareunia, pelvic pain, abnormal menstruation, painful defecation (dyschezia) and even hematuria.

SPRMs may be used as a therapeutic alternative. It improves the symptoms by its effects:
- Suppression of ovulation
- Antiproliferative effect on endometrium

- Reducing abnormal uterine bleeding
- Regression of ectopic endometrial tissues
- Improvement in pelvic pain
- Short courses asoprisnil, found to be effective in reducing nonmenstrual pelvic pain and dysmenorrhea
- However, long-term effects of SPRMs on the endometrium are awaited and it under evaluation.

Endometriosis, dysfunctional uterine bleeding and SPRMs: Mifepristone has been shown to reduce pain and induce regression of endometriosis.

Leiomyoma of the Uterus and SPRMs

Fibroids are the most common (20–30%) benign tumors of the uterus. Fibroids are the hormone-dependent tumors, including estrogen and progesterone. Symptomatic fibroid(s) need to be treated. Women with heavy menstrual bleeding due to fibroids may be treated medically when size of the fibroids are small (<3 cm) and there is no distortion of the cavity (NICE-2007).

SPRMs are helpful in such cases. **Ideal choice of a SPRM** should be that it has progestogenic effect on the endometrium and antiprogestogenic effect on the fibroid.

- **Mifepristone** was used for the treatment of fibroids in reduced doses between 12.5 mg and 50 mg daily. There was reduction in uterine fibroid volume by 40–50%. Many women became amenorrheic. The other important benefits of mifepristone are: significant improvements in quality of life, reduction in anemia.

Intrauterine fetal death: In late IUFD, induction of labor in a woman with an unscarred uterus is done using a combination of mifepristone and a prostaglandin preparation (misoprostol). The addition of mifepristone appeared to reduce the time interval, compared to the use of prostaglandin alone.

Contraindications of SPRMs

UA is currently not recommended because of its health concern.

Mifepristone is contraindicated with confirmed or suspected ectopic pregnancy or undiagnosed adnexal mass, chronic adrenal failure, concurrent long-term corticosteroid therapy. It is not to be given to a patient with history of allergy to mifepristone, hemorrhagic disorders or concurrent anticoagulant therapy.

Adverse effects: Most of the adverse reactions are mild. The common adverse effects are: nausea, hot flushes, headache, vertigo, acne, sweating, muscle pain and tiredness.

Safety of Long-term Use of SPRMs

SPRMs have different effects on endometrium. **Agonist and antagonist** functions of SPRMs on individual tissue especially on endometrium are different. Manifestations of such effects are variable on endometrium. The mechanism of action of SPRMs is not clearly understood. **Endometrial cancer** has been observed as a risk factor for long-term use of SPRMs. This is due to the effect of unopposed estrogen on endometrium. It is not always possible to identify a high-risk woman taking SPRM to develop endometrial carcinoma. Woman on SPRM may need endometrial biopsy at an interval (while on SPRM, for a long-term period).

Adverse effects for the use of ulipristal acetate are:
- Severe asthma uncontrolled by oral glycocorticoids
- Hepatic dysfunction
- Hereditary problems—galactose intolerance

SPRMs may have a role in the treatment of woman with breast cancer.

It is recommended to perform LFT at least once a month for any woman under therapy and to stop therapy when the transaminase levels are >2 times the upper limit of the normal.

Suggested Reading

1. Bouchard P, Chabbert-Buffet N, Fauser BC. Selective progesterone receptor modulators in reproductive medicine: pharmacology, clinical efficacy and safety. Fertil Steril. 2011;96:1175–89.
2. Chabbert-Buffet N, A Pintiaux A, Bouchard P. The imminent dawn of SPRMs in obstetrics and gynecology. Mol Cell Endocrinol. 2012;358:232–43.
3. Chwalisz K, Perez MC, DeManno D, et al. Selective progesterone receptor modulator development and use in the treatment of leiomyomata and endometriosis. Endocr Reviews. 2005;26:423–38.
4. Wilkens J, Critchley H. Progesterone receptor modulators in gynaecological practice. J Fam Plann Reprod Health Care. 2010;36:87–92.

Section 3: Infertility and Assisted Reproductive Technology (ART)

Section Outline

- Ch. 19. Current Concept in Physiology of Ovulation
- Ch. 20. Infertility Evaluation and Management
- Ch. 21. Female Infertility
- Ch. 22. Male Infertility
- Ch. 23. Assisted Reproductive Technology (ART)
- Ch. 24. Reproductive Outcome in Women with Advanced Maternal Age
- Ch. 25. Anti-Mullerian Hormone in Reproductive Biology
- Ch. 26. Fertility Management Strategies for Low Responder
- Ch. 27. Surrogacy

Current Concept in Physiology of Ovulation

Q.1 Regarding folliculogenesis and ovulation:
a. Follicular development and differentiation takes about 85 days
b. Anti-Müllerian hormone (AMH) supports monofollicular development
c. First phase of follicular growth (60 days) is gonadotropin sensitive
d. Elevated and static level of estradiol is essential for ovulation
e. Menstrual cycle and ovulatory cycle are the same

Ans. a. T b. T
c. F d. F
e. F

GERM CELL MIGRATION AND POPULATION IN THE GONADS

Germ cells are endodermal in origin. The germ cells migrate from the yolk sac to the genital ridge along the dorsal mesentery between 30 days and 40 days. The germ cells undergo a number of rapid mitotic divisions and differentiate into oogonia. The number of oogonia reaches its maximum at 20th week numbering about **7 million**. The mitotic division gradually ceases and majority enter into the prophase of first meiotic division and are called ***primary oocytes***. These cells when surrounded by flattened granulosa cells, are called ***primordial follicles***. At birth, there is no more mitotic division and all the oogonia are replaced by primary oocytes. The estimated number of primary oocytes, at birth is about **2 million. At puberty**, some **400,000** primary oocytes are left behind, the rest become atretic. During the entire reproductive period, **some 400** are likely to ovulate. Germ cells degeneration start in intrauterine life and it continues throughout the childhood and the child-bearing period. As a result, only few follicles with ova can be detected in menopausal women.

The phases of follicular growth, maturation and ovulation are discussed under the following heads.

Folliculogenesis:
- Follicular growth and maturation
- Emergence of dominant follicle (DF) and ovulation
- Follicular atresia
- Endocrine (estradiol) control of ovulation
- Difference in menstrual cycle and ovulatory cycle

- Events in ovulatory cycle
  ♦ Endocrine
  ♦ Biophysical
- Events in nonovulatory cycle.

Follicular Growth and Atresia

Follicular growth and atresia is a continuous process, from intrauterine life to the age of menopause. This process is not interrupted by pregnancy, ovulation or by combined oral contraceptive therapy.

Initial recruitment, growth and development of primordial follicles are not under the control of any hormone (including gonadotropins). It is dependent upon a variety of factors that are produced locally (autocrine and paracrine mechanism). These are transforming growth factor β (TGF-β) subfamily of proteins, activins, inhibins, growth hormone and AMH.

After a certain stage (>2 mm in size), the growth and differentiation of primordial follicles are under the control of follicle-stimulating hormone (FSH). Unless the follicles are rescued by FSH at this state, they undergo atresia. FSH also induces luteinizing hormone (LH) receptors on the granulosa cells of the DF.

Follicular Growth, Maturation and Emergence of Dominant Follicle

The cohort of growing follicles undergoes a process of development and differentiation which takes about 85 days and it spreads over 3 ovarian cycles. It is not clear as to how many and which of the primordial follicles amidst several thousands are recruited in a particular cycle. It is presumed that about 20 antral follicles (around 5–10 per ovary) proceed to develop in each cycle.

The cohort of follicles are recruited after puberty, as they become sensitive to gonadotropins. It is presumed that growth hormone (GH), insulin growth factor-I (IGF-I), androgen and also some other unknown growth factors play their role to make the follicles sensitive to gonadotropins. The cohort of follicles are recruited during last 20 days out of the total 85 days (3 ovarian cycles) of follicular growth and differentiation.

Each of these primordial follicles will compete for maturation under the influence of pituitary gonadotropins. Ultimately one will be successful for final maturation, leading to ovulation. The rest of the follicles will undergo the process of atresia beginning on D8.

Process of follicular growth and maturation: Primordial follicle → primary follicle → preantral follicle → antral follicle → preovulatory phase of Graafian follicle → final maturation and ovulation (Fig. 19.1).

Every 80 days cohort of follicles are recruited under the influence of GH, IGF-1 and androgens. Time interval from follicular recruitment, maturation, atresia or final phase of ovulation, is nearly 80 days. The entire process is divided into first phase of gonadotropin resistance (60 days) and second phase of gonadotropin sensitivity (20 days), coinciding with the late luteal phase of previous cycle (Fig. 19.2).

Role of AMH in follicular development: AMH inhibits initial recruitment of primordial follicles into the pool of growing follicles. It also decreases responsiveness of follicles to FSH. AMH plays an important role for monofollicular development and ovulation. It also prevents premature depletion of the follicular pool.

The probable mechanisms for monofollicular development and ovulation:
- All the primordial follicles that reach the preantral stage, produce AMH.
- AMH inhibits further growth of primordial follicles by decreasing the responsiveness of follicles to FSH.
- The growth of DF is however uninhibited as the DF has maximum number of FSH receptors, and it produces less AMH.
- Usually only one DF grows to maturity rest become atretic.

Endocrine Control of Ovulation

The primary endocrine control of ovulation is through estradiol (E2). Neither the pituitary nor the hypothalamus has the primary role, though estradiol is the outcome of hypothalamic-pituitary ovarian axis function.

The cyclicity of ovulation and menstruation depends upon the following sequence endocrine events where ***estradiol (E2) plays the dominant role:***
- Estradiol level must decline in the late luteal phase.
- Estradiol level must rise in the midmenstrual or midfollicular phase.
- Follicular microenvironment must be E2 dominant (follicular androgens must be converted to estrogen with the help of enzyme aromatase).

As early as days 5–7, one follicle out of so many, becomes dominant and undergoes further maturation. The granulosa cells of the DF have the maximum number of FSH receptors. The rest of the follicles become atretic by D8.

The selection of DF depends primarily on FSH. However, the FSH action is modulated by autocrine and paracrine action of many other factors.

Basically the selection of dominant follicle is explained under the two categories of supports:
1. ***Gonadotropic axis support:*** FSH, LH, E2, inhibin, activin and AMH.
2. ***Somatotropic axis support*** is GH, IGF-I, sex hormone binding globulin (SHBG), insulin growth factor binding protein (IGFBP) and TGF-β.

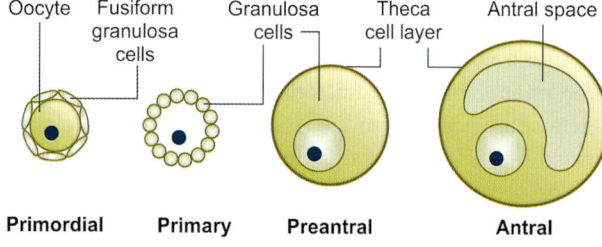

Fig. 19.1: Phases of follicular growth and maturation.

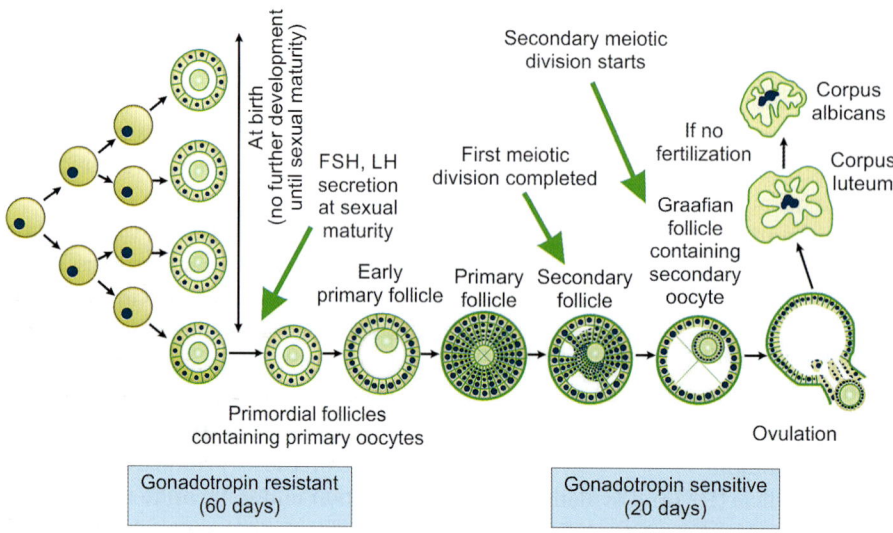

Fig. 19.2: Follicular growth-gonadotropin sensitivity-maturation and ovulation.
(FSH, follicle-stimulating hormone; LH, luteinizing hormone)

Therefore, *when analyzed critically, the menstrual cycle and ovulatory (follicular growth, maturation, ovulation and atresia) cycle are not the same but are different to some extent.* This understanding is essential for the management of dysovulatory subfertility.

Menstrual Cycle and Ovulatory Cycle

- *Menstrual cycle:* Begins on D1 of the preceding cycle and ends on D1 of the subsequent cycle
- *Ovulatory cycle:* Begins on the late luteal phase (D21–D28) of the preceding menstrual cycle and ends in the early luteal period of the existing cycle.

The entire period of ovulatory cycle can be divided into five distinct phases:

1. Late luteal (postovulatory: D21–D28) phase
2. Early follicular phase (menstrual: D1–D4)
3. Midfollicular phase (D5–D6)
4. Late follicular phase (D7–D14)
5. Early luteal (D15–D21)

Important sequence of events in the late luteal phase are:
- Decline in E2 level
- Decline in inhibin level
- Rise in FSH level
- Recruitment of fresh follicles.

Endocrinological and Biophysical Events in the Three Different Follicular Phases of an Ovulatory Cycle

Early follicular phase	
Endocrinologic events	**Biophysical events**
Adequate FSH level →	- Follicular growth
	- Proliferation of granulosa cells
	- Induction of receptors for FSH followed by LH
	- Aromatase activity
Optimum LH →	E2 synthesis and further follicular growth
Midfollicular phase	
- Rise in E2 levels	- Recruitment of dominant and co-dominant follicles
- Decline in FSH levels (negative feedback of rising E2)	- Induction of LH receptors in the granulosa cells of the dominant follicle by FSH
- Rise in LH levels than FSH	- Follicles become more LH responsive

Important events for selection of dominant follicle (in midfollicular phase) are:

- *Estrogen dominant follicular microenvironment* (privileged follicle).
- *Induction of LH receptors* in the granulosa cells of the DF. Luteinizing hormone receptor induction is essential for (i) midcycle LH surge to induce ovulation, (ii) luteinization of the granulosa cells to form corpus luteum, and (iii) secretion of progesterone.

- *Rise in estradiol levels*—establishing negative feedback effect on FSH (suppression). This results in less competent follicles to undergo atresia. The additional events are:

Late follicular phase	
Endocrinologic events	**Biophysical events**
- Peak and plateau levels of E2	- Growth of dominant follicle(s)
- Rise in LH level and its surge	- Completion of oocyte meiosis
- Further decline in FSH level	- Ovulation
	- Luteinization of granulosa cells
	- Secretion of progesterone

Important Endocrinological Events in the Process of Ovulation

- There is induction of LH receptors in the DF by FSH.
- There is shift of dominant follicular control from FSH to LH since the midfollicular phase.
- LH in the late follicular phase causes follicular atresia other than the DF. This keeps multifollicular ovulation and multiple pregnancy under check. Multiple pregnancy is common after induction of ovulation.
- LH surge occurs when E2 level reaches a peak (100 pg/follicle) and is sustained for 48–50 hours.
- Peak level of LH should be 75–100 ng/mL.
- Duration of LH surge is about 24 hours. It has a crescendo → peak → decrescendo pattern.
- Progesterone within the follicle inhibits oocyte maturation inhibitory factor (OMIF). This event initiates release of the first polar body. Thus, the oocyte becomes haploid and fertilizable.
- Actual process of ovulation is induced by perifollicular leukocyte activation. The leads to matrix dissolution by production of specific enzyme including plasminogen activator. Absence of the enzyme leads to luteinized unruptured follicle syndrome.
- Rise in estradiol (E2) in follicular phase is controlled by FSH (early) and by LH (late follicular phase) → peak (D10–D11) levels (100 pg/mature follicle) → plateau level of E2 for 48 hours → positive feedback on pituitary LH → LH surge (any time within next 48 hours) → ovulation (within next 34–36 hours).
- The basic prerequisite in ovulatory cycle is the fluctuating levels of E2. If for any reason, the E2 levels become static, anovulation is the rule [as in polycystic ovarian syndrome (PCOS)].
- Attenuated LH surge may lead to ovulation with a dysmature egg. This egg is unsuitable for fertilization.
- Unscheduled LH surge (when the granulosa cells are not yet matured), leads to premature luteinization of granulosa cells and release of a 'progeric' egg. This egg is unsuitable for fertilization.
- Premature luteinization of granulosa cells leads to defective formation of corpus luteum. This makes the luteal phase defective.

Flowchart 19.1: Events leading to failure of ovulation.

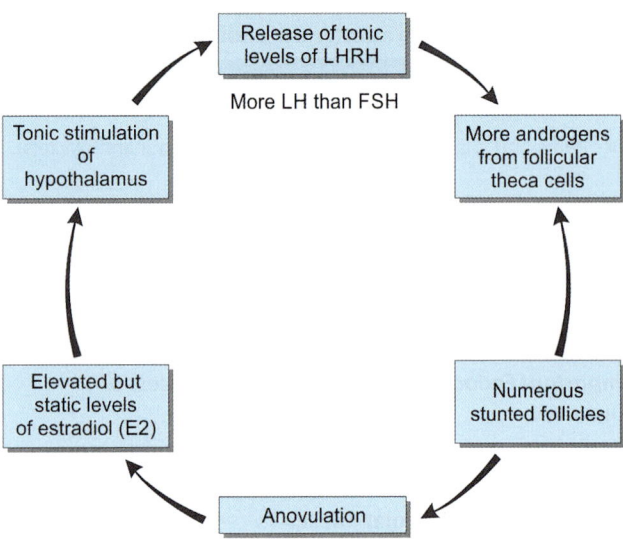

(LHRH, luteinizing hormone-releasing hormone; LH, luteinizing hormone, FSH; follicle-stimulating hormone)

- Androgenized follicular microenvironment leads to follicular atresia (as in PCOS).

Events in Nonovulatory Cycle

Static levels of estradiol → tonic stimulation of hypothalamus → release of tonic (levels) of luteinizing hormone-releasing hormone (LHRH) → more LH than FSH secretion → elevated but static levels estrogen (E2) → an ovulation (characteristic of PCOS).

Ovary, secreting the fluctuating level of estrogen (E2), is considered the band master of endocrine orchestra for a normal ovulatory cycle. When levels of E2 become static anovulation is the sequelae.

Suggested Reading

1. Anasti JN, Kalantaridou SN, Kimzey LM, et al. Human follicule fluid vascular endothelial growth factor concentrations are correlated with luteinization in spontaneously developing follicles. Hum Reprod. 1998;13(5):1144–7.
2. Demura R, Suzuki T, Tajima S, et al. Human plasma free activin and inhibin levels during the menstrual cycle. J Clin Endocrinol Metab. 1993;76(4):1080–2.

Chapter 20: Infertility Evaluation and Management

INTRODUCTION

Infertility is a medical as well as social problem. Infertility does not cost life. But it perpetuates a devastating emotional and social trauma on the couple. Ultimately, it results in dissatisfaction, dejection and despair in the couple.

During the last two and a half decades, there has been a marked increase in the prevalence of infertility world over and so also in India. Overall incidence of infertility in India is 15–20%. For understanding, infertility is classified into four simple types (Flowchart 20.1).

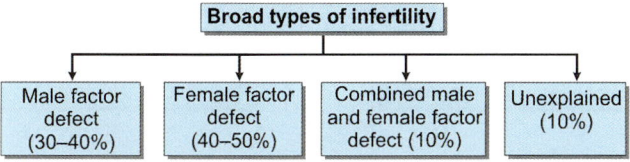

Flowchart 20.1: Broadly infertility can be classified under the following types.

EVALUATION OF INFERTILE COUPLES

Basic Parameters for Evaluation of an Infertile Couple

- **Inspection:**
  - Female partner: Obesity, hirsutism, acne → polycystic ovarian syndrome (PCOS)
  - Male partner: Scanty or absence of mustache and beard, presence of gynecomastia → Klinefelter's syndrome.
- **Interrogation:**
  - Female partner
  - Male partner
  - Both the partners.

Female partner menstrual history
- Amenorrhea
- History of mumps, sexually transmitted infections (STIs)
- Oligomenorrhea.

Male sexual dysfunction
- Loss of erection
- History of orchitis, STIs
- Loss of libido

- **Examination of both the partners**

Female partner	Male partner
◆ General physical examination	◆ General and systemic examination and examination of genitalia—penis, urethra, testis (volume), epididymis and the vas deferens
◆ Systemic examination	
◆ Pelvic examination	

- **Basic investigations**
  - Semen analysis
  - Ovulation detection/confirmation
  - Assessment of
    - Tubal patency
    - Tuboperitoneal factors (endometriosis)
    - Ovarian reserve (if history suggests *See* Ch 21, 26).

Following clinical evaluation, all infertile couples are broadly categorized into three groups:

1. **Easily treatable conditions**
   - ◆ *Female partner:* Ovulation dysfunction, tough hymen, mild endometriosis
   - ◆ *Male partner:*
     - Mild oligospermia
     - Phimosis
2. **Not easily treatable conditions**
   - ◆ *Female partner*
     - Premature ovarian failure, pelvic adhesions due to tuberculosis
     - Advanced pelvic endometriosis, uterine synechiae
   - ◆ *Male partner*
     - Azoospermia
     - Asthenospermia/teratospermia.

   There may be ***multiple defects*** in one or both the partners. Examples are—seminal defect (male partner) with tubal block or adenomyosis (female partner). There may be multiple defects in the one partner again, e.g., tubal block with uterine synechiae.

3. **Unexplained infertility** (*See* Ch 23): Couples having apparently no defect, in either partner, based on basic evaluation parameter, belong to the unexplained group of

infertility. Prognosis of these couples is somewhat better as compared to other two groups mentioned before. However, better prognosis is expected provided (a) age of the female partner <35 years, (b) duration of infertility is <7 years, and (c) menstrual cyclicity is regular.

Women having regular cyclical periods seldom suffer from ovulatory dysfunction, whereas women having delayed periods or having oligoamenorrheic cycles, usually have anovulation or oligoovulation. This is the common presentation of woman having polycystic ovarian syndrome (PCOS) (*See* Ch 8).

PATIENT CATEGORIZATION AND MANAGEMENT PROTOCOL

Five types of treatment options are available:
1. Medical
2. Surgical
3. Assisted reproductive technology (ART)
4. **Combination treatment:** (a) Surgical and medical, (b) surgical followed by ART, (c) medical followed by ART, and if nothing works
5. Adoption.

Medical treatment: Women with PCOS or with unexplained infertility may be benefitted with induction of ovulation (clomiphene citrate).

Surgical treatment: Surgery for improvement of infertility may be:
- **Obligatory:** As in cases with narrow introitus (Fenton's operation), uterine synechiae (hysteroscopic adhesiolysis), fibroid uterus where no other cause for infertility present (myomectomy—laparoscopy/laparotomy).
- **Complementary:** Laparoscopic ablation of endometriotic implants, ovarian drilling (LOD) or hysteroscopic septal resection.

Combination of therapy may improve the results of infertility.

Surgical (laparoscopic) and/or medical (long-acting GnRH-A) treatment of advanced endometriosis may be effective. Similarly, ART preceded by surgical or medical treatment is more rational for fertility restoration in advanced stages of endometriosis.

Summary: Infertility management protocol should be outlined based on the cause(s). Judicious planning may help in achieving an acceptable outcome.

Management Options for Couples with Multiple Defects

Corrections of multiple defects are seldom successful. Prospect of achieving spontaneous pregnancy is remote in such a couple having multiple defects. The options available for them are:
- ART with or without gamete donation (*See* Ch 23).
- Surrogacy (*See* Ch 27).
- Adoption.

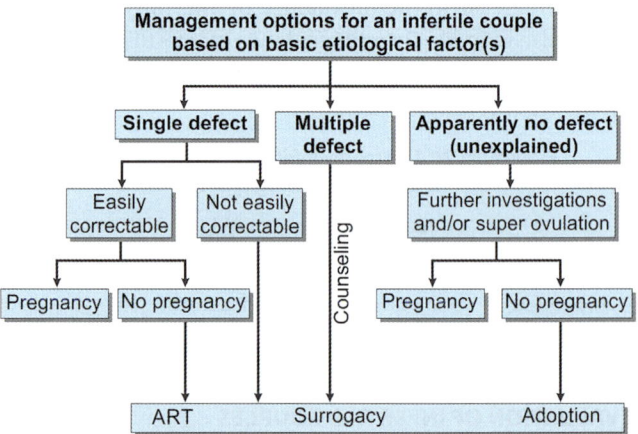

Suggested Reading

1. Jacobson TZ, Duffy JM, Barlow D, et al. Laparoscopic surgery for subfertility associated with endometriosis. Cochrane Database Syst Rev. 2010;1:CD001398.
2. Practice Committee of the American Society for Reproductive Medicine. Effectiveness and treatment for unexplained infertility. Fertil Steril. 2006;86(5 Suppl 1):S111-4.

Chapter 21: Female Infertility

Q.1 Regarding female infertility:
a. Antral follicle count >6 using TVS indicates adequate ovarian reserve
b. High levels of AMH indicates poor ovarian reserve
c. Abnormal endometrial perfusion may be a factor for unexplained infertility
d. Premature LH surge results in poor quality of oocyte
e. In ART cycle, younger the patient more the number (>3) of embryo to be transferred

Ans.
a. T b. F
c. T d. F
e. F

OVULATORY DISORDERS

Nearly 30–40% of infertile women suffer from the problem of ovulatory dysfunction.

Ovulatory dysfunction may be due to: (a) failure to release (ovulate) an egg, or (b) inability to produce fully matured eggs.

Classification of Ovulatory Disorders (WHO)
- Hypogonadotropic hypogonadism (hypothalamic-pituitary failure)
- Hypothalamic-pituitary dysfunction
- Hypergonadotropic hypogonadism—premature ovarian failure (POF).

Women need to be evaluated for the underlying pathology causing anovulation. Unless the underlying pathology is detected and corrected the main problem of ovulatory dysfunction could not be overcome even by therapy. The common underlying pathologies are:
- Thyroid dysfunction both: (a) hypothyroidism, (b) hyperthyroidism
- Hyperprolactinemia
- Weight disorders: (a) Excessive weight loss, (b) Excessive weight gain (obesity)
- Polycystic ovarian syndrome (PCOS)
- Pituitary tumor
- Adrenal disease
- Galactorrhea.

Physiology of Ovarian Cycle in Menstruation and Ovulation

Principle events are
- ***Recruitment of a group of follicles:*** It takes about 85 days for a group of primordial follicles (15–20) to grow.
- ***Selection of dominant follicle:*** Out of so many follicles rescued by FSH, dominant follicle is the one that has the maximum number of FSH receptors and has the dominant estrogenic follicular micro-environment (high estradiol: androgen ratio).
- ***Ovulation:*** Sustained high level of estradiol along with LH surge principally triggers ovulation.
- ***Formation of corpus luteum:*** Once conception occurs, there is luteal-placental shift (8–10 weeks). Thereafter, secretion of progesterone continues from the placenta.

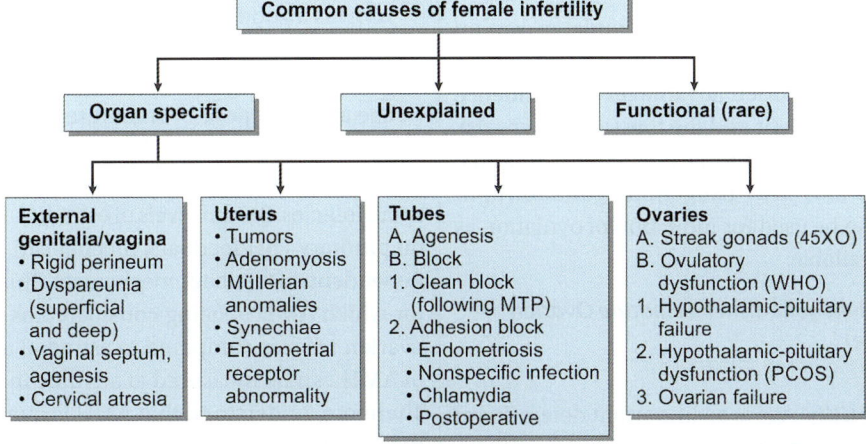

Fertile window: It is the 6 days interval ending on the day of ovulation (not after ovulation). Sperm survive up to 2–3 days in normal cervical mucus, but eggs survive for less than 24 hours. Generally a woman remains fertile between D10 and D17 of the menstrual cycle. Daily intercourse, during the window period, increases the probability of pregnancy.

Ovulatory disorders may be due to:
- Anovulation (complete absence of ovulation)
- Oligoovulation (infrequent ovulation).

Women having abnormal menstrual history (amenorrhea, oligomenorrhea, polymenorrhea or dysfunctional uterine bleeding) often suffer from ovulatory dysfunction. Successful treatment of ovulatory disorders depends on the correct identification of the underlying pathology for anovulation.

Management of Ovulatory Disorders

Hypogonadotropic Hypogonadism

(WHO Category-1)

This group of women is associated with (H-P failure) low level of serum FSH, LH and estradiol. Common causes of hypogonadotropic hypogonadism are: (a) Pituitary adenomas, (b) Craniopharyngioma and other factors like, (c) stress, anorexia, excessive exercise, extreme weight loss (BMI < 16 kg/m^2) or congenital hypothalamic failure—Kallmann syndrome.

Investigations
- Serum levels of FSH, LH, GnRH and serum estradiol are estimated.
- MRI study is done for the detection of central nervous system pathology.

Management issues: Single most important and effective treatment for this group of women with low BMI (<16 kg/m^2) is counseling and to encourage weight gain with good diet and nutrition.

Leptin is deficient in such women suffering from anorexia and exercise induced amenorrhea. Exogenous leptin restores ovulation in these women.

Pulsatile GnRH every 60–90 minutes stimulates ovarian physiology for ovulation. Success rate of pulsatile GnRH therapy is high (90%). The added advantages are incidence of monofollicular development and the low subsequent risk of ovarian hyperstimulation syndrome (OHSS). The multiple pregnancy rates are also low. Exogenous gonadotropin (FSH and LH) can also be used for induction of ovulation as GnRH is not easily available.

Hypergonadotropic Hypogonadism (Premature Ovarian Insufficiency or Failure)

(WHO Category-3)

Women's age and fertility: Age is an important determinant as fertility declines with advancing age. Many women are getting married in late 30s or early 40s. However, significant decline occurs in oocyte quality and quantity as the women enters late 30s, though it begins in early 30s. Primary ovarian insufficiency (failure) is the cessation of ovarian function prior to the age of 40 years. It is characterized by primary or secondary amenorrhea with elevated serum gonadotropin levels. However, ovarian failure is fortunately is a rare entity. Premature ovarian failure could be due to several reasons.

Causes of premature ovarian insufficiency (failure)
- Abnormal chromosomal pattern (45XO Turner, 47XXX) causing accelerated follicular atresia
- Pure gonadal dysgenesis
- Infections (HIV, mumps, tuberculosis)
- Iatrogenic: Radiation, chemotherapy, surgery (oophorectomy, excessive ovarian drilling)
- Metabolic: Galactosemia
- Autoimmune disorders (polyglandular autoimmune syndrome)
- However, 5–10% of women with POF achieve pregnancy and deliver successfully.

This indicates, women should be assessed for ovarian reserve before planning management.

ASSESSMENT OF OVARIAN RESERVE

Ovarian reserve tests are to assess the quantity as well as the quality of primordial follicles present in the women's ovary. These tests are done to determine how the ovaries will respond to therapy (ovulation induction). In other words, it is the assessment of the reproductive potential of the woman.

The tests are:
- ***Estimation of basal level of serum FSH*** on D3 and again on D10 following clomiphene citrate challenge test (CCCT): 100 mg orally each day from D5–D9: values >10 IU/L (more than 2SD) indicates poor ovarian reserve.
- ***Basal (D3) serum estradiol level*** > 70–80 pg/mL, poor ovarian reserve.
- ***Serum inhibin B (D5):*** Reduced inhibin B levels (less than 40 pg/mL) are observed in woman with advanced age.
- ***Serum anti-Müllerian hormone (AMH):*** Levels of serum AMH is a good predictor of ovarian stimulation response. Its level also comes with the direct proportion of antral follicle count (AFC). Levels of AMH (1 ng/mL) declines with age and with poor ovarian reserve. Levels of AMH can be measured any time in the menstrual cycle.

AMH: It is produced by the granulosa cells of the preantral small follicles. Serum levels of estradiol and inhibin B depend on pituitary FSH feedback mechanism. Level of AMH is not dependent on feedback mechanism. This is one of the reasons for which AMH is being considered as a better predictor of ovarian reserve compared to estradiol and inhibin B. Levels of AMH can be measured at anytime in the menstrual cycle. Therefore, understood that AMH is qualitative whereas AFC is a quantitative marker of ovarian reserve.

AFC is done by using TVS in early follicular phase in both the ovaries. AFC more than 7 (2-10 mm size) reflects adequate ovarian follicular reserve. AFC decreases with age. AFC reflects the primordial follicle pool in the ovary. AFC, less than 4 indicates poor ovarian reserve and there is poor response to ovarian stimulation (IVF).

Management Options for Ovarian Insufficiency (WHO Category-3)

- **Chance of conception from autologous cycles is remote** though spontaneous recovery of ovarian function (5-10%) and pregnancy has been reported.
- **Pretreatment with high dose estrogen and progesterone** or gonadotropin releasing hormone agonist (GnRH agonist) followed by ovulation induction with clomiphene or exogenous gonadotropins.
- **Pretreatment with corticosteroids** followed by induction ovulation with exogenous gonadotropins.
- **Therapy with dehydroepiandrosterone (DHEA)**: 25 mg three times daily for 5-6 months is thought to increase oocyte pool and successful pregnancy.
- **In vitro fertilization (IVF)** is an option with autologous oocyte, whenever available.
- Women in this group have few follicles left, which are unresponsive to chronically elevated levels of FSH. The above mentioned treatment regimens suppress the elevated level of FSH. The follicles are then reactivated with induction of new receptors. These receptors then respond to stimulation protocols for folliculogenesis and ovulation.
- **IVF with donor's oocyte** may be an option.
- **IVF and embryo transfer.**
- **Adoption.**

Hypothalamic-Pituitary Dysfunction (WHO Category-2)

Hypothalamic-pituitary dysfunction: Polycystic ovarian syndrome (PCOS) is the most common cause of ovulatory dysfunction.

Diagnostic criteria of PCOS (Rotterdam ESHRE/ASRM-2018)

1. Oligoovulation or anovulation (clinically presenting as oligomenorrhea or amenorrhea)
2. Hyperandrogenemia (clinical and/or biochemical)
3. Polycystic ovarian changes (other etiologies of hyperandrogenism like androgen secreting tumors, congenital adrenal hyperplasia) are to be excluded.

Presence of any two of the three above mentioned conditions fulfill the diagnostic criteria of PCOS.
Emphasis is given on the **far reaching consequences** of PCOS in all ages.

Two significant long-term consequences are:
1. **Metabolic syndrome**
   - Diabetes
   - Dyslipidemia—mostly in insulin resistant PCOS women
   - Hypertension (cardiovascular and coronary artery disease).
2. **Thrombophilic syndrome**
   - Coronary artery disease
   - Recurrent miscarriages.

Management issues in PCOS (irrespective of age)
- Early detection and prevention
- Change in lifestyle
- Calorie restriction
- Weight reduction.

Weight loss is essential while intending for fertility improvement. Weight loss can be achieved by exercise, decreased calorie consumption and lifestyle modification. Weight loss can also be achieved by pharmacologic agents and/or by surgery.

Significant **biochemical abnormalities** observed in PCOS are: Hyperinsulinemia (insulin resistance), hyperandrogenemia, hyperprolactinemia, hyperglycemia, hyperlipidemia, hypersecretion of LH and low serum SHBG levels. **Management of women PCOS can be optimized under three groups**—mild, moderate and severe, depending on their clinical, biophysical and biochemical presentation:

Group A (mild): Usually, these women are nonobese (normal BMI) and nonhirsute. Often they have delayed menstrual cycle. USG reveals ovarian size either normal or slightly enlarged but there is no thecal hyperplasia.

Management options: These groups respond well with clomiphene citrate. Depending upon the other investigations, they may need adjuvant therapy like bromocriptine, eltroxin or dexamethasone.

Group B (moderate): These women present with features of mild hirsutism (excess androgen levels) and mild obesity. Often these women suffer from oligomenorrhea. On transvaginal sonography (TVS), these women presents with enlarged ovaries with peripherally arranged cysts with stromal hyperplasia.

Management options
- Women still respond well with clomiphene citrate.
- However, better option for them is clomiphene citrate combined with insulin sensitizing agents like.
- **Metformin (oral biguanide)**, 500 mg three times a day for a period of 3-6 months.
- **Rosiglitazone (thiazolidinediones):** Rarely used, as it is a category 'C' drug in pregnancy.

Metformin acts by several mechanisms (*See* Ch 8).

Evidences are still lacking to support the therapy of metformin alone for ovulation induction. Combination of therapy of clomiphene with metformin is commonly recommended. There is no randomized control trial yet to support the continuation of metformin in pregnancy in women with PCOS in order to prevent miscarriage. However, metformin unlike thiazolidinedione group (rosiglitazone) appears safe when used during pregnancy especially in women with gestational diabetes mellitus (GDM). It is particularly recommended in patients with glucose intolerance. Metformin in this group of women, has been shown to improve ovulation rate though clinical pregnancy rate remains same.

Group C (Severe): These women are typically obese (BMI >25), stocky build. They have the family history of diabetes mellitus, they often suffer from secondary amenorrhea. They also present with the features of HAIR-AN syndrome. HAIR-AN syndrome is characterized by—hyperandrogenemia, insulin resistance and acanthosis nigricans. Transvaginal ultrasonography reveals—typical PCOS changes and ovarian stromal hyperplasia.

Management: Besides the general management issues, the specific management options for induction of ovulation are:
- Insulin sensitizing agents
- Clomiphene citrate plus metformin
- Insulin sensitizing agent plus ovarian drilling
- Aromatase inhibitors (letrozole, anastrozole) for induction of ovulation in clomiphene resistant women proved successful in 66–80%. Main concern with the use of letrozole is possible association of fetal congenital anomalies, though no such increased association has been observed when letrozole was compared with clomiphene citrate.

Gonadotropin (hMG/FSH): Anovulatory PCOS women, who fail to ovulate with oral medications, may be considered for exogenous gonadotropins. Women need to be monitored carefully. Low initial dose of FSH are generally given. Ovulation triggering with hCG is given when one or two follicles are 16–18 mm diameter. A serum E2 level per mature follicle of 100–150 pg/mL is optimum for monitoring.

Women with PCOS when treated with exogenous gonadotropin, run the high-risk of multiple pregnancy (36%), OHSS (4.6%) and cycle cancellation (10%). These complications are due to high number of antral follicular development.

Sequential use of clomiphene or aromatase inhibitors and exogenous gonadotropins is an alternative to avoid the complications of gonadotropin use. Combined treatment of GnRH agonist for down regulation followed by exogenous gonadotropins (hMG/FSH) is an alternative. The regimen may overcome the problems of premature luteinization of ovarian follicle and inadequate luteal phases. Women with PCOS may also require IVF.

Surgical treatment: Women with clomiphene resistant PCOS can be treated surgically by ovarian drilling. This surgical procedure reduces the ovarian androgen production and promotes ovulation. This procedure also minimizes the complications of exogenous gonadotropin therapy (multiple gestation and OHSS). Usually, laparoscopic drilling is done at 3–4 sites per ovary using electrodiathermy or laser. Results are similar to the use of exogenous gonadotropins. Cumulative ovulation rate within one year following laparoscopic ovarian drilling (LOD) is 52%. However, patients should be carefully selected for ovarian drilling.

Current Research and Management Options for Women with PCOS

Women who fail to respond with conventional management may be considered for other modes of therapy.
- Collection of immature oocytes using TVS
- *In vitro* maturation of these immature oocytes using an appropriate media
- Freezing the immature oocytes for future use.

Summary of Management Options for Women with PCOS

- ***First line management*** may be clomiphene citrate with or without adjuvant therapy insulin sensitizing agents.
- ***Clomiphene resistant women*** may be treated with exogenous gonadotropins with or without down regulation.
- ***Surgical management:*** LOD is an effective alternative in clomiphene citrate (CC) resistant cases. It is as effective as exogenous gonadotropins and has less complications compared to gonadotropins.
- ***Collection of immature oocytes*** for *in vitro* maturation and freezing for future use are the currently available options.

TUBAL FACTORS FOR INFERTILITY

Tubal factor is responsible for 25–40% of infertile women. The common causes tubal blocks are:
- Pelvic infections (PID) due to (a) *C. trachomatis, N. gonorrhoea*, (b) Tuberculosis, (c) Salpingitis isthmica nodosa. Risk of tubal block is as high as 75% after three episodes of PID
- Tubal polyps
- Mucus debris
- Pelvic endometriosis
- Previous tubal surgery or sterilization
- Tubal endometriosis.

Incidence and severity of pathology for tubal block rise with each episode of pelvic infection

Tuberculous salpingitis: Genital tuberculosis is almost always secondary to systemic tuberculosis. Common primary sites are lungs, lymph nodes, bones or gastrointestinal tract. Tubal affection of tuberculosis is almost 100%. Tubercular endosalpingitis (most common), interstitial salpingitis and perisalpingitis may occur (Fig. 21.1). Diagnosis of genital TB could be made by investigations for detection of systemic TB (*See* Dutta's Textbook of Gynecology, 8th Edition, p. 117). Menstrual blood or endometrial tissue for TB-PCR has got high sensitivity (85–95%). Tissue biopsy with endometrium or laparoscopically obtained peritoneal tubercles can be made. Genital TB has got poor reproductive outcome even following treatment. Failure of implantation and increased miscarriage rates are the consequences. Risks of ectopic pregnancy are high

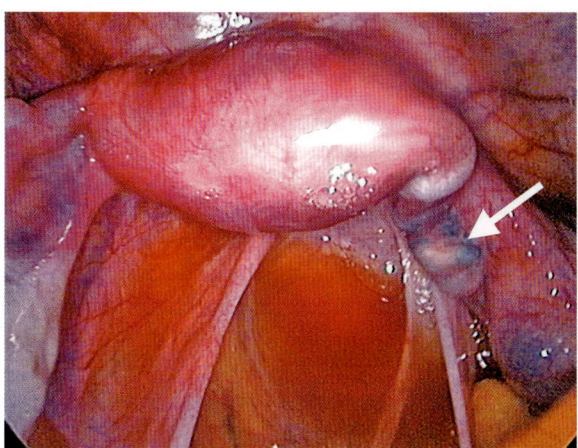

Fig. 21.1: Tuboperitoneal factors for infertility. Laparoscopic view of the pelvis showing bilateral tubal block due to tubercular salpingitis (based on laboratory tests). Dye is seen retained within both the tubes: tubes are dilated and adhesions are formed (arrow).

Courtesy: Dr H Ray, Patna

even if they conceive. Following successful chemotherapy, pregnancy can be achieved with the help of assisted reproductive technology (ART).

Tubal Patency Tests

Side and site of tubal block can be diagnosed by hysterosalpingography, laparoscopic chromopertubation, falloposcopy or with sonohysterosalpingography (less invasive).

Management Options for Tubal Factors for Infertility

In view of progressive success rate of ART, the place of tubal reconstructive surgery is gradually becoming less and less. However, there may be few situations where tubal reconstructive surgery may have a place.

Proximal tubal block is may be due to tubal mucosal adhesions, amorphous debris, cornual fibroid, fibrosis due to tuberculosis or mucosal polyp. It may be overcome with tubal cannulation under hysteroscopic guidance. A soft cannula is passed into the tubal ostia and a guidewire passed through contrast media (dye) is injected. Tubal patency (spillage of dye) could be seen simultaneously with laparoscopy. Successful pregnancy rate of proximal tubal cannulation is 20–40%.

Midtubal block is mainly due to tubal sterilization. Regret is not uncommon in India due to accidental death of all the children or that of the male child. Reversal of tubal sterilization can be done by laparotomy or by laparoscopy either by naked eye or by microsurgical procedures. Pregnancy rates following microsurgical procedure of tubal reconstructive surgery is around 60–80%. Risk of ectopic pregnancy is high (10%). The success of tubal reversal procedure depends on the following issues:
- Site of anastomosis—isthmic-isthmic or ampule-ampullary—better prognosis
- Lesser the interval between tubal sterilization and reversal procedure better the outcome
- Final reconstructed tubal length > 4 cm gives better result
- Lesser the tubal damage (use of rings or clips), better the outcome
- No other pelvic pathology.

Distal tubal block: It may be due to infection, adhesion formation with PID, endometriosis or previous surgery. Young patient with mild adhesions, normal tubal mucosa, may be considered for reconstructive surgery. Different surgical procedures are done depending on an individual patient. Tubal surgery may be—salpingolysis, adhesiolysis, salpingostomy, fimbrioplasty or resection-anastomosis.

Advantages of tubal surgery
- One time procedure
- Couple may attempt conception every month without further intervention
- May conceive more than once with a single surgery
- Avoid the risks of IVF like OHSS, multiple pregnancy.

Disadvantages of tubal surgery
- Surgical complications like infection, bleeding, anesthesia
- Risk of ectopic pregnancy
- Success depends significantly on surgeon's expertize.

Summary of tubal surgery
- Tubal surgery may be considered in young women after previous tubal sterilization or in women with mild disease at the distal tubal segment.
- Tubal surgery may tried for proximal tubal block (hysteroscopic tubal cannulation and balloon tuboplasty). Nearly 80% of cases obstruction can be relieved.
- In women having genital tuberculosis, surgery should be withheld. IVF-ET may be employed following antitubercular therapy when endometrium becomes free from disease.
- Elderly women (age >37 years) with tubal pathology should be considered for IVF.
- Women with complicated tubal occlusive disease are considered for IVF.
- ***Hydrosalpinx:*** IVF better option (following tubal clipping or salpingectomy).

IVF VERSUS REVERSAL OF TUBAL STERILIZATION

Intrauterine pregnancy rates following reversal of sterilization range between 31% and 92%. This is particularly high in women that they had been sterilized with microsurgical techniques.

IVF was originally developed to overcome the tubal factors for infertility. The success rate of IVF and ET on an average is 30–35% per IVF cycle (*See* Ch 23). In a women with intrauterine pregnancy following reversal of tubal sterilization, the rates of miscarriage and multiple pregnancy are lower compared to IVF. Ectopic pregnancy rates after surgical reversal (2–10%) are not acceptable. Women with age over 40 years, reversal of sterilization achieves a good intrauterine pregnancy (40–70%). It is about 90% in age (<40), whereas, success with IVF decreases after that age with a live birth rate of per treatment cycle is low (5.4%). Tubal anastomosis has significantly higher cumulative pregnancy rates for women <37 years compared to IVF, but no significant difference over 37 years.

PERITONEAL FACTORS FOR INFERTILITY (FIG. 21.1)

Endometriosis: Infertility management in women with endometriosis is complex. The pathophysiology of infertility in a woman with pelvic endometriosis has been (*See* Ch 10) observed due to multiple factors. It is mainly due to anatomic distortions, adhesions, associated endocrinopathy, presence of inflammatory mediators having gametotoxic effects or due to implantation failure.

Laparoscopy remains the gold standard for the diagnosis of endometriosis. It has the added benefit of therapy at the same time.

Management options: Determinant factors for the management are: (1) Age of the patient, (2) Stage of the disease (ASRM), (3) Severity of symptoms, (4) Results of previous therapy and (5) Location of the disease.

Hormonal suppression of endometriosis has hardly any effect on the outcome of endometriosis related infertility.

Laparoscopy: Ablation of endometriotic implants, adhesiolysis in mild and minimal pelvic endometriosis can significantly improve pregnancy rates. Intrauterine insemination (IUI) with ovarian stimulation is effective to improve fertility in women with minimal to mild endometriosis. Laparoscopic treatment of moderate endometriosis including removal of endometrioma can improve fertility status. Women may need ovulation induction with clomiphene citrate with or without exogenous gonadotropins. No randomized controlled trials or meta-analysis are available to support that surgical excision in cases with moderate to severe endometriosis, which enhances the pregnancy rates. However, majority of women with moderate to severe pelvic endometriosis are considered for IVF. Laparoscopic surgery is indicated prior to IVF as adhesions or endometrioma would interfere with oocyte retrieval. IVF may be the option after laparoscopic surgery, as a first line therapy depending upon the individual woman. Controversy remains as regard the ovarian reserve following ovarian surgery for endometrioma. Most recent evidence suggests for direct IVF without prior surgery.

UTERINE FACTORS FOR INFERTILITY

Uterine factors may be associated with infertility in about 10–15% of cases. *The pathology responsible for infertility are*: Submucous fibroids, uterine synechiae, congenital uterine malformations (unicornuate uterus, uterine septum, bicornuate uterus or uterine agenesis) or uterine polyps (Table 21.1).

Müllerian duct malformations may be responsible for infertility in about 10–37% of cases. These cases are often associated with urogenital malformations (40%). Müllerian malformations are also associated with recurrent early pregnancy loss.

Diagnosis of uterine cavity abnormalities can be made with hysteroscopy (gold standard), combined hysteroscopy and laparoscopy, hysterosalpingography, transvaginal ultrasonography (3D), sonohysterography or with magnetic resonance imaging (MRI). MRI is more informative compared to sonography for diagnosis of uterine malformations, fibroids and adenomyosis.

Management options: Surgical corrections improve obstetric outcome in few cases. Rudimentary horns are to be removed. Hysteroscopic metroplasty (septum resection) significantly improve the obstetric outcome.

Submucosal myomas and interstitial myomas impair fertility due to several reasons (*See* Dutta's Textbook of Gynecology, 8th Edition, p. 225) and mainly due to distortion of the endometrial cavity and poor implantation.

Surgery: Myomectomy (laparoscopic and/or hysteroscopic procedure) is recommended as a part of infertility treatment. Whether a myoma, not distorting the endometrial cavity, should be removed or not is not yet known.

Uterine synechiae: Overzealous curettage damaging the basal layer of the endometrium results in uterine wall adhesion formation with subsequent development of fibrosis. Endometrial tuberculosis, myomectomy, cesarean section, all may have the similar effect and can cause intrauterine adhesions

Table 21.1: Place of surgical interventions before ART.

Pathology	Treatment /Surgery	Method
Tube		
■ Hydrosalpinx	Salpingectomy/proximal tubal occlusion	Laparoscopically
Intrauterine		
■ Polyp (s)	■ Polypeptomy	
■ Adhesions	■ Synecholysis	Hysteroscopically
■ Septum	■ Resection	
■ Submucous fibroid	■ Myomectony	
Pelvis		
■ Pelvic endometriosis	Conservative surgery	Laproscopically

or Asherman's syndrome. Women usually give the history of surgical intervention. She usually presents with the problems of secondary amenorrhea, scanty period, secondary infertility or recurrent pregnancy loss. Diagnosis can be confirmed by hysterosalpingography or better with hysteroscopy. Intrauterine adhesions could be complete or partial.

Management: Adhesions could be released with hysteroscopic resection. Menstrual function and fertility status could be restored. Women suffering from synechiae due to endometrial tuberculosis usually have poor prognosis.

Postoperative management includes hormone therapy (estrogen and progesterone) for fresh endometrial growth. Combined therapy with hormones and placement of an IUCD to prevent re-adhesions may also be done. This therapy may be continued for 2–3 cycles.

UNEXPLAINED INFERTILITY

This group includes the couples in whom the basic infertility investigations have been completed and the reports revealed normal semen parameters, evidence of ovulation, patient fallopian tubes and there is no other obvious cause for infertility. Couples with unexplained infertility need counseling. They should be reassured that nearly 20% of such women will conceive in the next 12 months and over 50% in the next 36 months. **Nearly 10–20% of couples are diagnosed with unexplained infertility.**

Possible Explanations for Unexplained Infertility

- *Reduced endometrial vascularity:* Doppler ultrasound based studies have revealed that there is reduced and abnormal endometrial perfusion in women with unexplained infertility. However, no therapeutic approach has been made based on this observation as yet.
- *Unexplained male and female factors:* Sperm mitochondrial dysfunction, aberrant spindle formation or premature zona hardening are the areas thought to be responsible. However, these need further study.
- *Role of infection:* Subclinical endometrial infections have been thought for poor implantation. *Chlamydia trachomatis, M hominis, U urealyticum* infections may be associated. Prophylactic antibiotics (doxycycline 100 mg twice daily of 3–4 weeks) may be given to the couples with unexplained infertility.
- *Endometrial receptivity:* Besides reduced endometrial vascularity, endometrial receptivity including pinopode formation, biochemical expression of integrin and optimum endometrial genetic expression (HOXA genes) are thought to be inadequate in women with unexplained infertility.
- *Immunological:* Whether antisperm antibodies and other antibodies like antiphospholipid antibodies, antithyroid antibodies have any role, need further study. Till date no screening is recommended for this purpose.
- *Luteinized unruptured follicle (LUF) syndrome* is a known cause of infertility (20%) in women with unexplained infertility. In this condition, the follicle grows but undergoes luteinization before it ruptures and releases the oocyte. Mostly it can be diagnosed by transvaginal ultrasonography. These women should undergo IVF where follicles are aspirated. The oocytes are retrieved and fertilized *in vitro*.
- *Unexplained pelvic pathology:* Detection of undiagnosed pelvic endometriosis, adhesions may be made by laparoscopy. Whether the laparoscopic procedure has got any distinct advantage as a routine needs to be evaluated.

Possible causes of unexplained subfertility
■ Elderly woman (age > 35 years)
■ Low ovarian reserve
■ Poor oocyte quality
■ Tubal function defects
■ Implantation failure
■ Fertilization defects
■ Endometriosis (Ch 10)
■ Adenomyosis (Ch 12)
■ Immunological

Management Options for Unexplained Infertility

Young women are be counseled and advised for expectant management. However, some patients may need indepth investigations including laparoscopy. Women with unexplained infertility are treated stepwise as follows:
- With clomiphene citrate or letrozole for 3–4 cycles
- Then exogeneous gonadotropins for 3–4 cycles
- Followed by IUI or ART (*See* Ch 23).

ART Options for Unexplained Infertility Include IVF and ICSI

Baseline ovarian cyst: Baseline ultrasound scan is done on D2 or D3 of the cycle. Basal endometrium should be thin (< 4 mm) and the ovaries should be normal (without any cysts). Presence of functional ovarian cysts (> 2 cm) on baseline scan and baseline serum estradiol >80 pg/mL is associated with decreased pregnancy rate following ovulation induction with gonadotropins. Gonadotropin requirements are high. Embryo qualities are also poor.

Management: Pretreatment use of oral contraceptive prior to GnRH agonist cycle is associated with decreased rate of cyst formation.

Controlled ovarian stimulation (superovulation) is done to produce more than one egg for the purpose of either ART or non-ART cycles. This principle enhances the possibility of conception in women. Baseline USG scan is done on D2/D3 to assess the antral follicle count and to exclude the presence of any ovarian cysts. Clomiphene citrate and gonadotropins are started for induction of ovulation. In superovulation protocols, gonadotropins are started on D2/D3 of menses. The dose of gonadotropins are monitored each day until D6/D7 depending upon response. Thereafter, serum estradiol levels and TVS are done to monitor the ovarian response. Gonadotropin dose may need to be increased by 50–100 IU/day every 2–4 days until an optimum response is observed.

TABLE 21.2: Patient categorization in terms of treatment outcomes.

Parameters	Favorable	Unfavorable
Age	<37 years	>37 years
Duration of infertility	<7 years	>7 years
Type of defect	Single, treatable	Multiple, untreatable
Baseline FSH level	<10 mIU/mL	>10–12 mIU/mL
Basal antral follicle count	>6	<6
Pelvic adhesions/chocolate cyst	Minimum or none	Dense
Uterine shape and size	Normal	Deformed/Distorted
Previous failed IVF	None	>3

Triggering of ovulation is done when at least two follicles of 17–18 mm diameter are seen and endometrial thickness is ≥ 8 mm. For non-ART cycles serum E2 and TVS are monitored. Cycle cancellation should be considered if serum E2 level of 1000–2500 pg/mL for 3 or more follicles of 16 mm or more, or ≥ 2 follicles of 16 mm size plus ≥ 2 follicles of 14 mm diameter or more are seen. ***For ART (IVF) cycles ultrasound, monitoring alone of follicles are sufficient.***

Results: Pregnancy rates of unexplained infertility varies widely in studies. This may be due to heterogeneity in treatment protocols and also with patients' age. Overall pregnancy rates for women with unexplained infertility with age < 40 years when grouped by treatment protocol are as follows:

- Clomiphene or letrozole treatment protocol/IUI 10–12% per cycle
- Gonadotropins/IUI 15–20% per cycle
- IVF 30–35%.

Women with age ≥ 40 years should be offered IVF as a initial and early treatment option. ICSI may be a treatment option for these groups of women with unexplained infertility. ICSI improves fertilization rates. However, studies have shown no difference in pregnancy rates or live birth rate when treatment results of IVF and ICSI were compared. For management of women with unexplained infertility, optimum treatment options available are: Clomiphene/IUI for 3–4 cycles, failing which superovulation regimen with IUI or they may be considered directly for IVF.

Luteal phase defect (LPD): During normal luteal phase adequate progesterone secretion by the corpus luteum is observed. This promotes adequate development of secretory endometrium for blastocyst implantation. ***LPD is an inevitable phenomenon in all ART cycles.*** Induction of ovulation using gonadotropins may cause LPD due to supraphysiological levels of estradiol along with GnRH agonist or antagonist therapy. LPD may cause implantation failure and is thought to account for 4% of infertility. Diagnosis of LPD is not based on uniform criteria. Low levels of midluteal serum progesterone (<5 ng/mL), endometrial histology >2 day out of phase or a shortened luteal phase <14 days are considered for the diagnosis.

Treatment for Luteal Phase Defect

Progesterone supplementation can be given via oral, intramuscular or vaginal route. Progesterone in a dose 25–50 mg daily IM is given. Micronized progesterone given orally has erratic absorption rate and decreased bioavailability. It is given best vaginally 200–600 mg daily. Vaginal and IM route has got similar effect. Progesterone therapy is begun 3–4 days following the hCG trigger or LH surge and it is continued for next 7–10 weeks, if pregnancy occurs. Role of progesterone therapy in a non-ART treatment cycle is not clear (Table 21.2).

Suggested Reading

1. Giudice LC. Clinical Practice. Endometriosis. N Engl J Med. 2010;362(25):2389-98.
2. Jacobson TZ, Duffy JM, Barlow D, et al. Laparoscopic surgery for subfertility associated with endometriosis. Cochrane Database Syst Rev. 2010;1:CD001398.
3. Kwan I, Bhattacharya S, Mc Neil A, et al. Monitoring of stimulated cycles in assisted reproduction (IVF and ICSI). Cochrane Database Syst Rev. 2008;(2);CD005289.
4. Lainas T, Zorzovilis J, Petsas G, et al. In a flexible antagonist protocol, earlier, criteria-based initiation of GnRH antagonist is associated with increased pregnancy rates in IVF. Hum Reprod. 2005;20(9):2426-33.
5. Pritts EA, Parkar WH, Olive DL. Fibroids and infertility: An updated systematic review of the evidence. Fertil Steril. 2009;91(4):1215-23.
6. Rotterdam ESHRE/ASRM-Sponsored PCOS consensus workshop group. Revised 2003 consensus on diagnostic criteria and long-term health risks related to polycystic ovary syndrome (PCOS). Fertil Steril. 2004;81(1):19-25.
7. Sunkara SK, Khairy M, El-Toukhy T, et al. The effect of intramural fibroids without uterine cavity involvement on the outcome of IVF treatment: A systematic review and meta-analysis. Hum Reprod. 2010;25(2):418-29.
8. Tulandi T, Martin J, Al-Fadhli R, et al. Congenital malformations among 911 newborn conceived after infertility treatment with letrozole or clomiphene citrate. Fertil Steril. 2006;85(6):1761-5.
9. Vercellini P, Somigliana E, Viganò P, Abbiati A, Barbara G, Crosignani PG. Surgery for endometriosis-associated infertility: A pragmatic approach. Human Reprod. 2009;24(2):254-69.
10. Welt CK, Chan JL, Bullen J, et al. Recombinant human leptin in women with hypothalamic amenorrhea. N Engl J Med. 2004;351(10):987-97.

Chapter 22: Male Infertility

Q. Regarding male infertility:
a. Leydig cells are the site of spermatogenesis
b. Varicocele repair improves male infertility
c. GnRH therapy is effective for an infertile male due to Kallmann's syndrome
d. Low volume and low levels of fructose in semen suggest vasal agenesis
e. Asthenospermia is an indication for intracytoplasmic sperm injection (ICSI).

Ans.
a. F   b. F
c. T   d. T
e. T

MALE FACTORS FOR INFERTILITY

Male infertility may be due to:
- Defective spermatogenesis
- Obstruction in the efferent duct system
- Failure to deposit sperm in the vagina
- Errors in the seminal fluid analysis.

Male reproductive organs are: Testes, epididymis, vas deferens, prostate, seminal vesicles, ejaculatory duct, bulbourethral glands and urethra.

Two important cells in the testes are: **Leydig cells** and the **Sertoli cells**. Leydig cells produce androgens. Sertoli cells line the seminiferous tubules and, are the site of spermatogenesis.

Luteinizing hormone (LH) stimulates leydig cells for the synthesis of testosterone. Follicle stimulating hormone (FSH) act on the Sertoli cells to stimulate spermatogenesis. It also stimulates Sertoli cells to produce androgen binding proteins (ABP) and inhibin-B. Spermatogenesis and sperm maturation need a high androgenic environment.

Spermatogenesis is controlled predominantly by the genes located on Y chromosome. Approximately, 75 days are required to complete the process of spermatogenesis (from spermatogonia stem cells to the mature sperm cells). Additional 12–20 days are needed for spermatozoa to travel the epididymis.

Basic semen analysis measures semen volume, sperm concentration, sperm motility and sperm morphology. WHO (2010) revised the normal values for semen analysis (*See* Dutta's Textbook of Gynecology, 8th Edition, p. 192).

MANAGEMENT OPTIONS FOR MALE INFERTILITY

- ***Medical treatment for male infertility*** (effective in few cases)
  - Infective causes (STIs)
  - Thyroid disorders
  - Endocrine causes (*See* Dutta's Textbook of Gynecology, 8th Edition, p. 189).

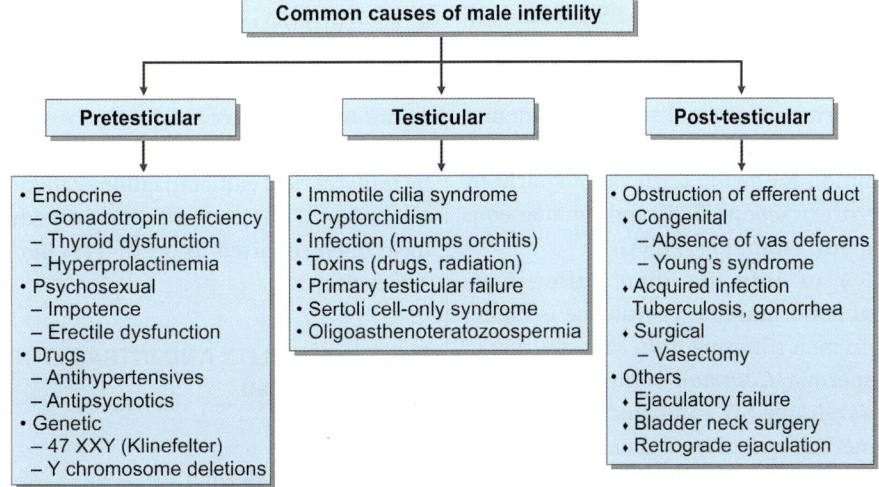

(*See* Dutta's Textbook of Gynecology, 8th Edition, p. 189)

- **Male infertility not due to azoospermia**
  - *Exogenous testosterone* should not be given for male subfertility because it decreases spermatogenesis due to negative feedback inhibition of the pituitary.
  - *Antioxidant food supplement:* Glutathione, carnitine and vitamin E do not affect semen parameters but administration of zinc and folic acid have been shown to be associated with improved sperm concentration and morphology.
  - *Varicocele repair:* It may affect male fertility due to rise in testicular temperature, reflux of toxic metabolites from left adrenal or left renal veins or due to high reactive oxygen species. Treatment is done by surgical repair (varicocelectomy) or percutaneous embolization. It is not certain that varicocele repair improves male fertility status. Varicocelectomy is recommended in grade 3 cases associated with infertility.
- **Male infertility due to azoospermia**
  Azoospermia classification and treatment: 1% of all men and 15–20% of infertile men are found to be suffering from azoospermia.
  - *Pretesticular azoospermia:* The important causes are hypogonadotropic hypogonadism. **Investigation to be done are:** Serum LH (↓), FSH (↓), testosterone (↓) levels. Pituitary imaging may be needed.
    Treatment options are: Pulsatile gonadotropin-releasing hormone (GnRH), human chorionic gonadotropin (hCG) and exogenous gonadotropin therapy.
  - *Testicular azoospermia:* Important causes are (*See* Dutta's Textbook of Gynecology, 8th Edition, p. 189) genetic (Y chromosome deletions), infections (mumps), primary testicular failure, oligoastheno-teratozoospermia and developmental (cryptorchidism).
    Management options
    - In individuals having hypergonadotropic hypogonadism (raised levels of FSH and LH), testicular biopsy is not helpful. Donor sperm may be considered.
    - Men having normal hormonal results—testicular biopsy may be done. If sperm is present in biopsy, ICSI is the option following retrieval of sperm by testicular sperm extraction (TESE) and percutaneous epididymal sperm aspiration (PESA).
    - About 5–15% of infertile men suffer from chromosomal abnormalities. Prevalence is higher in (10–15%) in men suffering from azoospermia or severe oligospermia. *Common abnormalities are:* Klinefelter's syndrome (47 XXY), microdeletions of Y chromosome. These men need genetic counseling as the microdeletions can be transmitted to the male offspring following *in vitro* fertilization (IVF)/ICSI.
  - *Post-testicular azoospermia:* Common causes are congenital absence of vas deferens (cystic fibrosis), obstruction due to infection (tuberculosis, gonorrhea) or vasectomy. About 40% of azoospermic men have obstructive pathology which again may be congenital bilateral absence of vas deferens (CBAVD) or infective etiology. Men with normal gonadotropin and testosterone level having low volume ejaculation should be tested for postejaculatory urine analysis.

Treatment: Men suffering from diabetes or past history of bladder neck or prostate surgery, suffer from the problem of retrograde ejaculation. Sperm received from neutralized urine of men can be processed for assisted reproductive technology (ART) or insemination. Men suffering from bilateral or unilateral vasal agenesis should have renal imaging as the association of renal agenesis is 10–25%. Men with CBAVD suffer seminal vesicle agenesis. So, they have low semen volume, low pH, and low fructose levels. Spermatogenesis is normal in such a male. About 75% of men with CBAVD have mutation of cystic fibrosis transmembrane regulator gene (CFTR). Men with CBAVD should have their female partner's carrier status tests done.

Vasectomy reversal: It can be done successfully and subsequent pregnancy rate is about 80–100%. Microsurgical methods of vasovasostomy or vasoepididymostomy are effective. The time interval between vasectomy and reversal is an important determinant for success of surgery and pregnancy. Longer the interval, poorer is the result.

INFERTILITY AND INTRAUTERINE INSEMINATION (IUI)

Indications

- Oligospermia (mild)
- Asthenospermia (mild)
- Immune factor (male and female)
- Male factor (impotency, hypospadias)
- Hostile cervical mucus
- Unexplained infertility.

Intrauterine Insemination

About 0.3–0.5 mL of washed, processed and concentrated motile sperm (5–10 million) is pushed into the uterine cavity by transcervical catheterization. Patient should be in bed for about 15–20 minutes after the procedure. Pregnancy rates have been reported to be 10–11% per cycle and 40% after 4–6 cycle.

MALE INFERTILITY AND INTRACYTOPLASMIC SPERM INJECTION (ICSI)

Indications

- Severe oligospermia
- Asthenospermia, teratospermia

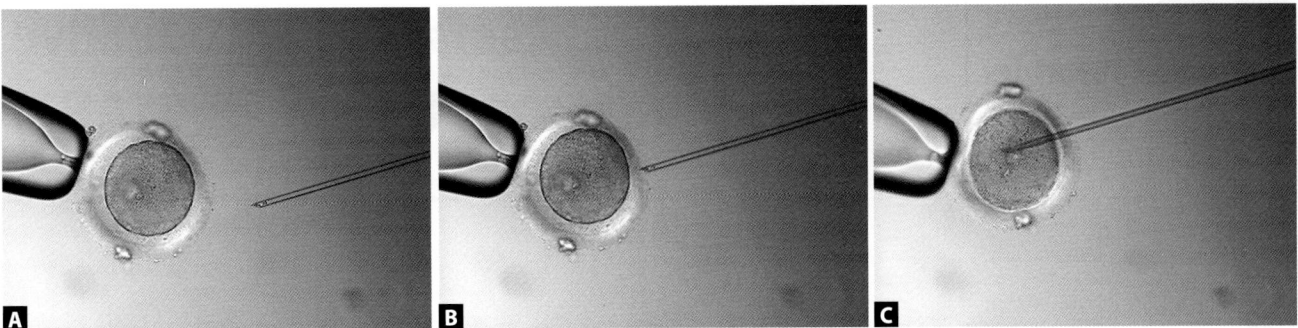

Figs. 22.1A to C: Intracytoplasmic sperm injection (ICSI) procedure: (A) The holding (left) and the injecting (right) pipettes are seen; (B) The oolemma is penetrated; (C) The injection pipette has reached nearly the center of the oocyte.

- Obstruction of efferent duct system (male)—obstructive azoospermia
- CBAVD
- Failure of IVF
- Unexplained infertility.

Methods of Sperm Recovery

- Microsurgical epididymal sperm aspiration (MESA)
- Percutaneous epididymal sperm aspiration
- Testicular sperm extraction
- Testicular sperm aspiration (TESA).

Fertilization rate of ICSI is about 70–80% and clinical pregnancy rate around 40%. Success rate of ICSI following sperm retrieval in obstructive azoospermia is 30–60%. Men with obstructive azoospermia need counseling as regard the transmission of genetic disorder to their offspring.

ICSI (Figs. 22.1A to C): ICSI is associated with higher congenital anomaly risk (4.2%) when compared with conventional IVF (2–3%).

Donor insemination: Men with azoospermia who do not desire ART, donor insemination is an effective alternative.

Suggested Reading

1. Practice Committee of American Society for Reproductive Medicine. Report on varicocele and infertility. Fertil Steril. 2008;90(5 Suppl):S247-9.
2. Practice Committee of American Society for Reproductive Medicine in Collaboration with Society for Male Reproduction and Urology. Evaluation of the azoospermic male. Fertil Steril. 2008;90(5 Suppl):S74-7.
3. Practice Committee of American Society for Reproductive Medicine; Practice Committee of Society for ART. Genetic considerations related to ICSI. Fertil Steril. 2008;90(5 Suppl):S182-4.

Chapter 23: Assisted Reproductive Technology (ART)

MCQs

Q.1 Regarding use of gonadotropin for controlled ovarian stimulation (COS):
a. Gonadotropin stimulation could be done either using follicle-stimulating hormone (FSH) or human menopausal gonadotropin (HMG)
b. Monitoring with serum estradiol levels with transvaginal ultrasound is essential in all assisted reproductive technology (ART) cycles
c. Less aggressive stimulation increases cycle cancellation rates
d. Pretreatment therapy with combined oral contraceptives (COCs) reduces pregnancy rates
e. Supportive treatment in women with polycystic ovarian syndrome (PCOS) may prevent ovarian hyperstimulation syndrome (OHSS)

Ans. a. T   b. F
c. F   d. F
e. T

Q.2 Use of gonadotropin-releasing hormone (GnRH) analogs and ART cycles:
a. GnRH agonists cause immediate down regulation
b. GnRH agonists long protocols have better pregnancy rates
c. GnRH antagonist use results of higher pregnancy rate
d. Daily dose GnRH agonists have higher pregnancy rate
e. GnRH analogs suppress premature luteinizing hormone (LH) surge

Ans. a. F   b. T
c. F   d. T
e. T

Table 23.1: Commonly used GnRH analogs.

GnRH analog	Route of administration	Dose
Agonists		
• Leuprorelin	• IM/SC	• 3.75 mg/vial, prefilled syringe once every 4 weeks
• Goserelin	• SC	• 3.6 mg in syringe applicator, once in every 4 weeks
• Nafarelin	• Nasal spray	• 200 µg/metered spray One spray in each nostril BID
• Buserelin	• Nasal spray	• 150 µg/metered spray One nasal spray QDS
	• Injection	• 1 mg/mL; 5.5 mL/vial; 200-500 µg SC/OD
Antagonists		
• Cetrorelix	• IM	• 250 µg OD
• Ganirelix	• IM	• 250 µg OD

Table 23.2: Commonly used gonadotropins in ART procedures.

Gonadotropin	Mode of administration
■ Human menopausal gonadotropin (hMG)	Injection
♦ Menotropin (FSH: LH = 1:1)	SC/IM
♦ Urofollitropin (purified hMG containing FSH)	SC/IM
■ **Recombinant gonadotropins**	Injection
■ Follitropin α (r-FSH)	SC/IM
♦ Lutropin α (r-LH)	SC
♦ Follitropin α with lutropin α (r- FSH/LH)	SC/IM
♦ hCG	SC/IM
♦ Recombinant hC	SC

Q.3 In ART cycles:
a. Blastocyst transfer has lower implantation failure
b. Three embryo transfer is optimum in women age, < 35 years
c. Embryo cryopreservation facilitates the multiple transfer cycles from single oocyte retrieval
d. Overall success rates of fertility treatment following *in vitro* fertilization (IVF) and embryo transfer (ET) is 35%
e. Live birth (LB) rate per cycle from donor oocyte depends on recipient's age

Ans. a. T   b. F
c. T   d. T
e. F

ART encompasses all the procedures that involve manipulation of gametes outside the body for the treatment of infertility. The procedures are exclusively carried out in tertiary care unit.

Currently Practiced ARTs
- *In vitro* fertilization and embryo transfer (IVF-ET)
- Intracytoplasmic sperm injection (ICSI)
- Intrauterine insemination (IUI).

By strict criteria of definition, IUI is not included under the heading of ART, as the procedure does not involve in direct retrieval of oocytes from the ovaries. However, extracorporeal male gamete manipulation and superovulation of the female partner is involved in this procedure. Considering these issues, majority of the IVF clinics consider IUI as one of the technologies of assisted reproduction. **Other procedures of ART** are—gamete intrafallopian transfer (GIFT), zygote intrafallopian transfer (ZIFT), subzonal insemination (SUZI) and peritoneal oocyte and sperm transfer (POST).

GnRH agonist: It has long half-life and increased receptor binding affinity. Initial 7 days of administration, GnRH agonist exerts a flare effect due to upregulation of GnRH receptors. This is followed by receptor desensitization resulting in fall in the level of gonadotropins (down regulation). Ultimately with prolonged use, GnRH agonist induces menopause-like state (low estradiol levels).

GnRH agonist are available either depot or daily use. Intramuscular/subcutaneous (IM/SC) or intranasal route can be used. The GnRH agonist protocols may be long or short. Long protocols may again be *long follicular or long luteal down regulation*.

In long luteal down regulation protocol, GnRH agonist is started in the luteal phase, D21 of the previous cycle (*See* Dutta's Textbook of Gynecology, 8th Edition, p. 207). After 10–14 days of GnRH agonist therapy on D2 of subsequent menstrual cycle (whichever is earlier), a pelvic ultrasound and serum estradiol levels are done to confirm suppression. Thereafter, gonadotropin stimulation is begun. *Use of single-dose depot GnRH agonist is associated with higher gonadotropin (dose and duration) requirement and has lower pregnancy rates when compared with daily GnRH agonist formulation*.

GnRH antagonist (Cetrorelix, ganirelix) (*See* Dutta's Textbook of Gynecology, 8th Edition, Ch 32, p. 442): GnRH antagonists have no agonist action. Suppression to GnRH receptor and desensitization effect is immediate. There is immediate suppression of FSH and LH. GnRH antagonist is started on D4–D7 of stimulation in ART cycles. This schedule reduces the risks of premature LH surge. This also allows endogenous FSH-mediated follicular recruitments prior to GnRH suppression.

GnRH antagonists: Protocols may be fixed or flexible.
- ***Fixed protocol*** uses the antagonist on D4, D5, D6 or D7 of stimulation irrespective of follicular growth
- ***Flexible protocol:*** Antagonist is used when the leading follicle has reached 12–16 mm or when serum estradiol level has reached above 600 pg/mL.

Table 23.3: Steps of assisted reproductive technology.

- Patient counseling and selection
- **Pituitary down regulation**
- Pretreatment therapy with COCs to synchronize follicular growth and to prevent ovarian cysts
- Controlled ovarian stimulation
  - GnRH analog down regulation followed by gonado-tropin stimulation
- Ovulation triggering with human chorionic gonadotropin (hCG) or GnRH agonist
- Oocyte retrieval
- Insemination (IVF or ICSI)
- *In vitro* embryo culture in nutrient media and incubation in CO_2 incubator
  - Embryo transfer (not more than 3) back into mother's uterus between D2 and D5 at the cleaving embryo (4–8 cell) stage or blastocyst stage (Fig. 23.2)
  - Cryopreservation of surplus embryos
- Luteal support mostly with micronized progesterone
- Serum β-hCG estimation D14 postembryo transfer.

Till date, there is no randomized control trial to establish the superiority of one protocol over the other. However, most of the centers have shifted to the antagonist protocol. ***Advantages are:*** (a) Shorter duration of therapy and (b) Simplicity of protocol.

Other protocols are flare, ultrashort, microdose and modified natural.

Comparison of GnRH Agonists to GnRH Antagonists

(*See* Dutta's Textbook of Gynecology, 8th Edition, Ch 32, p. 442)
Use of GnRH antagonist is associated with lower duration of stimulation, lower dose of gonadotropins and reduced rates of OHSS. According to 27 randomized controlled trials (RCTs), both the regimens have similar rates of production of good quality embryos. However, clinical pregnancy rates are higher by 4.7% in agonist compared to antagonist cycles.

What is Early LH surge? How it Causes Premature Follicular Luteinization?

Due to high estradiol level in early follicular phase (as a consequence of gonadotropin stimulation), early LH surge occurs. GnRH agonist or antagonist is used to suppress it. Spontaneous ovulation prior to oocyte retrieval is observed in about 16% of nonsuppressed cycles. Premature LH surge occurs usually 5–7 days after starting follicular stimulation. Overall premature luteinization has been observed in 7–35% of cases. The possible mechanism of premature luteinization are: (a) Incomplete pituitary desensitization, (b) increased receptor sensitivity of granulosa cells to LH, (c) innate poor responder and (d) total amount of progesterone secreted from multiple follicles equals to the late follicular phase.

The main ***disadvantage of premature luteinization*** is endometrial advancement. Adverse effect on quality of oocyte or embryo has not been remarkably observed.
The different measures to overcome the problems of premature follicular luteinization are:
- Triggering ovulation at the appropriate time
- Using less aggressive stimulation protocols
- Cryopreservation of oocytes and embryos
- Use of antiprogesterone (mifepristone) at the time when hCG is given (less commonly used procedure).

Follicular growth and maturation: Initial growth of preantral and small antral follicles is independent of any hormone. Small antral follicles > 2 mm become responsive to FSH stimulation. The follicles become recruitable in the late luteal phase of the cycle. Preceding ovulation, FSH induces the receptors for LH on the granulosa cells once the antral follicle attains the size of 10 mm or more. At that state, LH can induce FSH-like actions on the granulosa cells (contrary to the 2-cell, 2-gonadotropin theory) and also stimulate the enzyme aromatase. Human menstrual cycles have two waves of follicular development. The ***first wave*** is the minor wave that occurs immediately after the ovulation in the preceding cycle. Once progesterone is available following ovulation, all the follicles, except the dominant one, undergo atresia. The subsequent wave is the ***major wave*** that occurs during the time of menstruation of the previous cycle. During this time, the dominant follicle is selected and other follicles are deprived of their growth. The follicle having the maximum number of FSH receptors and higher level of E2—androgen ratio in the follicular microenvironment is recruited as the dominant one. The dominant follicle is recruited by the cycle D6 or D7 which coincides with an estradiol rise that inhibits FSH.

Controlled ovarian stimulation (COS): Synchronous growth of dominant and codominant follicle(s) is achieved by gonadotropin stimulation. The main hormone in this process is the FSH. Most investigators suggest that the optimum number of retrieved oocytes in a given cycle is between 5 and 15. The optimal level of estradiol at the time of hCG administration is between 70 and 140 pg/mL per follicle. Estradiol monitoring ***may not be that essential in the ART cycle. Ultrasound monitoring alone may be adequate to maximize pregnancy and live birth rates.***

Cycle cancellation in normal responders occurs in up to 6% of the cycles because of inadequate response. Cycle cancellation increases with advancing age and is decreased with ovarian reserve. It can be minimized by increasing the dose of gonadotropins. However, maximum upper limit of gonadotropin dose is 450 IU beyond which no benefit is observed.

Gonadotropin stimulation could be done either using FSH or with HMG: A systematic review of 14 RCTs found no significant differences between HMG and urinary FSH in rates per cycle pregnancy, multiple pregnancy, miscarriage, ovulation or hyperstimulation. However, risk of OHSS was less with FSH compared to HMG. Similarly, no significant difference in the outcome was observed when urinary FSH was compared with recombinant FSH.

However, recent studies have shown that HMG use is associated with higher androgen and lower progesterone levels on the day of hCG trigger for ovulation. This indicates a more favorable endocrine profile with HMG compared to FSH.
Less aggressive stimulation reduces cycle cancellation rate: The problems of premature luteinization and lower pregnancy rates are encountered when more aggressive FSH stimulation protocols are used. ***COCs given for 28 days prior to GnRH analogs, can give some benefits.*** It helps in cycle regularity, synchronizes follicular development, prevents premature LH surge, reduces the incidence of ovarian cysts and hyperstimulation syndrome. More importantly, ***it reduces the cycle cancellation.***

Therapy schedule of COCs for antagonist cycles: COS is to begin 2–5 days after stopping of COCs (irrespective of menses). For long agonist protocols, the agonist overlaps the last 5 days of COC pills followed by start of COS on D2 or D3 of withdrawal bleeding. ***COCs pretreatment during GnRH agonist cycles is associated with higher pregnancy rates.***

Supportive medications have been used with some benefits. Prophylactic antibiotics (doxycycline or azithromycin) are of help when subclinical infection is thought of. Glucocorticoids during peri-implantation period may improve pregnancy rates in women with autoimmune disease, assisted hatching or with advanced age. Metformin has been shown to prevent ovarian hyperstimulation (OHSS) in PCOS patients and is of benefit.

Growth and maturation of oocyte and ovulation (Figs. 23.1A and B): In natural cycle, meiosis-I is completed just before ovulation. The oocyte will extrude the first polar body and the oocyte-cumulus complex will detach from the ovarian wall and ovulation will occur.

Ovulation triggering in ART: It is done when at least two follicles are 17–18 mm or larger in diameter (but <24 mm), with endometrial thickness 8 mm or more is observed. Recombinant hCG 250 μg SC or urinary hCG 10,000 IU is given. When there is the risks of OHSS, GnRH agonist can be given in place of hCG in antagonist protocol or recombinant LH can be given for hCG in agonist protocol.

Oocyte retrieval is performed by transvaginal ultrasound-guided needle aspiration. Each follicle is punctured and the follicular fluid is aspirated. In Kolkata, Institute of Reproductive Medicine protocol, intravenous conscious sedation is used. Prophylactic antibiotic (augmentin and metronidazole) is given. Oocyte retrieval is usually done 34–36 hours after the hCG injection. Luteal support is started after embryo transfer.

In vitro fertilization insemination: 100,000–800,000 motile sperm/mL per oocyte is used. Processed sperm are incubated in media for 3–4 hours for sperm capacitation and acrosome reaction. Before insemination, retrieved oocytes are cultured in media.

Embryo culture: Assessment of embryo development is done after 15–20 hours of insemination or ICSI. Fertilization is characterized by the presence of two pronuclei and extrusion of second polar body. After another 24–30 hours, embryos are examined for cleavage. ***First embryo cleavage*** occurs about 21 hours after the fertilization, subsequent divisions occur every 12–15 hours up to the 8 cell stage on 3rd day of embryo development. Compaction to form the 16 cell morula occurs on 4th day of embryo development. Blastocyst formation with differentiation of inner cell mass and trophectoderm is completed on D5 or D6.

Blastocyst transfer is observed to have lower implantation failure, higher pregnancy rate and higher live birth rate (32–42%) than cleavage stage transfer.

Embryo Morphology and Selection of Embryo for Transfer

Cleavage stage embryo with normal development is characterized by—early cleavage (2 cells) on D1, 4 cells on D2, and 8 cells on D3. ***About 10% or less number of blastomeres should have fragmentation***.

The ***blastomere size*** should be regular and there should be no multinucleation. Scoring of blastocysts: ***Scale 1 (worst) to scale 6 (best)***, is done by Gardner and Schoolcraft. The trophectoderm in a grade 6 blastocyst has completely escaped or hatched from the zona. Similarly, the ***inner cell mass is graded from A to C*** depending upon tightness and cellularity (A is the best). Trophectoderm is graded from A to C based on cohesiveness and cellularity (A is the best) (Figs. 23.2A to D).

Morphological Assessment of Embryo Quality

A good quality embryo is considered with the following morphological characters:
- All the blastomeres' size and shape should be almost equal
- Blastomeres should occupy almost whole of the space within the zona pellucida
- There should be no multinucleation
- The blastomeres should appear transparent with clear cytoplasm (less fragmentation).

Number of embryos to be transferred: It is not a uniform one. Current guidelines indicate 1–3 embryos to be transferred depending on age of the patient. This is done to

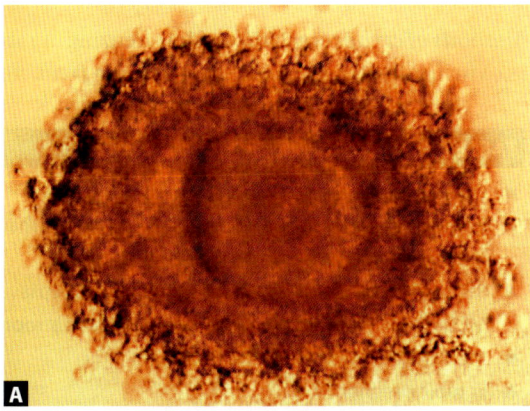 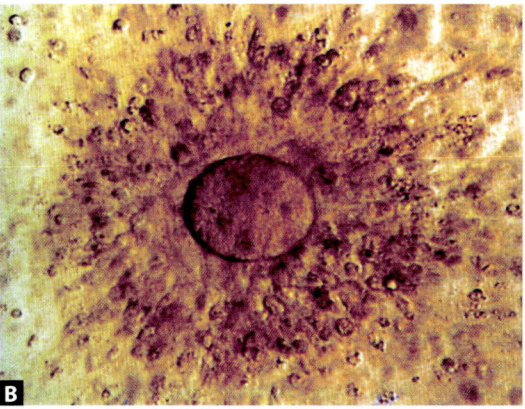

Figs. 23.1A and B: (A) ***Very immature oocyte:*** Tightly packed cumulus and corona, granular ooplasm, presence of germinal vesicle and absence of first polar body (FPB); (B) ***Mature oocyte:*** Well-expanded cumulus, sun burst-like corona, clear ooplasm and FPB in perivitelline space (PVS).

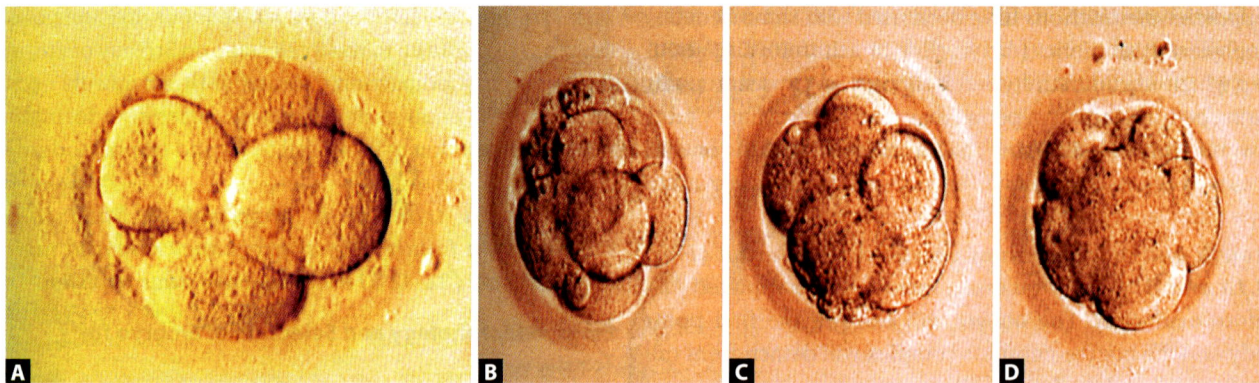

Figs. 23.2A to D: Embryos are divided into four types depending upon the extent of fragmentation. **Type-A** is the best and **Type-D** is the worst.
Type-A: Minimal volume of fragmentation associated with one blastomere.
Type-B: Localized fragmentation mainly occupying the periphery of the blastomeres.
Type-C: Small fragmentation speckled in all the blastomeres over the embryo.
Type-D: Large volume of fragmentation in all the blastomeres.

TABLE 23.4: Factors determining the treatment outcomes of ART.	
Factor(s)	Outcomes
Age	Advance age of the woman reduces fertility and ART success
Past obstetric history	Prior pregnancy increases the success rate
Ovarian reserve	AMH and AFC can predict the response rate of COS
Number of oocytes	Higher the number of oocytes retrieved (15–20), higher the live birth rate
Embryo quality	Better the embryo quality higher the live birth (LB) rate
Number of embryo transferred	Double embryo transfer increases LB rate and multiple births

avoid risks of multiple pregnancies and the complications thereof. Single embryo transfer should be considered for younger patients (age <35 years). Usually, these women have large quantity of good quality embryos. Otherwise, two embryo transfers may be optimum. For women with advanced age, maximum number of cleavage stage embryo transfer could be three (age >35 years) (Table 23.5).

Embryo transfer procedure: It is aimed to deliver the embryos transcervically, safely in an atraumatic manner, within the endometrial cavity for implantation. It is performed using a soft catheter. It is done to deposit the embryos at a level of about 0.5–1.0 cm below the uterine fundus. Transfer under ultrasound guidance may be helpful. Currently, multiple meta-analysis have shown ultrasonography (USG)-guided ET improves clinical pregnancy rates and implantation rates. Most centers now do the ET under USG guidence.

Cryopreservation of Embryos/Oocytes

Embryo cryopreservation can be done at (a) pronuclear, (b) cleavage stage and also at (c) blastocyst stage.

Benefits

- Multiple transfer cycles from single oocyte retrieval
- Pregnancy rates following cryopreserved embryos are nearly similar or marginally less
- Fertility treatment can be optimized significantly
- Reduces treatment cycle complications, OHSS, and failure rates.

Like any other treatment, ART procedures carries certain risks. ART procedures are associated with some short-term and long-term complications for the mother and the baby (Table 23.6).

Methods of cryopreservation: Slow freezing or rapid freezing (or vitrification) are two methods. **Slow freezing** protocols

TABLE 23.5: Number of embryo transfer [American Society for Reproductive Medicine (ASRM-2013)].	
Age (years)	Embryo transfer
<35	1 (maximum 2)
35–37	2 (maximum 3)
38–40	3 (maximum 4)
41–42	5

TABLE 23.6: Adverse effects of ART treatment.
- Ovarian hyperstimulation syndrome
- Complications following oocyte retrieval: hemorrhage, infection, injury to adjacent viscera
- Risks following surgical procedures of sperm retrieval (PESA, MESA, or TESA): Infection, bleeding, testicular atrophy
- Multiple pregnancy
- Ectopic pregnancy
- Congenital malformations of children
- Borderline ovarian tumor.

take longer time and concentration of cryoprotectants is less. ***Vitrification*** uses high concentration of cryoprotectants and rapid cooling. It is less expensive and has higher postthaw embryo survival. Embryo thawing is done by brief exposure to air and warm water followed by rehydration. ***Pregnancy rates following frozen embryos are lower compared to fresh transfer cycles.*** This again may be due to embryo selection as best embryos are selected for fresh transfer.

Endometrial preparation for frozen embryo transfer (FET): In natural cycle, no exogenous treatment is needed for the recipient. Transfer is timed to spontaneous ovulation. Otherwise estradiol supplementation is started in early follicular phase and is continued for 13–15 days till endometrial thickness of 8 mm is obtained. Endometrial thickness is measured with transvaginal ultrasound. Progesterone supplementation begins 48–72 hours prior to transfer of cleavage state embryo. Blastocysts are thawed 5–6 days prior to transfer. GnRH agonists are sometimes used in medicated cycles to prevent premature LH surge, which may affect the endometrial maturation adversely.

Luteal support: LH is essential for morphological development and functional activity of the corpus luteum. Corpus luteum is the main source of progesterone. Progesterone is essential for endometrial growth, implantation and early pregnancy growth and maintenance. During the ART procedures ovarian stimulation protocol is used (discussed above). There is formation of multiple corpora lutea, which produce excessive amount of steroid hormones. LH secretion is reduced due to negative feedback mechanism of the steroid hormones. There is premature luteolysis. Therefore, progesterone replacement therapy is essential in the luteal phase to improve the live birth rate. This is no significant difference between the different routes of progesterone supplementation through vaginal route is preferred by many.

Success rates of fertility treatment: Overall success rates are follows—clomiphene citrate (CC) and timed intercourse (TI): 3–17%; IUI, CC and IUI: 10–14%; Gonadotropins and IUI: 15–20% and IVF success: clinical pregnancy rate/cycle for age <35 years: 31–46%.

Donor Oocyte

Indications of pregnancy from donor oocytes
- Woman with ovarian failure
- Poor ovarian response to stimulation
- Poor oocyte quality (as in advanced age)
- Repeated failure of fertilization
- Failure of implantation after multiple ART
- Inherited genetic disorders.

Live birth (LB) rate per cycle of donor oocyte IVF are 50% regardless of the recipient's age. Oocyte recipient needs to undergo endometrial preparation (described above). At present, donor oocytes must be used to create embryos during the retrieval cycle (as oocyte freezing is considered experimental till date).

ART is accepted as an useful and a relatively safe procedure for the couples with infertility. Complications (both short-term and long-term) are not uncommon (Table 23.6). Success rates of ART vary significantly among the centers. Many a times, the reasons for unsuccessful outcomes are unclear. Unsuccessful outcomes, often have a devastating negative impact both psychologically and financially upon the couple and the family members. Healthcare professionals providing ART treatment should understand the limitations of the treatment and the result. The couple should therefore be counselled appropriately before, during and after the course of treatment.

Suggested Reading

1. Abbara A, Jayasena CN, Christopoulos G, Narayanaswamy S, Izzi-Engbeaya C, Nijher GM, et al. Efficacy of Kisspeptin-54 to Trigger Oocyte Maturation in Women at High Risk of Ovarian Hyperstimulation Syndrome (OHSS) During In Vitro Fertilization (IVF) Therapy. J Clin Endocrinol Metab. 2015;100(9):3322-31.
2. Blake DA, Farquhar CM, Johnson N, et al. Cleavage stage versus blastocyst stage embryo transfer in assisted conception. Cochrane Database Syst Rev. 2007;4:CD002118.
3. Centers for disease controls and prevention (2016). 2007 assisted reproductive technology success rates [online] CDC website. Available from http://www.cdc.gov/art/ART 2007/PDF/Complete.2007_ART.pdf.
4. Cissen M, Wely MV, Scholten I, Mansell S, Bruin JP, Mol BW, et.al. Measuring Sperm DNA Fragmentation and Clinical Outcomes of Medically Assisted Reproduction: A Systematic Review and Meta-Analysis, PLoS One. 2016;10;11:e0165125.
5. Daya S. Follicle-stimulating hormone and human menopausal gonadotropin for ovarian stimulation in assisted reproductive cycles. Cochrane database Syst Rev. 2009;1.
6. Fleming R, Seifer DB, Frattarelli JL, Ruman J. Assessing ovarian response: antral follicle count versus anti-Müllerian hormone. Reprod Biomed Online. 2015;31:486-96.
7. Hansen M, Kurinczuk JJ, Milne E, de Klerk N, Bower C. Assisted reproductive technology and birth defects: a systematic review and meta-analysis. Hum Reprod Update. 2013;19(4):330-53.
8. Hargreave M, Jensen A, Toender A, Andersen KK, Kjaer SK. Fertility treatment and childhood cancer risk: a systematic meta-analysis. Fertil Steril. 2013;100(1):150-61.
9. Kwan I, Bhattacharya S, Woolner A. Monitoring of stimulated cycles in assisted reproduction (IVF and ICSI). Cochrane Database Syst Rev. 2021;12;4:CD005289.
10. La Marca A, Sunkara SK. Individualization of controlled ovarian stimulation in IVF using ovarian reserve markers: from theory to practice. Hum Reprod Update. 2014;20:124-40.
11. Leung ASO, Dahan MH, Tan SL. Techniques and technology for human oocyte collection. Expert Rev Med Devices. 2016;13:701-3.
12. Malizia BA, Hacker MR, Penzias AS. Cumulative live-birth rates after in vitro fertilization. N Engl J Med. 2009;360(3):236-43.

13. Martins WP, Vieira CVR, Teixeira DM, Barbosa MAP, Dassunção LA, Nastri CO. Ultrasound for monitoring controlled ovarian stimulation: a systematic review and meta-analysis of randomized controlled trials Ultrasound Obstet Gynecol. 2014;43:25–33.
14. Pandian Z, Marjoribanks J, Ozturk O, Serour G, Bhattacharya S. Number of embryos for transfer following in vitro fertilisation or intra-cytoplasmic sperm injection. Cochrane Database Syst Rev. 2013 29;2013:CD003416.
15. Sunkara SK, Rittenberg V, Raine-Fenning N, Bhattacharya S, Zamora J, Coomarasamy A. Association between the number of eggs and live birth in IVF treatment: an analysis of 400 135 treatment cycles. Hum Reprod. 2011;26:1768-74.
16. Tso LO, Costello MF, Albuquerque LE, Andriolo RB, Macedo CR. Metformin treatment before and during IVF or ICSI in women with polycystic ovary syndrome. Cochrane Database Syst Rev. 2014:18;2014(11):CD006105.
17. Vaisbuch E, de Ziegler D, Leong M, Weissman A, Shoham Z. Luteal-phase support in assisted reproduction treatment: real-life practices reported worldwide by an updated website-based survey. Reprod Biomed Online. 2014,28:330–5.
18. Van der Linden M, Buckingham K, Farquhar C, Kremer JA, Metwally M. Luteal phase support for assisted reproduction cycles. Cochrane Database Syst Rev. 2015;7:CD009154.
19. Xiao JS, Su CM, Zeng XT. Comparisons of GnRH antagonist versus GnRH agonist protocol in supposed normal ovarian responders undergoing IVF: a systematic review and meta-analysis. PLoS One. 2014;12;9:e106854.
20. Youssef MA, Abou-Setta AM, Lam WS. Recombinant versus urinary human chorionic gonadotrophin for final oocyte maturation triggering in IVF and ICSI cycles. Cochrane Database Syst Rev. 2016;4(4):CD003719.

Chapter 24: Reproductive Outcome in Women with Advanced Maternal Age

Women with advaned age, face difficulties to conceive. Once conceived, often face complications during pregnancy and also in delivery. All over the world average age of childbearing has steadily increased. With the assistance in reproduction, many women can get the choice of having a baby even in the advanced age. Moreover it is established that advanced maternal age is associated with the higher risks of adverse maternal and perinatal outcomes.

Generally women with age < 35 years are considered in the category of advanced age. Medical literature considered the term as "very advanced maternal age" (VAMA) to those women who are aged 45 years or more at the time of delivery.

Q.1 How is the prospect of conception for the women with advaned age?
Ans:
- Spontaneous conception for women with advanced age is less. It is rare for women with very advanced maternal age (≥48 years)
- It is observed that 78% of women with VAMA delivering, had conceived following assisted reproductive technology (ART)
- Health hazards of ART are many (discussed below). But the important issues are:
    - *Maternal:* Failure of the procedure may be on repeated occasions and
    - *Family members:* Due to its adverse impact on family economy and the psychology.

Q.2 What are the risks on maternal health during the period of conception and there after?
Ans. It is commonly due to the procedure of ART.
- Ovarian hyperstimulation syndrome (*See* Ch 23)
- Miscarriage
- Ectopic pregnancy
- Pre-eclampsia
- Preterm labor
- Development of maternal medical disorders are higher
- Obesity
- Venous thromboeblism
- Increased need of thromboprophylaxis
- Increased risks of maternal admission

Q.3 What are the effects on perinatal morbidity?
Ans:
- Perinatal morbidities are increased. Morbidities are more depending upon the gestational age and the period of preterm birth
- Lower the gestational age (<32 weeks), higher the morbidities
- Pregnancies with multiple fetuses are associated with higher risks
- Combined together, the problem of preterm birth with LBW (FGR), the risks are increased.

Q.4 What is the impact on perinatal mortality in such women with VAMA?
Ans:
- Absolute rate of stillbirth and perinatal death is increased (1.87%) when compared with a young woman (0.55%)
- Perinatal mortality rates 2–4 times higher in such women with VAMA
- Preterm and SGA babies are the main cause for stillbirths and neonatal deaths
- Associated fetal genetic, chromosomal and structural abnormalities are higher
- Higher risks of admission at neonatal intensive care unit (NICU)
- Neonates from singleton pregnancy are less likely to suffer perinatal morbidity than multifetal pregnancy.

Q.5 What are the health risks of assisted reproductive technology (ART) following conception?
Ans: The woman is at significantly higher risks of developing the following medical complications:
- Gestational diabetes mellitus (GDM 20%)
- Gestational hypertension
- Pre-eclampsia
- Abnormal placentation
- Cesarean delivery
- Complications related to placenta
    - Placenta previa
    - Placental abruption
    - Placenta previa and accreta
- Postpartum hemorrhage (PPH 25%)
- More need of blood transfusion
- Admission to intensive care unit (ICU 33%)
- Prolonged hospital stay.

Q.6 What are the fetal and neonatal complications?
Ans:
- Genetic and chromosomal abnormalities
- Structural malformations
- Fetal growth restriction (FGR)
- Low birth weight babies (< 2500 gm)

- Preterm newborns
- Stillbirths
- Increased perinatal loss

Q.7 How best the women with VAMA should be managed during the course of pregnancy?

Ans: Essential management issues are:
- Early diagnosis of pregnancy
- First trimester anomaly scan with PAPP-A, hCG and USG for NT and multimarker screening (*See Clinics in Obstetrics, Ch 10, 57*)
- USG anomaly scan at 20–22 weeks
- Serial assessments of fetal size, amniotic fluid volume, and umbilical artery Doppler evaluation from 28 weeks onwards
- Low dose aspirin from 14 weeks of gestation
- To monitor fetal movement counting since 26 weeks till delivery
- Woman need to be discussed balancing the benefits and risks of pregnancy continuation and waiting spontaneous labor and delivery versus the **benefits and risks of induction of labor or planned cesarean delivery.**

Q.8 How the risks of fetal trisomy and other congenital anomalies are related to maternal age following spontaneous conception and following ART?

Ans:
- Trisomy 21 (Down Syndrome) is the most common chromosomal abnormality. Down syndrome is directly related to advanced maternal age. Risk for Down syndrome, following spontaneous conception at maternal age of 30, 40 and 45 are: 1/952, 1/106 and 1/30 respectively
- Pregnancy following donor embryos, it is related to the age of the donor. The live birth rate of cases with trisomy 21 to woman of VAMA is significantly lower than 1/35, probably due to the use of younger donor embryos
- Confirmation of diagnosis needs invasive prenatal testing (amniocentesis or chorionic villous sampling). Non-invasive perinatal testing (NIPT) may be an alternative to invasive testing (*See Clinical in Obstetrics, Ch 57*). Detection rate of NIPT is 99% for down syndrome. It has no risk of pregnancy loss. However women are explained that any positive NIPT result needs confirmation with invasive diagnostic testing.

Q.9 What the different assisted reproductive technologies (ART) are available for conception of women with very advanced age?

Ans:
- Chance of spontaneous conception for such women is rare
- Conception following autologous embryos is also rare
- Live birth rate for women aged older than 46 years following autologous embryos reported was 0%
- Assisted conception may be possible following egg donation (majority)
- Donor sperm have also been used
- Embryo transfer—mostly two embryo transfer is done in majority
- Women having multiple embryo transfer had multiple pregnancy.

Suggested Reading

1. Arya S, Mulla Z, Plavsic S. Outcomes of women delivering at very advanced maternal age. Womens Health (Larchmt). 2018;27:1378-84.
2. Carolan M, Davey M, Biro M, Kealy M. Very advanced maternal age and morbidity in Victoria, Australia: a population based study BMC Pregnancy Childbirth. 2013;27;13:80.
3. Carolan M. Maternal age ≥45 years and maternal and perinatal outcomes: a review of the evidence. Midwifery 2013;29:479-89.
4. Chaudhary S, Contag S. The effect of maternal age on fetal and neonatal mortality. J Perinatol 2017;37:800-4
5. Dildy G, Jackson G, Fowers G, Oshiro B, Varner M. Very advanced maternal age: pregnancy after age 45. Am J Obstet Gynecol 1996;175:668-74.
6. Fitzpatrick K, Tuffnell D, Kurinczuk J, Knight M. Pregnancy at very advanced maternal age: a UK population-based cohort study BJOG. 2017;124:1097-06.
7. Laufer N, Simon A, Samueloff A, Yaffe H, Milwidsky A, Gielchinsky M. Successful spontaneous pregnancies in women older than 45 years. Fertil Steril. 2004;81:1328-32.
8. Morris J, Wald N, Mutton D, Alberman E. Comparison of models of maternal age-specific risk for Down syndrome live births. Prenat Diagn. 2003;23:252-8
9. Schwartz A, Many A, Shapira U. Perinatal outcomes of pregnancy in the fifth decade and beyond - a comparison of very advanced maternal age groups. Sci Rep 2020;10:1809.
10. Waldenström U, Cnattingius S, Vixner L, Norman M. Advanced maternal age increases the risk of very preterm birth, irrespective of parity: a population-based register study; BJOG. 2017;124:1235-44.

Chapter 25: Anti-Mullerian Hormone in Reproductive Biology

- Anti-Mullerian hormone (AMH) is a member of the transforming growth factor beta (TGF-β) family.
- AMH is produced by the granulosa cells of the preantral and small antral follicles up to 6 mm diameter.
- It is also secreted by the sertoli cells of the fetal testis.
- In male, AMH causes regression of the Mullerian duct system.
- AMH is detectable in a female fetus as early as 36 weeks of gestation.
- Levels of AMH progressively rise after birth and reach its highest level after puberty. It decreases progressively with age and is undetectable at menopause. Serum AMH levels are found to correlate strongly with the number of antral follicles of the ovary.
- Level of AMH is taken as indicator of ovarian reserve.
- Serum levels of AMH are cycle-independent and can be measured at any phase of menstrual cycle. This is a distinct advantage compared to estimation of serum FSH and estradiol (E2). Inhibin (A and B) is secreted by the granulosa cells. Inhibin regulates FSH secretion through negative feedback response to the pituitary.
- AMH levels can vary in certain clinical situations.
- Long-term (>1 year) use of combined oral contraceptives (COCs) or GnRH analog can lower the levels of AMH. However, these changes are reversible.
- AMH reduces follicular sensitivity to FSH.
- Currently normal levels of plasma AMH has been considered as 1–3 ng/mL. Levels between 0.7 ng/mL and 0.9 ng/mL are considered as low normal while levels <0.3 ng/mL is recognized as low. Level >3 ng/mL is considered very high and may be a diagnostic marker for PCOS women.
- **Physiological functions of AMH**:
  a. Prediction of ovarian reserve
  b. Prediction of ovarian response to a stimulation protocol
  c. For diagnosis of granulosa cell tumors of the ovary
  d. Diagnosis of polycystic ovarian syndrome (PCOS)
- **AMH is an important biomarker and its role in reproductive endocrinology is multiple.**

Q.1 What are the different parameters to assess ovarian reserve?

Ans. Different parameters for assessment of ovarian reserve are:
1. Levels of cycle D3 serum FSH
2. Cycle D3 serum levels of estradiol
3. Levels of AMH
4. Basal serum inhibin B
5. Antral follicle count (AFC) using TVS and
6. Ovarian volume measurement (OVM).

The following values indicate poor ovarian reserve and response:
- D3 serum FSH > 10–15 IU/L
- D3 serum estradiol > 60–80 ρg/mL
- Serum AMH low value: 0.2–0.7 ng/mL (<1 ng/mL)
- Basal serum inhibin B (<40 ρg/mL)
- AFC using TVS <3 from both the ovaries
- Ovarian volume <3 cm^3

Of all the parameters as mentioned above AMH and AFC have high accuracy for prediction of poor ovarian response.

Q.2 How are the different values of AMH clinically correlated?

Ans. Values of AMH above and below the optimal range are viewed and interpreted carefully.

Values below the optimal range suggest low antral follicular pool and poor reproductive ability. Values above the optimal range suggest polycystic ovarian syndrome (PCOS). These women are having high antral follicular count. These women run the higher risk of ovarian hyperstimulation syndrome (OHSS).

The role of AMH as a prediction of ovarian reserve and ovarian responsive to FSH:
Reproductive ability of a woman is strongly correlated with the chronological age as well as the ovarian reserve. Women with advanced age are considered as poor responder due to depleted follicular pool. Combined together, age (≥ 36 years) and reduced ovarian reserve (AFC < 5–7 follicles) and lower levels of AMH (<0.5–1.1 ng/mL) are associated with poor reproductive outcome. Decreased AMH levels indicate reduced antral follicle count, hence reduced ovarian reserve. It is independent of the woman's age.

The correlation of AMH levels and ovarian responsiveness: Controlled ovarian stimulation has a strong positive correlation with the number of oocyte retrieval. AMH can predict quantitative ovarian response. AMH can be a guide for selection of stimulation protocol (in respect of an individual patient.)

TABLE 25.1: AMH and AFC for categorization of treatment protocol.

Low ovarian reserve: AFC: < 5 AMH: < 1 ng/mL	Normal ovarian reserve: AFC: 5–15 AMH: 2–5 ng/mL	Higher ovarian reserve: AFC: > 15 AMH: > 5 ng/mL
Minimizing treatment burden	Maximizing success rate	Minimizing OHSS risk
▪ GnRH antagonist protocol ▪ Maximal FSH stimulation	▪ Antagonist/Agonist protocol ▪ Average FSH stimulation	▪ Antagonist protocol ▪ Minimizing FSH stimulation

The main advantage with this approach is AMH level can optimize the response and can avoid the over-response and the complications like ovarian hyperstimulation syndrome (OHSS).

Levels of AMH can be correlated with optimum ovulation stimulation protocols. Pretreatment AMH values can guide to design the protocol. The commonly used optimal treatment protocols are:
a. Long agonist,
b. Antagonist, and
c. Flare protocol.

A. **Women with poor ovarian reserve** (AMH < 1 ng/mL)
   Options may be: GnRH agonist with gonadotropins (FSH) and hCG for oocyte maturation and luteal phase support.
   Women with low AMH have low risk of OHSS. These women could be treated with long-acting gonadotropins, and hCG safely.

B. **Women with normal ovarian reserve** (AMH 2–5 ng/mL).
   These women are preferably considered for antagonist-based protocol. Risks of OHSS are there but some extent small.

C. **Women with high ovarian reserve** (AMH > 5 ng/mL). These women are considered for antagonist-based protocol. These women run the higher risks of OHSS compared with the previous two categories.

Based on the results of AMH, patient's response to ovarian stimulation protocol varies. Patients are classified as: (a) Normal responder, (b) Hyper-responder or (c) Poor responder.

AFC (antral follicular count) denotes ***quantity*** (number of follicles) and AMH indicates ***quantity*** of follicular response. Table 25.1 illustrates the practical utility of AMH and AFC for categorization of treatment protocol.

Suggested Reading

1. Chakraborty BN. Individualization of controlled ovarian stimulation. In Clinics in Reproductive Medicine and Assisted Reproductive Technology. CBS Publisher and Distributors Pvt Ltd, New Delhi; 2018. pp. 222–34.
2. Franchin R, Mendez Lozano DH, Frydman N, et al. Anti-Mullerian hormone concentrations in the follicular fluid of the preovulatory follicle are predictive of the implantation potential of the ensuing embryo obtained by in-vitro fertilization. J Clin Endocrinol Metab. 2007;92:1796–802.
3. Kwee J, Schat SR, McDonnell J, et al. Evaluation of anti-Mullerian hormone as a test for the prediction of ovarian reserve. Fertil Steril. 2008;90:737–43.
4. La Marca, Sighinolfi G, Radi D, et al. Anti-Mullerian hormone (AMH) as a predictive marker in Assisted Reproductive Technique (ART). Hum Reprod Update. 2010;16:113–30.
5. Nardo LG, Christodolok D, Gould D, et al. Anti-Mullerian hormone levels and antral follicle count in women enrolled in IVF cycles: relationship to life style factors, chronological age and reproductive history. Gynecol Endocrinol. 2007;23:486–93.
6. Templeton A, Morris JK, Parslow W. Factors that affect outcome of in-vitro fertilization treatment. Lancet. 1996;348:1402–6.

Fertility Management Strategies for Low Responder

The decline in female fecundity with age is well-documented. Spontaneous conception is low in women over the age of 45 years. Deliveries after the age of 45 years are only 0.2%. It is documented that oocyte depletion accelerates after the age of 37 years. Moreover, ovarian response to stimulation in older women with low ovarian reserve is poor. This is due to the increased resistance of the ovaries to gonadotropin stimulation even with a high dose.

Factors for poor response of ovaries to gonadotropin stimulation:
- Age is an independent and significant determinant
- Body weight
- Body mass index (BMI)
- Size and count of antral follicles (≥ 2–11 mm). A count of < 5 follicles of 2–5 mm diameter has been suggested as a poor responder
- Basal hormonal levels are also used to predict the response. D3-FSH > 10 IU/mL; inhibin B (low), serum estradiol (high) and anti-Müllerian hormone (AMH) (low)—suggest poor response.

MANAGEMENT ISSUES

Gonadotropin stimulation for poor responders may produce more follicles when given 300–400 IU or even 600 IU of FSH per day.

Stimulation may done with fixed high dose FSH or with step-down protocol depending upon the response. Maximum dose of gonadotropin (FSH) used with the effective response is 450 IU/day.

GnRH agonists (GnRH-a) in the treatment of poor responders:
- ***Long GnRH-a protocol:*** Resulted in increased number of oocytes, improved clinical pregnancy rate per embryo transfer compared to conventional stimulation. Therefore, long GnRH-a protocol was found superior in terms of efficacy in low responder patients. However, in many patients with poor response, resulted in excessive ovarian suppression with GnRH-a. Consequently, hormonal stimulation was excessively prolonged with increased cost and duration of treatment. The ovarian unresponsiveness was very high.
- ***Step down GnRH-a protocol:*** Excessive ovarian dampening due to long GnRH-a made this protocol less popular. This supported the concept of a step down GnRH-a with the low dose (mini-dose) protocol. Mini-dose is found superior to standard agonist dose in terms of oocyte yield and cycle outcome.
- ***GnRh-a 'stop' protocol:*** Pituitary recovery and resumption of gonadotropin secretion following GnRH-a treatment usually takes up several weeks. Use of 'ultrashort protocol' was effective to suppress the endogenous LH secretion when GnRH-a (leuprolide acetate 0.1 mg/day from cycle day 21 reducing to 0.05 mg/day upon down regulation) was using to the stop protocol. The ultrashort protocol was stopped after 5 days. There was no premature LH surge. This forms the basis of 'stop protocol' or discontinuous GnRH protocol. This 'stop protocol' showed favorable results in terms of both cost effectiveness and clinical outcome.
- ***Short GnRH-a protocol:*** Patients who failed to multifollicular growth with long GnRH protocol were considered for a short protocol with short and ultrashort regimens. It had the advantages of the initial agonistic stimulatory effect of GnRH-a non-endogenous FSH and LH secretion which is also known as flare-up effects.

Advantage is that it eliminates excessive ovarian suppression due to prolonged agonist use. Pituitary desensitization generally achieved within 5 days of treatment. Patients are protected from premature LH surge. This protocol was considered favorable for the poor responder woman.

The limitations of the protocol was that its efficacy were not judged in prospective randomized controlled trials in comparison to standard long protocol. The live birth rate in flare-up group was found low (3.8%) when compared to the standard long protocol (25%).

Adverse effects of flare-up protocol with GnRH-a was LH secretion and development of increase androgen levels in the follicular environment. This is detrimental to the process of folliculogenesis and meiosis leading to poor oocyte formation and reduced rate of fertilization and implantation. Early follicular use of GnRH-a (flare-up protocol) resulted in increased levels of LH, E2, androgens and progesterone compared to the mid-luteal group of GnRH-a use.

To improve the ill effects of flare-up GnRH-a use, the following measures could be taken:
- Pretreatment use of oral contraceptive pills (OCPs)
- Use of progestin (norethisterone) before the use of gonadotropin stimulation

- Dose reduction of GnRH-a to minimize the flare (micro-dose flare).
- **GnRH antagonists in the treatment of poor responders:** Its use has an immediate effect (within 6 hours) of dose-related suppression of gonadotropin release and resulted in comparable therapeutic efficacy compared to agonists. GnRH antagonist is administered in the late follicular phase to suppress the LH surge.

  Other advantages are:
  - It avoids the 'flare-up' of LH
  - Shortens the overall treatment protocol
  - Reduces the risk of ovarian hyperstimulation syndrome (OHSS)
  - Reduces the menopausal side effects of the woman.

  The dose schedule may be fixed or flexible depending upon the response. In the beginning of controlled ovarian stimulation (COS), the pituitary is fully responsive to GnRH pulses.

  This allows more natural follicular recruitment without any inhibitory effect of GnRH-a. This antagonist protocol for poor responders also permit the use of clomiphene citrate (CC) with or without gonadotropin stimulation. Owing to the synergistic effect, the requirement of gonadotropin may be less and so also the concomitant cost. There is some modest improvement in oocyte retrieval, embryo transfer and clinical pregnancy rates.

- **Role of androgens:** Human follicular growth and development is regulated by different endocrine and paracrine factors that develop the favorable follicular microenvironment. Same amount of androgens from theca cells are produced and this small amount contributes to the follicular environment.

- **Role of follicular androgens in folliculogenesis:**
  - Reduces follicular apoptosis and responsiveness to gonadotropin
  - Enhance the action of FSH for follicular growth and maturation.

  This concept encouraged the use of dehydroepiandrosterone (DHEA) for women with diminished ovarian reserve. The woman is given 75 mg of DHEA daily for an average of 4–5 months. With this concept, aromatase inhibitors were used to block the intraovarian androgen conversion to estrogens. Few studies support the beneficial effects of DHEA or aromatase inhibitors for women with diminished ovarian function. However, it needs authentication with prospective randomized control trials.

- **Role of human growth hormone (hGH):** Results are conflicting with the role of hGH when used in women with poor responders. Few studies showed improvements in follicular responsiveness and pregnancy rates.

- **Pre-treatment with oral contraceptive pills:** It is suggested that use of OCPs may increase the pregnancy rates of IVF specially in the poor responders.

The suggested mechanisms are:
- Induction of estrogen receptors in the follicle and sensitization
- Suppression effect on the pituitary with either alone or in combination with GnRH agonists
- Improvement of local (intraovarian) growth factors
- Changes in the endometrium.

Cycle outcomes of gonadotropin stimulation with prior hypothalamic-pituitary suppression with OCP with or without GnRH-a were improved in terms of oocyte retrieval, embryo transfer, embryo quality and clinical pregnancy rates. However, more published data are needed to support the observation.

- **Low-dose aspirin:** It was used to improve follicular vascularity. However, available evidence does not support its use in the poor responder women undergoing IVF.

Aneuploidy screening: Women with advanced age produce oocytes with inadequate reserves of energy. Energy produced by mitochondrial DNA, is necessary for oocyte maturation, meiosis and process of disjunction. Mitochondrial dysfunction (due to related pathology), can lead to an increase in nondisjunction, abnormal chromatid separation and higher rates of oocyte apoptosis. Because of this reason oocytes retrieved during ART procedures may be biochemically or chromosomally defective. Chromosome abnormalities are the important cause of embryo wastage. Preimplantation genetic screening (PGS) confirmed this association for women aged >35 years.

SUMMARY

- Treatment strategies for low responder or women with diminished ovarian reserve are difficult and at times frustrating.
- Development of any definitive treatment strategy is difficult as there is a paucity of any large-scale prospective randomized controlled trials (RCTs).
- High dose gonadotropins (300–450 IU of FSH daily) for women with diminished ovarian reserve or poor ovarian response are useful to yield a maximum number of oocytes.
- Long GnRH-a protocol—might be the protocol of choice when ovarian reserve is low and the response is poor. Mini-dose (low dose) agonist down regulation is found useful to increase ovarian responsiveness.
- Short (micro-dose) flare—GnRH-a protocol. It is found beneficial. Pretreatment of OCPs uses can prevent the adverse effects of LH and excess androgen secretion. OCP use prevents the high LH which is due to the endogenous gonadotropin flare-up effect.
- GnRH antagonists—results in immediate suppressive gonadotropins release. COS for follicular recruitment is done with the inhibitory effect of GnRH-a. Clomiphene citrate alone or combined with gonadotropins (synergistic effects) result in higher oocyte yield.

- Stop protocol: In some failed cases of long or short GnRH-a regimen, agonist administration can be withdrawn and gonadotropin stimulation is continued. No LH peak was observed and clinical outcomes were found favorable.
- ART treatment is recommended for women with declining years of fecundity. In addition to diminished ovarian reserve and poor response, other associated factors have been a challenge. Poor oocyte quality (aneuploid oocytes and embryos), uterine factors and women's psychological stress are also the hindrances.
- Use of donor oocyte has been considered the successful alternative.

Suggested Reading

1. A-Mizyen E, Sabatini L, Lower AM, et al. Does pretreatment with progesterone or OCPs in low responders followed by the GnRH-a flare protocol improve the outcome of IVF-ET? J Assist Reprod Genet. 2000;17(3):140-6.
2. Cedrin-Durnevin I, Bständig B, Herve F, et al. A comparative study of high fixed-dose and decremental-dose regimens of gonadotropins in a minidose GnRH-a flare protocol for poor responders. Fertil Steril. 2000;73(5):1055-6.
3. Chuang CC, Chen CD, Chao KH, et al. Age is a better predictor of pregnancy potential than basal FSH levels in women undergoing IVF. Fertil Steril. 2003;79(1):63-8.
4. Craft I, Gorgy A, Hill J, et al. Will GnRH antagonists provide new hope for patient considered 'difficult responder' to GnRH-a protocols? Hum Reprod. 1999;14(12):2959-62.
5. Kovacs P, Barg PE, Witt BR. Hypothalamic-pituitary suppression with OCPs does not improve outcome in poor responder patients undergoing IVF-ET cycles. J Assist Reprod Genet. 2001;18(7):391-4.
6. Laufer N, Simon A, Samueloff A, et al. Successful spontaneous pregnancies in women older than 45 years. Fertil Steril. 2004;81(5):1328-32.
7. May-Panloup P, Chretien MF, Jacques C, et al. Low oocyte mitochondrial DNA content in ovarian insufficiency. Hum Reprod. 2005;20(3):593-7.

Chapter 27: Surrogacy

The term 'surrogate mother' or 'surrogate' is usually used for a woman who carries and delivers a baby on behalf of another couple. The couples who are intending to parent a child resulting from a surrogate pregnancy are referred as **"commissioning parents"**. Surrogacy can be either *'traditional'* or *'gestational'*.

TRADITIONAL SURROGACY

Traditional (partial, natural or straight) surrogacy uses the eggs of the surrogate mother and the sperm of the commissioning father. The procedure can be performed in an IUI clinic or at home. The baby in such a case is genetically related to the surrogate mother and the commissioning father. The surrogate mother has to leave her biological baby to the commissioning mother who knows that her husband has fathered the child with another woman.

GESTATIONAL SURROGACY (FULL OR IVF SURROGACY)

This method needs in vitro fertilization procedures. The sperm and the oocyte from the commissioning couple are fertilized in vitro and the embryo is transferred to the surrogate mother. The surrogate host is not genetically related to the baby. Gestational surrogacy is an expensive procedure and it takes longer time. Success rate of the procedure is low.

Both the surrogacy procedures (Traditional and Gestational) may be:
1. **Commercial:** The commissioning couple compensates the surrogate mother for her service (this may be illegal in many countries such as in the UK).
2. **Altruistic:** The surrogate mother desires to carry the child for reasons other than financial gain.

   In a surrogacy procedure, a woman agrees to bear a child for another woman or couple and surrenders the baby at birth to the commissioning couple.

Alternative option of surrogacy is adoption. Surrogacy provides an opportunity for couples to have a child with some genetic contribution of their own.

Specific Situations to Suggest Surrogacy

- Congenital absence of uterus: Mayer-Rokitansky-Küster-Hauser (MRKH) syndrome
- Women with surgically removed uterus (hysterectomy)
- Uterine shape has been distorted and deformed (fibroid or adenomyosis and Müllerian abnormalities)
- Uterine synechiae
- Renal and cardiac pathology
- Recurrent unexplained miscarriage
- Repeated IVF failure due to unknown causes.

Other extended indications are: Married woman seeking surrogacy for career plan.

> **Ethical issues and the dilemmas of surrogacy**
> - The surrogate mother may desire to keep the child with her
> - Non-acceptance of the child after birth—both by the surrogate mother and the commissioning parents
> - Psychological effects on all involved in the arrangement
> - Dilemmas of surrogacy whether it should be commercial or not?
>
> The protagonists think that commercial surrogacy allows freedom of choice for both parties. Antagonists think moral value of child-bearing and the parent–child relationship suffers. Children should not be treated as commodities and that moral values of parent and child cannot be sold or abandoned.

Procedure of Gestational Surrogacy

- The procedure involves creation of an embryo by IVF.
- The embryo results from the union of gametes (sperm and egg) derived from the infertile couple.
- The infertile couple is the genetic or biological parents (commissioning couple).
- Surrogate mother (surrogate host) may be a friend or relative or she may be unknown to the commissioning couple.
- Endometrial preparation in the surrogate before embryo transfer is needed.
- This procedure is also known as **IVF surrogacy** or **full surrogacy.**
- In India at the moment, there are few practical problems as well as legal considerations that need modifications. It is suggested that the agreement of surrogacy between the surrogate host and the commissioning couple should be signed in the presence of a lawyer. After all, the commissioning couple is the biological parents of the child.

LAW AND SURROGACY

The legal frameworks of surrogacy vary in each country depending upon the ethical and social values of individual country.

The countries where commercial surrogacy is allowed: USA (not all the states), Israel.

The countries where altruistic surrogacy is allowed: Australia, UK.

Surrogacy arrangements are not legally enforceable. Therefore, the parties draw up a written agreement clarifying their feelings on all the areas of conflict, either through an agency or a solicitor.

Legal Status of the Child and Indian Parental Order

The surrogate is always the legal mother. The status of the legal father is more complicated depending on his status. However, when the treatment was done in a licensed clinic and the surrogate mother has no partner, the child will be legally fatherless. Parental order is obtained by application to the court. The criteria to be fulfilled are as below:

- A parental order cannot be given until 6 weeks after birth. The surrogate mother and the commissioning father need to sign a parental responsibility agreement so with the birth of the baby (in the hospital) to check the period until a parental order is obtained.
- *Couple counseling:* All parties in the surrogacy arrangement must be counseled to have clear understanding about the implications of surrogacy.

Criteria for Obtaining a Parental Order

- The baby must be genetically related to one or both of the commissioning parents.
- The commissioning couple must be over 18 years of age and are married.
- The surrogate parents must consent to the order and consent cannot be given until 6 weeks after birth.
- The payments for reasonable expenses must be paid for the surrogacy arrangements.
- In UK, one or both of the commissioning parents must be living and baby must reside with them. Surrogacy registration in the UK remains complex and unsatisfactory as yet.

Health Risks of the Surrogate Mother

The generally an agreed criterion exists to reduce health risks of the surrogate mother.

This covers the traditional surrogacy and the IVF surrogacy also. The potential surrogate mother must be in good mental and physical health. She should not have any known risk factors like obesity, any addiction and should be in her reproductive age (ideally <35 years).

Consent

In the eyes of the law, the developing fetus is a part of the woman's baby. A surrogate mother, therefore, has the right to accept or refuse any medical procedures during the pregnancy. The decisions as regards ultrasound scanning or serum screening for trisomy 21, amniocentesis, chorionic villus sampling for chromosomal abnormalities, should be made. All these need prior discussion and counseling. Decisions also need to be made about the preferred place and mode of delivery.

Postpartum Care of the Mother and the Baby

The parental responsibility arrangement needs to be signed (if not done earlier) by the surrogate mother. Once the court has granted a parental order, the responsibilities for the newborn pass solely to the commissioning parents.

The immediate postpartum period is a time of great emotional upheaval in a surrogacy arrangement. Midwifery support is essential in handling the surrogate by the commissioning parents.

Recommendations of Indian Council of Medical Research (ICMR)

- Assisted reproductive technology (ART) clinic should play no role in commercial surrogacy program.
- Surrogate must surrender all parental rights.
- Surrogate should have not more than five children in her life (including her own children).
- Procedures to be done only at ICMR recommended clinics.
- Birth certificate to have names of the genetic parents.

CONCLUSION

Care of surrogate pregnancy involves care of the surrogate mother according to her need. The obstetrician also provides care for the interest of the unborn baby. Pregnancy counseling is the key to successful surrogacy arrangements.

Suggested Reading

1. British Medical Association. What is surrogacy? [online] Available from www.bma.org.uk/ap.nsf/ Content/Consideringsurrogacy?OpenDocument&Highlight=2,surrogacy.
2. Human Fertilisation and Embryology Authority. Code of Practice. 7th edition. London: HFEA; 2007. [online] Available from www.hfea.gov.uk/en/371.html.
3. Jadva V, Murray C, Lycett E, MacCallum F, Golombok S. Surrogacy: the experiences of surrogate mothers. Hum Reprod. 2003;18:2196–204.
4. Reilly DR. Surrogate pregnancy: a guide for Canadian prenatal health care providers. CMAJ. 2007;176:483–5.

Section 4: Contraception

Section Outline

- Ch. 28. Advances in Contraception including Contraceptive Measures Following Treatment of GTD
- Ch. 29. Long-acting Reversible Contraceptives
- Ch. 30. Male and Female Sterilization
- Ch. 31. Safe Abortion Service and WHO Guidelines

Chapter 28: Advances in Contraception including Contraceptive Measures Following Treatment of GTD

ADVANCES IN CONTRACEPTION

Q.1 What is the significance of knowing advances in contraception?

Ans. Advances in contraceptive research contribute greatly to better health and healthcare. Progressive research in this field has made contraceptive measures more safe and effective for all the ages of clients. It is also essential that the healthcare providers should also know 'what is new' so that they can communicate with the clients more effectively.

Q.2 How the service of the healthcare providers is important?

Ans. A holistic approach brings the well-informed clients together for good quality services. Contraceptive care providers need to be well-informed, skilled and competent to communicate the clients sympathetically and should also deal the complication if any develops.

INTRAUTERINE CONTRACEPTIVE DEVICES (IUCDs)

Q.3 What are the new directions for the use of IUCDs (IUDs)?

Ans. The modern IUDs (CuT380 A, Multiload 375 and LNG-IUD) are safe, effective and quickly reversible. They can be used for long-term contraception. They are also cost-effective. CuT380 A is supplied free of cost by the Government of India through family planning program. CuT380 A can be used for ≥10 years, and Multiload 375 and LNG-IUD for 5 years each. They can be used to delay pregnancy or even to end childbearing (Figs. 28.1A to C).

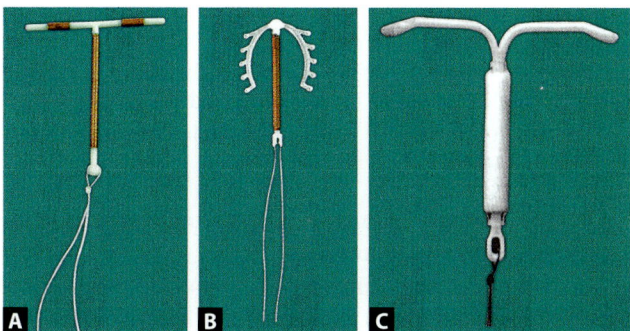

Figs. 28.1A to C: (A) CuT380 A; (B) Multiload 375; (C) LNG-IUD.

- Effectiveness of IUDs is similar to that of female sterilization.
- *Failure rate:* LNG-IUD: 1 in 1,000 women; CuT380 A: 3–8 in 1,000 women.

Q.4 What are the other advantages of using IUDs?

Ans.
- In reality most women can use IUDs safely and effectively
- Including women who are breastfeeding
- Other advantages are:
  Women can use IUDs:
  - Without any tests for sexually transmitted infections (STIs), including human immunodeficiency virus (HIV)
  - Without any blood tests or laboratory tests
  - Without cervical cancer screening
  - Without breast examination.

Q.5 What is the current guidance to the use of IUDs in women with STIs?

Ans.
- Women who are at risk of HIV or are infected with HIV can safely use IUDs.
- Women having gonorrhea and chlamydia or purulent cervicitis are not recommended for the use of IUDs.

Q.6 What are advances in contraception as regard to the use of IUDs?

Ans.
- Refusing women IUDs in the absence of laboratory tests for STIs, blood tests, would deny benefits to a great majority of women.
- There is no significant increase in infertility associated with IUD use, which has been observed.
- About 72–96% women conceived within a year after the removal of IUDs.

Q.7 What is the medical eligibility criteria for contraceptive use?

Ans. According to WHO, categories for temporary methods are described in Table 28.1.

TABLE 28.1: The medical eligibility criteria for contraceptive use.

Category	With clinical judgement	With limited clinical judgement
1.	Use method in any circumstances	Yes (use the method)
2.	Generally use method	Yes (use the method)
3.	Method is not usually recommended unless other more appropriate methods are available or acceptable	No
4.	Method not to be used	Do not use the method

Q.8 What is the current guidance to IUD users having HIV (medical eligibility criteria category 2 and 3; WHO 2008)?

Ans.
- A woman with HIV (not AIDS) can have Cu-IUDs or hormonal IUD inserted.
- A woman having AIDS on highly active antiretroviral therapy (HAART) and is clinically well can have IUD inserted.
- IUD insertion is not recommended for women with AIDS and not on HAART (WHO category 3).
- However in all the situations the woman must be urged to use condoms along with IUD.

Q.9 Compared to the worldwide use of IUDs, which country has the maximum use of IUDs?

Ans. Most IUD users are in China (60%), thereafter eastern Europe and central Asia (11%) and other Asia (12%).

Q.10 What is the place of immediate postpartum insertion of IUCD (PPIUCD)?

Ans. Immediate postpartum insertion of IUCDs is safe. It can be inserted as:
- *Post-placental:* Immediately following delivery of the placenta (following vaginal or cesarean delivery).
- *Early postpartum* (<48 hours) before the woman leaves the hospital following childbirth.

Q.11 What is the importance of PPIUCD?

Ans. Postpartum insertion of IUCD is encouraged in India as a measure of population control. Risk of unplanned and unintended pregnancy is high during the period following completion of exclusive breastfeeding. Majority of women resume menstruation, ovulation and sexual activity during this period. As such in India, unmet need of contraception in the postpartum period is still there. Currently, the rate of institutional delivery has increased significantly (70%). While in hospital postpartum women have opportunity to use it without coming to the hospital for the second time. At that time the family planning, health workers have easy access to these women for counseling during the antenatal as well as postpartum period. PPIUCD is proved to be safe, effective and convenient for long-term use.

Q.12 What is the concern with breastfeeding in woman with HIV?

Ans.
- Risks of mother-to-child transmission (MTCT) for HIV infection with breastfeeding is 30%.
- Lactational amenorrhea may be an option for contraception in women with HIV.
- Exclusive breastfeeding carries lower risk of HIV transmission (MTCT) as compared to mixed feeding.
- Exclusive breastfeeding is the preferred feeding option for HIV exposed infants up to < 6 months of age (National guidelines 2011).
- Exclusive replacement feeding should be done only when AFASS criteria is fulfilled (A: Affordable, F: Feasible, A: Acceptable, S: Sustainable, S: Safe).
- Mother is counseled and helped to make her own choice regarding the use of exclusive breastfeeding or exclusive replacement feeding.

COMBINED ORAL CONTRACEPTIVES (COCs)

Q.13 What is the current guidance for the missed pills while the woman is on COCs or the pill?

Ans. **Missed pills:** Normally, there is return of pituitary and ovarian follicular activity during the pill-free interval (PFI) of 7 days. Breakthrough ovulation may occur in about 20% cases during the time. Lengthening of PFI due to omissions, malabsorption, or vomiting either at the start or at the end of a packet, increases the risk of breakthrough ovulation and, therefore, pregnancy.

Management: When a woman forgets to take **one pill** (late up to 24 hours), she should take the missed pill at once and continue the rest as schedule. There is nothing to worry.

When she **misses two pills or more** she should take 2 pills on each of the next 2 days and then continue the rest as scheduled. Extra precaution has to be taken for next 7 days either by using a condom or by avoiding sex. Alternatively, a new pack can be started and a barrier method to be used additionally for a week. If she misses any of the **7 inactive pills** (in a 28-day pack only) she should throw away the missed pills. She should take the remaining pills one a day and start the new pack as usual. Failure of withdrawal bleeding during the pill free interval, pregnancy should be excluded with medical tests. COCs are not teratogenic when taken accidentally in early pregnancy.

Q.14 What are the risks of missed pills and pregnancy?

Ans. Women who are late starter and/or missed pill in the third week, run the higher risks of failure and pregnancy. This is due to speeded development and growth of follicles resulting in ovulation and pregnancy. There are some women who are biologically active in this response.

Q.15 What about the ultra dose pills and shortening the hormone free interval?

Ans. Ultra dose pills contain ethinyl estradiol (EE) 15 µg and gestodene 60 µg. It is quiet effective but have more risks of break through bleeding. Withdrawal bleeds are more.

Shortening the hormone free interval is done using hormone pills for 24 days and nonhormone pills for 4 days. This reduces the amount of withdrawal bleeding both in the amount and duration.

Q.16 Does the woman need to have menstruation to start the pill?

Ans. Woman can start the pill at any time when it is certain that she is not pregnant.

Q.17 Who are the women suitable for COCs?

Ans. Nearly all healthy women are found safe and suitable for COCs irrespective of marital status or parity.

Q.18 What examination she needs to have before using COCs?

Ans. Women who are clinically fit and otherwise healthy, can begin COCs:
- Without a pelvic examination
- Without any routine blood or laboratory tests
- Without cervical cancer screening
- Without breast examination.

Q.19 What are the extended and continuous use of COCs?

Ans. Taking the pills for 12 weeks without a pause followed by 1 week of no pills (break) is the *extended use* of pills. Whereas taking the pills without a break at all is called *continuous use*.

Q.20 What are the advantages and disadvantages of extended or continuous use of the pills?

Ans. *Advantages*
- Women have vaginal bleeding only for four times a year or no bleeding at all.
- Reduce the problems of premenstrual tension syndrome, dysmenorrhea, heavy bleeding and mood changes.

Disadvantages
- Irregular bleeding may occur initially
- More pills need to be used.

Q.21 How the pill effectiveness is affected?

Ans. Drug interactions are the important areas that often alter the pill effectiveness.
- *Drugs that reduces pill effectiveness are:* Rifampicin, griseofulvin, barbiturates, ritonavir and topiramate.
- *Anticonvulsants:* Carbamazepine, phenytoin, primidone.

The drugs induce hepatic enzymes to cause enhancement in metabolic degradation of pills.
- Drugs that reduces the absorption of EE.
  - *Broad-spectrum antibiotics:* Ampicillin, ciprofloxacin, doxycycline.
  - *Others:* Fluconazole, ofloxacin, tetracycline, triazole.

Q.22 How she can avoid the failure rate in such a situation?

Ans. She is to be counseled:
- If these drugs are for short-term use she can use a back-up method along with COCs.
- When these drugs are used for long-term, she may use a different method (progestin injectables, CuT380 A or LNG-IUD).

Q.23 What is the guidance regarding the hormonal contraception for the women with HIV?

Ans. The main concerns are:
- Risks of acquiring HIV
- Progression of disease
- HIV transmission
- Adverse interaction with HAART.

Current situation and guidance is as below:
- Regarding acquisition—no additional risk has been observed.
- Regarding progression of the disease, mixed observation has been mentioned.
- Risks of infectivity, evidence is limited and conflicting. So more study results are awaited.
- Drug interactions with HAART [nucleoside reverse transcriptase inhibitors (NRTIs), nonnucleoside reverse transcriptase inhibitors (NNRTIs)] do not reduce the efficacy of Depo-Provera® (DMPA).

Centchroman (Saheli): Ormeloxifene is a nonsteroidal compound with potent antiestrogenic and weak estrogenic properties. It works preventing implantation of the fertilized ovum. It has noncontraceptive use also (*See* Dutta's Textbook of Gynecology, 8th Edition p. 410).

IMPLANTS

Q.24 Discuss about the implants used as the next generation.

Ans. The implants of the next generation are:
- One rod system: Nexplanon (etonogestrel 68 mg) (Fig. 28.2)
- Two rod system:
  - JADELLE® (Levonorgestrel) (Fig. 28.3)
  - Sino-implant (Zarin)

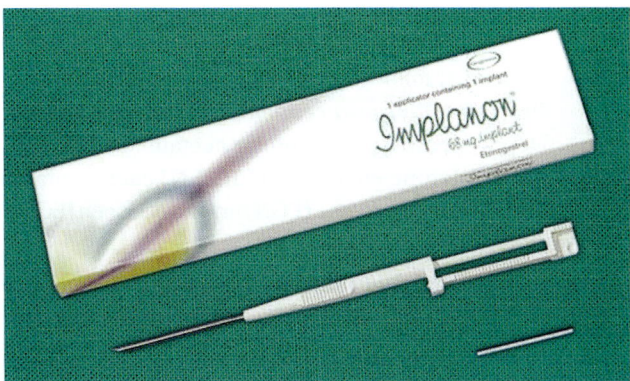

Fig. 28.2: IMPLANON® implant.

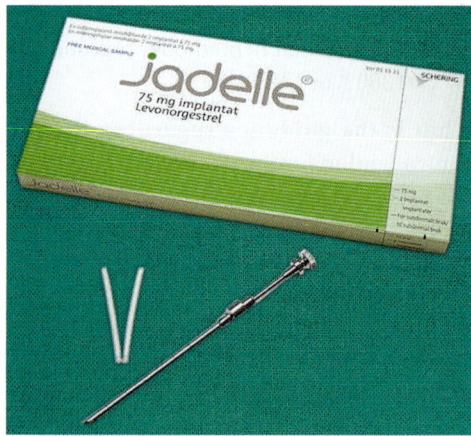

Fig. 28.3: JADELLE® implant.

- Six-capsules (Norplant)
- These implants are safe, highly effective and quickly reversible
- Duration of use is 3–5 years
- Ease of insertion (1–2 min) and removal (2–3 min).

Q.25 What are the special issues with the use of the new generation of implants?
Ans. The new generation implants are safe and suitable for nearly all women including adolescents and breastfeeding (> 6 weeks) and women with anemia.
- Implants are more effective than injectables and pills. Effectiveness is comparable to sterilization.
- Women with implants can be almost certain not to get any unintended pregnancy for up to 3–5 years.
- It releases the hormone about 60 µg gradually reduced to 30 µg per day over more than 3 years. It inhibits ovulation in 90% of cases for the first year. It has got the other effects to suppress the endometrium and to make the cervical mucus thick as well.
- Women with HIV, AIDS on antiretroviral (ARV) therapy can safely use implants.
- Women with HIV, AIDS should be urged to use condoms also.
- Provision should be there to ensure routine, regular follow-up and reliable removal services.

Progestin only contraception (PGN only injectables): Depot medroxyprogesterone acetate (DMPA) and norethisterone enanthate (NET-EN) each contains hormone progesterone (PGN) and no estrogen (EGN). DMPA is widely used.

Q.26 What is new about DMPA (Antara)?
Ans.
- DMPA reinjection schedule is unchanged but the grace period or the extended period has been permitted for the late clients (WHO-2008). Schedule injection is at 3 months interval and grace period of 4 weeks has been added.
- Average delay in pregnancy is there for 7 months, since the last injection.
- **Sayana press (medroxyprogesterone acetate):** Injection 104 mg is available in a prefilled syringe single dose injector. It is given SC into the anterior thigh or abdomen every 3 months (12–14 weeks).
- Depo-subQ provera 104 (Unijet) contains 104 mg of DMPA. It is given SC at every 90 days.

Q.27 What is the effect on bone mineral density (BMD) with the use of DMPA?
Ans. There is slight decrease in BMD with its use but it is reversible. Decreased BMD should not limit its use.

Q.28 Is there any contraindication of its use?
Ans. Contraindications are very few:
- Breastfeeding < 6 weeks of birth
- Severe high BP (systolic ≥ 160 mm Hg or diastolic ≥ 100 mm Hg)
- Ischemic heart disease
- History of prior stroke
- Arterial cardiovascular disease
- Severe liver disease, breast cancer.

Q.29 What is the place of PGN-only injectables for women with HIV?
Ans.
- Women with HIV or AIDS on ARV can safely use PGN-only injectable.
- They should use condoms also.

Q.30 What are the long-acting reversible contraceptives (LARCS)?
Ans. *See* Ch 29.

TRANSCERVICAL STERILIZATION

Q.31 What are the different methods for transcervical sterilization?
Ans.
- Quinacrine pellet is a sclerosing agent used to block the tubes. Failure rate is 2–3/100 WY.
- Essure is a microcoil (spring-like). It is used hysteroscopically and placed within the cornual end of the fallopian tube.

VASECTOMY

(See Ch 30, Figs. 30.3A and B)

Q.32 What is the current scenario of vasectomy as a permanent method of male contraception?
Ans. It is a very effective method but neglected and under utilized due to misconceptions.

Q.33 What are the advantages of vasectomy over tubectomy?
Ans. Advantages of vasectomy are:
- It is a quicker method
- Safe
- Cheaper and

- Associated with faster recovery and above all it is a highly effective method (failure rate is 0.2 per 100 couples). It needs 3 months delay or 20 ejaculations to become effective.

Q.34 What is the over all prevalence rate of vasectomy throughout the globe?
Ans. It is performed in Bhutan (13.6%), Australia/New Zealand (11.8%), China (6.7%) and India (1.0%).

Q.35 Is there any health risk associated with vasectomy?
Ans. Generally-there is nothing such.
- Does not cause impotence
- No increased risk of testicular cancer
- No increased risk of cardiovascular disease
- Risk of prostate cancer is likely to be noncausative.

CONTRACEPTIVE MEASURES FOLLOWING TREATMENT OF GESTATIONAL TROPHOBLASTIC DISEASES (GTD)

- **After evacuation of molar pregnancy**: Women should wait for the normalization of hCG (which usually becomes negative by next 8–9 weeks). Thereafter she is advised to avoid pregnancy for another at least 6 months.
- **After a partial molar pregnancy**, women should avoid pregnancy until two consecutive hCG levels, done at 4 weeks interval, are normal.
- **Women who had chemotherapy for GTD**, should avoid pregnancy for 1 year after the completion of treatment.

Options for Methods of Contraception
- Long-acting reversible contraception are superior.
- Compared to other methods, advantages of **long-acting reversible contraceptives (LARC):** (progesterone only implants), are superior, when used after GTD.
- Most methods of contraception can be safely used with the exception of intrauterine contraception (IUC).
- IUC may be used once hCG levels have been normalized.
- Emergency contraception (EC) is needed for unprotected sexual intercourse. CU-IUD may be used when the hCG levels are falling.
- Hormonal contraception can be started immediately after uterine evacuation for GTD.
- Women who have been treated with methotrexate, should be advised that effective contraception to be used for at least 3 months after treatment. This is in view of the teratogenic effects of the medicine.
- Combined hormonal contraception (CHC) should be avoided by women in the presence of antiphospholipid syndrome (APS).
- Tubal occlusion method should ideally be done, some times after surgical evacuation for GTD.
- Barrier methods (male and female) can be used after evacuation of GTD.
- Use of fertility awareness methods (FAM) may be difficult to follow as the signs and symptoms of fertility and ovulation are too variable, following treatment of GTD.
- There is no evidence that any method of contraception increases the risk of GTD.

Suggested Reading
1. Balachandran K, Salawu A, Ghorani E, Kaur B, Sebire NJ, Short D, et al. When to stop human chorionic gonadotrophin (hCG) surveillance after treatment with chemotherapy for gestational trophoblastic neoplasia (GTN): a national analysis on over 4,000 patients. Gynecol Oncol. 2019;155:8–12.
2. Ireson J, Jones G, Winter MC, Radley SC, Hancock BW, Tidy JA. Systematic review of health-related quality of life and patient reported outcome measures in gestational trophoblastic disease: a parallel synthesis approach. Lancet Oncol. 2018;19:e56–64.
3. The Faculty of Sexual and Reproductive Healthcare. Contraception After Pregnancy. FSRH Guideline Executive Summary. London: FSRH; 2021.

Chapter 29: Long-acting Reversible Contraceptives

Current trends in contraceptive use: Majority of women in India presently use user-dependent method. These are COCs, condom (male), withdrawal, natural family planning, and emergency pill.

Overall prevalence of use in different methods of contraception in India (WHO-2015): COCs (3.9%); IUCD (2%), and female sterilization (39%).

Use of long-acting reversible contraceptives (LARCs) in India is very low. The pregnancy rates are extremely low with all LARCs. Use of user-dependent methods ends with much higher rates of unplanned pregnancy than with the LARCs. This is due to inconsistent use of the user-dependent methods (COCs due to missing pills, condoms due to incorrect and inconsistent use, withdrawal methods and the emergency contraceptive pills).

Currently available LARCs are: Intrauterine contraceptive devices (IUCDs), IUS (LNG-IUS), implants (Implanon). POP, injectable contraceptive and the nursing.

LARCs: They are long-acting reversible contraceptive and, once fitted, the user needs not to do any thing more until the method has expired. It is a user-independent method. For the sake of convenience, use of user-independent contraceptive methods are becoming more popular than the user-dependent method. Unless a method is properly selected, it cannot be used correctly and consistently. Knowledge has changed regarding the use of contraceptive methods.

IUCDs: They are safe, effective and suitable for majority, of all ages. Current understanding as regard to the use of IUCDs, are: the risk of ectopic is no longer any higher rather it is reduced when compared to a woman not using any method. The return of fertility following removal of IUCD, is immediate. IUCD does not cause infertility.

With IUCD use, the risks of endometritis is <1%, up to 20 days after insertion. Thereafter the risk of PID is no longer high compared to a women not using any IUCD. IUCD could be used by sexually active women of any age. There is no lower age limit of IUCD user. Moreover IUCD should be offered to women regardless of their parity status and mode of delivery. Another advantage of IUCD use is that it can be inserted at any time of the menstrual cycle, provided the woman is reasonably certain that she is not pregnant. Moreover, for woman with HIV, IUCD does not increase the risk of viral shedding. IUCD can be used immediately following first and second trimester abortion or following delivery (post-placental or transcesarean). The special advantage of post-placental insertion is that, woman is protected from unplanned pregnancy by the time she goes home. Women with *Chlamydia* infection should be treated with antibiotics before insertion. CuT 380A and CuT 380S are more effective, safe and minimal side effects. Compared to other IUCDs, failure rate is <2%. Any copper IUCD fitted at the age of 40 years can be left *in situ* until menopause. The intrauterine system (LNG-IUS) is highly effective with many other health benefits. It inhibits implantation and 75% of women have ovulation. LNG-IUS is to be replaced every 5 years. Women, using it near the age of menopause (40 years), can continue it till menopause.

Implants: Implanon, the single rod system is inserted subdermally, on the inner side of the arm. Its efficacy is similar to sterilization procedure. It is replaced after 3 years. It is extremely safe. Common contraindications are: active liver disease, breast cancer, current venous thromboembolism and migraine with aura. Menstrual bleeding patterns are commonly altered. Bleeding is unpredictable (50%), prolonged (20%), and at times, there may be amenorrhea (20%). This may be cause of discontinuation in about 43% of women. Combined oral contraceptive may be added to implant to improve the bleeding abnormality.

PROGESTOGEN-ONLY INJECTABLE CONTRACEPTIVE (POIC)

Two injectables are commonly used. Depo-provera (medroxyprogesterone acetate) and NET-EN (norethisterone enanthate) are available. DMPA is administered IM, are at the interval of 3 months and NET-EN is used at the interval of 2 months. Both of these POICs are safe and highly reliable method of contraception.

Menstrual irregularly is in the form of irregular bleeding and even amenorrhea are common. There is no evidence of depression, acne, or breast disease. Some women may gain weight. There may be delay in returning to ovulation after stoppage of its use. Both of them cause suppression for ovulation. Bone density may be slightly reduced and it is reversible.

NuvaRing: It is a soft, flexible, transparent ring of 54 mm diameter and 4 mm thick. It is made of evatane. It releases ethinyl estradiol 15 μg/day and etonogestrel 120 μg/day. It has the lowest estrogen content. It prevents ovulation. The ring has to be inserted inside the vagina by the woman. It is to be removed after 3 weeks. Another ring is to be inserted after a week when she gets her withdrawal bleeding.

Contraindication of its use are the same as for combined pill. NuvaRing has high efficacy and failure rate is <1% per 100 women a year. The menstrual cycle pattern is better even when serum estrogen levels are low.

Common side effects are vaginal discharge (3%) and expulsion (6%). The device must be kept in a fridge including during transport. Once dispensed, it must be used by 4 months time to maintain its effectiveness. Among the LARCs available NuvaRing is the most expensive.

With progressive knowledge and understanding, use of effective contraception has increased to prevent unplanned pregnancy. Uses of less reliable and user-dependent methods of contraception are being replaced with long-acting reversible methods of contraception which are user-independent also. Long-acting contraceptive including IUCDs can be used safely by a sexually active woman irrespective of age and mode of delivery.

Suggested Reading

1. Faculty of Sexual and Reproductive Healthcare. UK Medical Eligibility Criteria for Contraceptive Use (UKMEC 2005/2006). London: FSRH; UK; 2006 [www.ffprhc.org.uk/admin/uploads/572_Infocards_common_ Methods.pdf].
2. Faculty of Sexual and Reproductive Healthcare Clinical Effectiveness Unit. Intrauterine Methods of Contraception. London: FSRH CEU; 2007 [www.ffprhc.org.uk/admin/uploads/CEUGuidanceIntrauterineContracepti onNov07.pdf]
3. Kulier R, Helmerhorst FM, O'Brien P, Usher-Patel M, d'Arcangues C. Copper containing, framed intra-uterine devices for contraception. Cochrane Database Syst Rev. 2006;(3);CD005347.
4. National Institute for Health and Clinical Excellence. Long-acting Reversible Contraception. Clinical Guideline 30. London: NICE; October 2005 www.nice.org.uk/nicemedia/pdf/cg030niceguideline.pdf.

30 Chapter — Male and Female Sterilization

FEMALE STERILIZATION

Q.1 Regarding female sterilization:
a. Laparoscopic method is quicker and should be done for all cases
b. Filshie clip application is effective for postpartum sterilization
c. Laparoscopic tubal occlusion should be done ideally by Filshie clip
d. Lifetime risk of failure of tubal occlusion is estimated to be 1 in 200.

Ans.
a. F; it is not suitable for all cases
b. F; failure rate of Filshie clip application (postpartum) is high compared to Pomeroy procedure by minilaparotomy
c. F; both Filshie clip or Falope rings (not only Filshie clip) should be the method of choice for laparoscopic tubal occlusion
d. T.

Q.2 Regarding male sterilization (vasectomy):
a. Compared to tubectomy, vasectomy has got more failure rates
b. Vas division or occlusion by clips or by diathermy is equally effective
c. It should be performed under local anesthetic whenever possible
d. Following vasectomy men should use effective contraception until azoospermic.

Ans.
a. F; vasectomy has got less failure rates (1 in 2,000) compared to tubectomy
b. F; clips has got unacceptably high failure rates and should not be used. Division along with fascial interposition or diathermy should be done
c. T.
d. T; azoospermia is to be checked by semen analysis after 16 weeks postvasectomy or after 20 ejaculations, till then men should use some form of contraceptive.

Q.3 Tubal occlusion for female sterilization:
a. Diathermy can be used as a primary method
b. Hysteroscopic method is very effective
c. Laparoscopic tubal sterilization needs general anesthesia
d. Tubal occlusion can be done any time during the menstrual cycle.

Ans.
a. F; diathermy cause more tubal damage, increases the risk of ectopic pregnancy and is more difficult to reverse if needed
b. F; effectiveness of this procedure is under evaluation
c. F; this procedure can be done under local anesthesia as an alternative to general anesthesia. It should be performed as a day care
d. F; it can be done so, provided the women have used an effective method of contraception up to the day of operation (see discussion below).

Case Selection

Q.4 Criteria to be fulfilled before regarding case selection for female sterilization:

Ans.
- Self-declaration by the client is accepted
- Client must be married (including ever married)
- Client's age is > 22 years but < 45 years
- The couple should have at least two children and the last child of age >1 year, unless sterilization is medically indicated
- Clients or their spouses/partners have not undergone sterilization in the past
- Client must be in a sound state of mind
- Mentally ill client must be certified by a psychiatrist and a statement should be given by the legal guardian/spouse regarding client's abnormal state of mind.

MALE AND FEMALE STERILIZATION

Management Options

Couple when requesting for sterilization, both the methods of vasectomy and tubectomy (tubal occlusion) should be discussed. Couple counseling and advice should cover details of information about the individual procedure.

Discussion about the other alternative long-term reversible methods of contraception [levonorgestrel-releasing intrauterine system (LNG-IUS) implants] with advantages, disadvantages and failure rates, should be made. Counseling must be done with up-to-date knowledge and it should be recorded.

Other Long-term Reversible Methods of Contraception

LNG-IUS, subdermal implants and copper intrauterine devices (IUDs) can work for 3–10 years depending upon the method. Some of these methods are as effective as tubal occlusion at the same time they have the benefit of reversibility. The cumulative rates of failure are as follows: Cu-T 380A at 12 years is 1.9/100 women; LNG-IUS is 1.1/100 after 5 years of typical use. These rates are comparable with tubal occlusion at the same time they have the benefit of reversibility. Currently, it is said that women should continue contraceptive use (once started) until up to a period of 2 years after menopause, if aged ≤ 50 years or one year if over 50 years (FPA-2001).

Tubal Sterilization (Occlusion)

Laparoscopic method of tubal occlusion is quicker. Compared to minilaparotomy, it has less morbidity. But surgeon need to be trained with this method. Postpartum sterilization procedure should be done by modified Pomeroy's method. Compared to laparoscopic method (Filshie clip or Falope ring) (Figs. 30.2A and B), modified Pomeroy's methods has got lower failure rates.

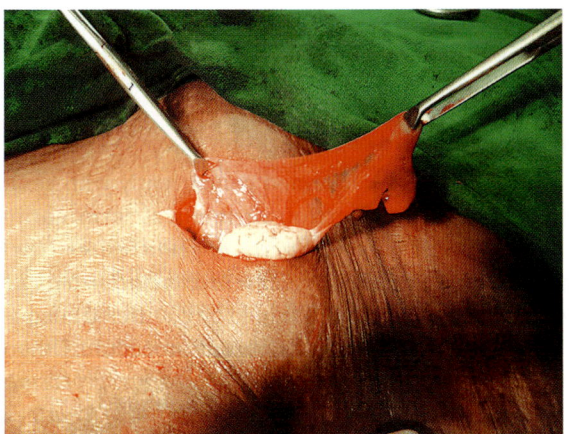

Fig. 30.1: Female sterilization (Pomeroy's method).

Minilaparotomy is the method of approach for an interval sterilization, though any effective surgical or mechanical method can be used.

Modified Pomeroy technique is the most widely used ligation technique. Absorbable sutures (chromic catgut) are used (Fig. 30.1). A loop of the tube is made near the mid portion (ampulla). The base of the loop is tied with chromic catgut suture. Finally, the loop is resected off (*See* Dutta's Textbook of Gynecology, 8th Edition, p. 416). Once the suture material is absorbed (10–14 days), the ends of the tubes fall apart. The chance of fistula formation is also less. However, the procedure removes 3–4 cm of the tube. The chance of reversal of the procedure is less compared to laparoscopic tubal occlusion method (Filshie).

Madlener technique: The tube loop is made. The base of the loop is crushed with a clamp or forceps. The base is then ligated with nonabsorbable suture material. This method has high failure rate.

Kroener technique: The entire fimbrial end of the tube is excised and removed. It is practically impossible to reverse the method.

Uchida technique (*See* Dutta's Textbook of Gynecology, 8th Edition, p. 416): This method is technically more difficult. It has high success rate but chances of reversibility are very low.

Laparoscopic Method of Tubal Sterilization (Occlusion)

Diathermy should not be used as method of tubal occlusion. Disadvantages are:
- More damage to the tube (with monopolar)
- Damage (burn) to other organs (bowel/bladder)
- Not easy to reverse
- Increased risk of subsequent ectopic pregnancy.

Hysteroscopic method of tubal occlusion is done by using 'Essure' (*See* Dutta's Textbook of Gynecology, 8th Edition, p. 424). This is a new method. It is found to have good success rates. But this method is still under evaluation.

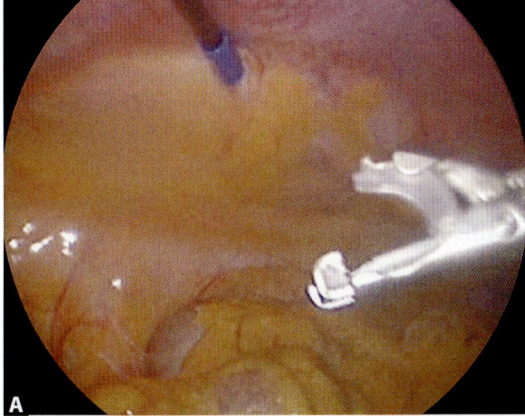
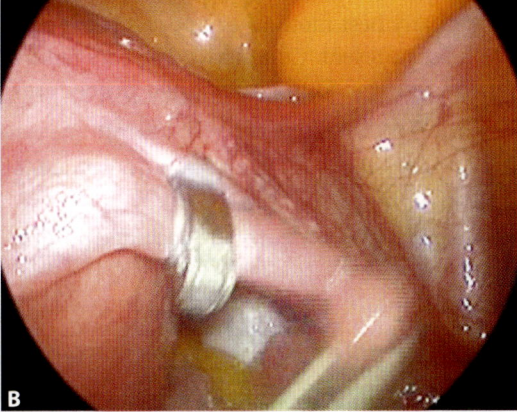

Figs. 30.2A and B: Laparoscopic method of female sterilization (using Filshie clip): (A) Filshie clip loaded applicator; (B) Filshie clip is applied over the Fallopian tube.

Laparoscopic Method of Sterilization

Any women opting for laparoscopic method of tubal occlusion should be informed about the chance of laparotomy, if there is any problem with laparoscopy. This is particularly in cases with obesity or with previous abdominal surgery. Laparoscopic tubal occlusion can be done with local anesthetic. General anesthesia is usually used and it is done on a day care basis. Failure rate of laparoscopic method is about 1 in 200. Failure rate of Filshie clip after 10 years is 2–3 per 1,000 procedure. Whenever there is failure of tubal occlusion (sterilization) method, the risk of ectopic pregnancy is high.

Timing of Tubal Occlusion

Tubal sterilization should ideally be done as an interval method (in between pregnancies). Tubal ligation (occlusion) when done in the postpartum or postabortal period, the risk of failure is increased. There is also increased rate of regret following these two periods.

Tubal occlusion should be done during the follicular phase of the menstrual cycle. The woman should be advised to use some contraceptive measures until the next menstrual cycle. On the other hand, if the woman has used any method of effective contraception up to the day of operation in that case tubal occlusion can be done anytime during the menstrual cycle. Routine curettage at the time of tubal occlusion to prevent a *luteal phase pregnancy*, is not recommended.

Laparoscopic tubal occlusion should be performed as a day care. Use of local anesthesia can be done. Occlusion of the tubes is done mechanically using either Filshie clip which is applied at right angle to the tube over the isthmic portion, at a place 1–2 cm from the cornu. The entire circumference of the tube must be encased.

Tubal occlusion by mechanical method (using clips or rings) is very painful compared to methods done with diathermy. This is due to local tissue necrosis and ischemia at the site of tubal occlusion. Topical instillation of local anesthesia (bupivacaine) to the fallopian tubes at the end of the procedure is effective to reduce the pain.

Failure of Tubal Sterilization

Despite the use of any best method or approach of tubal sterilization, failure is present. Cumulative 10 years failure rate after sterilization was found 16.6/1,000 procedures Collaborative Review of Sterilization (CREST) study.

Q.5 What are the various reasons for failure following tubal sterilization?

Ans.
- Fistula tract development of the occluded portion of the tube
- Ends of the tube can reconnect spontaneously (recanalization)
- Tubes may be occluded incompletely (partially)
- There may be slippage of the occlusive device
- Application of the occlusive device over a wrong anatomical structure (round ligament)
- Failure of recognition of pregnancy that has already taken place *(luteal phase pregnancy)*.

Luteal phase pregnancy is defined when conception occurs unknowingly in the same menstrual cycle in which the sterilization operation is performed. Luteal phase pregnancies are estimated to occur in about 2–3/1,000 interval procedures. Therefore, it is a must, before the operation, to exclude the possibility of a preexisting pregnancy. However, a negative pregnancy test does not exclude the possibility of a luteal phase pregnancy. Routine curettage at the time of tubal occlusion, to prevent luteal phase pregnancy, is not recommended.

Luteal phase ectopic pregnancy can be caused iatrogenically by occluding the tube before the blastocyst has passed the site of occlusion.

If the woman has a copper intrauterine contraceptive device (IUCD) or LNG-IUCD *in situ*, it should be removed at the next period.

Whenever any method of tubal occlusion fails, the resultant pregnancy may be an ectopic pregnancy. The overall incidence of ectopic pregnancy following tubal sterilization ranges from 4.3 to 76.0% depending upon the method used to occlude or destroy the tube. Tubal occlusion with bipolar diathermy has much higher (27 times higher) rate of ectopic pregnancy.

Concurrent Method of Sterilization

Sterilization can be performed concurrently with cesarean delivery, induced abortion or medical termination of pregnancy. *In India majority of female sterilization procedures are concurrently done in association with all the above procedures.* Women should be counseled adequately beforehand at least a week prior to any procedure. Otherwise the woman regret (3–10%). *In Indian set-up, regret is mainly due to the death of a child, particularly that of a male child. In developed countries, regret is mainly due to the desire of a child with a new partner.* Failure rate of sterilization following concurrent procedure is high compared to an interval procedure.

Long-term Risk of Tubal Occlusion

There have been a report of significant *abnormal uterine bleeding* among women who have undergone tubal sterilization compared with a nonsterilized control group. There have been a debate, whether the *post-tubal sterilization syndrome exists or not?*

CREST study found the risk of hysterectomy to be higher among these women compared to general population. However, there is no evidence to suggest that tubal occlusion leads to the problems that necessitate hysterectomy. It may be possible that *alteration in ovarian blood supply by the occlusion method is the cause for abnormal uterine bleeding*.

VASECTOMY

Methods of Vasectomy

No-scalpel vasectomy is the optimum method to perform. It was developed by Li Shun Quiang of China in 1991. This method has low complications. Only ***division of the vas*** is not an acceptable technique because it results in failure. This method should be accompanied by ***fascial interposition or diathermy*** (*See* Dutta's Textbook of Gynecology, 8th Edition, p. 415).

Li's method takes less time. Complications are also low. ***Common complications of vasectomy using scalpel method are:*** Injury to testicular blood vessels, bleeding, hematoma formation, infection and pain.

Methods of Vas Occlusion (Figs. 30.3A and B)

- Ligation with absorbable (catgut) or nonabsorbable sutures (silk or cotton).
- Coagulation using monopolar or bipolar energy source. This method make reversal more difficult as damage to vas is much more.
- Application of clip.

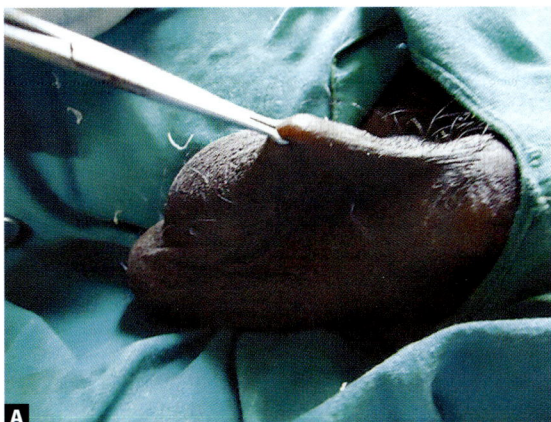

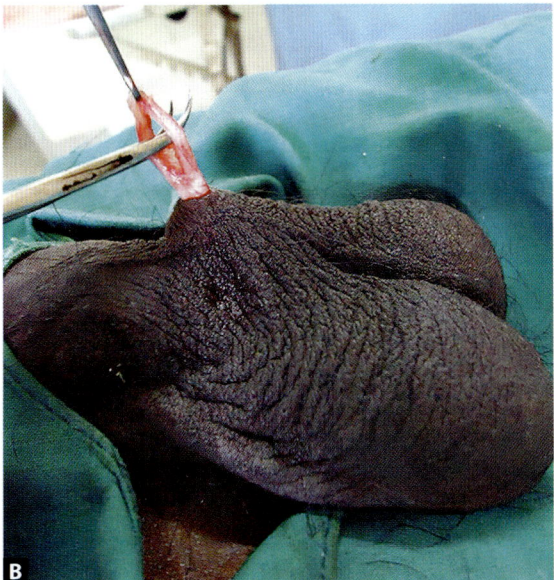

Figs. 30.3A and B: No scalpel vasectomy: (A) Holding the vas with ringed clamp; (B) Dissection of the vas with forceps.

Fascial interposition is done to reduce the risk of recanalization and the subsequent failure rates. Usually, a 2–3 cm segment of the vas is excised during the procedure. One end of the vas (usually the distal end) is allowed to fall back into the wound. The spermatic fascia is interposed over the defect so that the two ends are in different tissue planes. This makes the possibility of recanalization between the two ligated ends far less.

Fascial interposition makes no scalpel vasectomy much successful.

Application of clips and excision method has got high failure rate. Vasectomy is usually performed under local anesthetic and it is found safe.

Postvasectomy Considerations

Histological examination of the excised portions of vas is not routinely needed (unless when there is any doubt about their identity). Following vasectomy, men should use an effective contraception until azoospermia has been confirmed. This is to confirm the clearance of stored spermatozoa down the vasectomy site. Usually, semen analysis is done 16 weeks after vasectomy. Men should use other birth control methods for at least 20 ejaculations. ***Association for voluntary sterilization*** recommended at least 15 ejaculations or semen analysis 6 weeks after the procedure. By that time most men become sterile.

In a small group of men (2–3%), nonmotile sperm may be present in the postvasectomy period. Presence of ≤ 10,000 nonmotile sperm/mL, 7 months after vasectomy was not associated with any pregnancy report. In such a situation, men can be given, ***special clearance*** to stop contraception.

Failure of Vasectomy

Pregnancy can occur even several years after vasectomy. The rate may low as 1 in 2,000 after clearance has been given.

Vasectomy failure is defined as the presence of spermatozoa on semen analysis or presence of a pregnancy.

Causes of Vasectomy Failure

- Surgeon failure (operator)
- Method failure (technical failure)
- Unprotected intercourse soon after vasectomy while residual sperm is still stored in the reproductive tract
- Spontaneous recanalization of the vas
- Occlusion of a wrong structure instead of the vas, inadequate occlusion of the vas (loose tie), or congenital duplication of one or both vas (rare).

Risks of Vasectomy

- ***Prostate cancer:*** Population based study with systematic review found ***no association*** between vasectomy and prostate cancer.
- ***Testicular cancer***: ***No increased risk*** has been observed, based on contact and case-control studies.

- ***Cardiovascular disease: No association*** has been observed between vasectomy and cardiovascular disease, atherosclerotic disease, hypertension, myocardial infarction or coronary artery disease.
- ***Chronic testicular pain*** may be observed months or years after vasectomy. The incidence of postvasectomy pain ranges from 12 to 52%.

Suggested Reading

1. Hillis SD, Marchbanks PA, Tylor LR. Higher hysterectomy risk for sterilized than nonsterilized women: findings from the US Collaborative Review of Sterilization. The US Collaborative Review of Sterilization Working Group. Obstet Gynecol. 1998;91(2):241-6.
2. Peterson HB, Xia Z, Hughes JM. The risk of pregnancy after tubal sterilization: findings from the US Collaborative Review of Sterilization. Am J Obstet Gynecol.1996;174(4):1161-8.

Chapter 31: Safe Abortion Service and WHO Guidelines

GUIDING PRINCIPLES

Care providers should be aware of local laws and reporting requirements. Within the national laws all norms, standards, and clinical practice related to abortion should be promoted and protected.

Principles of Health Care

- Treating all women equally regardless of age (including ethnicity, religion, marital and socioeconomic status).
- Abortion care is delivered in a respectful manner with the provision of all the information.
- The information should be complete, accurate, and easy to understand.
- Should maintain the dignity, privacy and confidentiality.
- Family planning is a human right.
- For the adolescents, minors and mentally disabled, parents to be involved.
- Decision-making must be informed and voluntary.
- Autonomy is maintained without any discrimination.

COUNSELING

Following information is provided to the women prior to the procedure:
- Specific method of abortion, advantages and disadvantages, and the potential risk factors of each method is to be discussed.
- Lab tests are done if it is available or as per countries guidelines. Lab tests are not the prerequisite for abortion service.
- Management of pain, bleeding or any other potential complication
- Period of rest: time to resume the normal activities including sexual intercourse
- Follow-up care: preventive measures against any unintended pregnancy
- Any legal or other reporting requirements.

Methods of Abortion (≤12 Weeks)

Medical Abortion

Advantages
- Avoids surgery
- Under the control of the woman and may take place at home

Disadvantages
- Takes time (hours to days) to complete abortion, and the timing may not be predictable
- Women experience bleeding and cramping pain
- Other side-effects (nausea and vomiting)
- May require more clinic visits than surgical methods
- May be preferred in the following situations: Presence of uterine malformations or fibroids, previous cervical surgery
- If the woman wants to avoid surgical intervention.

Contraindications
- Allergic reaction to one of the drugs
- Chronic adrenal failure or inherited porphyria
- Suspected ectopic pregnancy

Caution and clinical judgement are required in cases of:
- Long-term corticosteroid therapy (including those with severe uncontrolled asthma)
- Hemorrhagic disorder
- Severe anemia
- Pre-existing heart disease or cardiovascular risk factors or unknown uterine scars.

Surgical Abortion

There is no known absolute contraindication for surgical abortion.

Advantages and disadvantages
- Quick procedure
- Complete abortion easily verified by evaluation of aspirated material
- Takes place in a healthcare facility
- Sterilization or placement of an intrauterine device (IUD) may be performed at the same time at the end of the procedure.
- May be preferred in the following situations:
  - If there are contraindications to medical abortion
  - If there are constraints for the timing of the abortion

Caution and clinical judgement are required in cases of:
- Any medical disorders in pregnancy (hemoglobinopathy in pregnancy)
- Congenital heart disease.

ASSESSMENT OF DURATION OF GESTATIONAL AGE

- Pregnancy is assessed by bimanual examination. Uterine size usually corresponds to the gestational age based

on the first day of last menstrual period. However, there are limitations to menstrual dating. In that situation ultrasonography is helpful.
- Suspected ectopic pregnancy or abnormal intrauterine pregnancy, e.g., spontaneous or missed abortion.

INVESTIGATIONS

The following tests, when available, may be performed on the basis of individual risk factors:
- Urine for pregnancy test
- Hemoglobin (Hb) or hematocrit estimation for suspected anemia
- Blood for ABO and Rhesus (Rh) testing. Rh-immunoglobulin should be available for Rh-negative women
- HIV testing/counseling
- Nasopharyngeal swab for RT-PCR, COVID-19
- Sexually transmitted infection (STI) screening (usually performed during the pelvic examination)
- Cervical cancer screening (performed during the pelvic examination)
- Other laboratory tests as indicated by medical history (kidney or liver function tests, etc.)
- Diagnostic ultrasound is indicated to confirm pregnancy dating or for the identification of location of the pregnancy.

Routine laboratory testing is not a prerequisite for abortion services. It mostly depends on clinician's decision.

DISCUSSING CONTRACEPTIVE OPTIONS

- Immediate initiation of contraception following abortion has been shown to improve continuation and at the same time reduce the risk of unintended pregnancy.
- Women is provided with post-abortion information and counseling (using WHO MEC wheel).
- Ovulation usually returns by 2–3 weeks following abortion. Risk of unplanned pregnancy is there unless an effective contraceptive method is adopted.

However, a woman's acceptance to a contraceptive method must never be a precondition for providing her abortion services.

PREVENTION AND CONTROL OF INFECTION

Since abortion procedures and care involves contact with blood and other body fluids, all clinical and support staffs who provide these services should understand and apply standard precautions for prevention and control of infection, This is both for their own protection as well as for the patients.

Standard precautions (universal precautions)
- One should avoid any direct contact with blood, body fluids, non-intact skin, and mucous membrane. This should be followed, regardless of the patient's presence of infection.
- This is done to minimize or eliminate the transmission of disease from the patient to health-care worker, or from health-care worker to patient.

PAIN MANAGEMENT

- Almost all women will experience some pain and cramping with abortion.
- Pain should be adequately treated to reduce the anxiety and discomfort.
- The amount of pain that women get with the procedure varies greatly.
- It is necessary to assess each individual woman's pain and manage it accordingly.

Pain Management Options

Surgical Abortion
- Analgesia nonsteroidal anti-inflammatory drugs (NSAIDs), e.g., ibuprofen 400–800 mg at least 30 min before the procedure
- Anxiolytics/sedatives (e.g., diazepam 5–10 mg)
- Local anesthetic (paracervical block using lidocaine usually 10–20 mL of 0.5–1.0%)
- Conscious sedation, deep IV sedation or general anesthesia in some cases (not routinely).

Medical Abortion
- Analgesia (NSAIDs, e.g., ibuprofen 400–800 mg)
- Anxiolytics/sedatives (e.g., diazepam 5–10 mg)
- Regional analgesia may be used in cases with mid-trimester termination.
- Adjuvant medications may also be provided, if indicated, for the side-effects of misoprostol (e.g., loperamide for diarrhea).
- **In cases with >12 weeks' gestation,** addition to NSAIDs one or more of the following may be needed.
  - Oral opioids
  - Intramuscular (IM) or intravenous (IV) opioids and paracervical block or epidural anesthesia.

Procedure to Administer a Paracervical Block
- Initial procedure is the same
- To stabilize the cervix with a tenaculum
- Slight traction is given to move the cervix and to see the smooth cervical epithelium. It is the site for infiltration of local anesthetics.
- Slowly injections of 2–5 mL of lidocaine into a depth of 1.5–2 cm at 2–4 points at the cervical/vaginal junction (**2 and 10 o'clock, and/or 4 and 8 o'clock**) is given.
- Aspiration is done before injecting the drug to avoid intravascular injection.
- The maximum dose of lidocaine in a paracervical block is 4.5 mg/kg/dose or generally 200–300 mg is injected.

WHO MEDICAL MANAGEMENT OF ABORTION GUIDELINES 2018

Management of abortion: Current recommendation on medical management of induced abortion.

Medical management of induced abortion at <12 weeks (first trimester) of pregnancy

Recommendations	Combination regimen (Recommended)	Misoprostol only regimen (Alternate)
Induced abortion <12 weeks	▪ Mifepristone 200 mg PO once ▪ Misoprostol (after 1–2 days) 800 µg B, PV or SL	Misoprostol 800 µg B, PV or SL

(B: buccal; PO: per oral; PV: per vaginal; SL: sublingual)

Recommend dose of 200 mg mifepristone is administered orally, followed 1–2 days later by 800 µg misoprostol administered vaginally, sublingually or buccally. The minimum recommended interval between use of mifepristone and misoprostol is 24 hours.

For the misoprostol-only regimen, recommend dose of 800 µg misoprostol is administered vaginally, sublingually or buccally.

Medical management of induced abortion at ≥12 weeks of gestation

Recommendations[b]	Combination regimen (Recommended)[a]	Misoprostol only regimen (Alternate)[c]
Induced abortion ≥12 weeks	▪ Mifepristone 200 mg PO once ▪ Misoprostol (after 1–2 days) 400 µg B, PV or SL every 3 hours	Misoprostol 400 µg B, PV or SL every 3 hours

(B: buccal; PO: per oral; PV: per vaginal; SL: sublingual)
a: Combination regimen is recommended because it is more effective.
b: Evidence suggests that vaginal route is the most effective. Consideration for patient and use suggest that use of all the routes including buccal administration are effective.
c: Repeat doses of misoprostol can be considered when needed to achieve success of the abortion process. In this guideline, no such maximum number of doses of misoprostal has been mentioned. Healthcare providers should use caution and clinical judgement to decide the maximum number of doses of misoprostol in pregnant individuals with prior uterine incision. Uterine rupture is a care complication. Clinical judgment and health system preparedness for emergency management of uterine rupture must be considered with advanced gestational age.

It is suggested to use of 200 mg mifepristone administered orally, followed 1–2 days later by repeat doses of 400 µg misoprostol administered vaginally, sublingually or buccally every 3 hours. The minimum recommended interval between use of mifepristone and misoprostol is 24 hours.

For the misoprostol-only regimen, we suggest the use of repeat doses of 400 µg misoprostol administered vaginally, sublingually or buccally every 3 hours.

Note: The use of a loading dose of misoprostol is not necessary. There is no advantage to the use of moistened over dry misoprostol.

Second trimester termination of pregnancy is more traumatic both physically and psychologically. Fetal autopsy following second trimester miscarriage revealed malformation 13% of cases.

Complications of Elective Abortion

In an elective case, with mortality rate is low: <1 death per 100,000 procedures. Risks of infertility or ectopic pregnancy are not increased. The complications of the procedure increase as the gestational age increases and specially in second trimester.

Medical Method of TOP in the Second Trimester

The methods used are: Mifepristone and misoprostol combined regimen or use of misoprostol only. Combined method is commonly used. It reduces the onset of induction and termination time. Use of hygroscopic dilators may further reduce the time- and procedure-related trauma.

Routes of misoprostol use: Oral route takes longer time to expulsion compared to vaginal or sublingual routes. PGE2, intracervical can also be used similar to misoprostol. Use of high-dose oxytocin IV in normal saline is also effective in 80–90% of cases.

Ethacridine lactate is an organic antiseptic. It activates decidua to release prostaglandins. It is instilled extra-amniotic with a Foley catheter. It is effective and safe. However, it takes longer time compared to misoprostol.

A levels should be monitored if possible. It usually declines by 90% on D8 of misoprostol use.

Ultrasonography is useful to detect any retained products of conception and it is a noninvasive procedure.

Surgical Method of Abortion in Second Trimester

Important indication is fetal anomaly or death, maternal medical disorders or others (see above). The commonly used method is D and E. Wide cervical dilation is needed before evacuation of the fetal parts. Pre-evacuation cervical ripening could be done by using hygroscopic dilators and/or misoprostol. Use of laminaria tent, helps cervical dilation. Sometimes multiple number of tents are needed over more time. Misoprostol can be added to supplement laminaria tents. A misoprostol 400 µg is given vaginally or buccally 3-4 hours prior to D and E. Mifepristone has also been used either alone or along with hygroscopic dilators. In second trimester termination of pregnancy at times fetal demise is induced prior to avert live birth. In those cases intracardiac KCL injections are given guided by USG.

Hysterotomy for an induced abortion is rarely done these days (*See* Dutta's Textbook of Obstetrics, 9th Edition, p. 527). This is a surgical procedure where a small vertical incised is made on the body of the uterus. Once the amniotic cavity is reached, the conceptus and the placenta are removed. The uterine cavity is thoroughly cleared. The uterus closed in layers.

Procedure of Evacuation

The operation may be done under IV anesthesia. Once cervical dilatation is sufficient enough, the amniotic sac is ruptured to drain the amniotic fluid. This induces the risk of amniotic fluid embolism. The fetus is extracted in parts with ovum forceps. With completed removal of the fetus, a large-bore vacuum curette is used to remove the remaining tissues.

Contraindications of Medical Abortion

Severe anemia until it is improved, chronic systemic disorders such as long-term systemic corticosteroid use, chronic adrenal failure, prolong anticoagulant use, inherited porphyria, severe renal pulmonary or cardiovascular disease. Methotrexate and misoprostol are both teratogens. Once these drugs are used, abortion process must be completed.

Side-effects, complications of medical or surgical abortion and their management

- **Pain:** Verbal support and reassurance can improve the pain. The presence of a support person is helpful. NSAIDs, such as ibuprofen is often helpful.
- **Bleeding:** Small amount of bleeding is common. If there is evidence of hemodynamic compromise, start IV fluids and oxytocic if needed. For profuse bleeding, blood transfusion, is required.
- **Fever** (repeated doses of misoprostol may cause temperature elevation): Antipyretic drugs, such as paracetamol may be given.
- **Nausea and vomiting:** It is mostly self-limiting. Reassurance and antiemetics (tab. Domperidone) is helpful.
- **Diarrhea:** Self-limiting; reassure and to give antidiarrheal medication if needed; encourage oral hydration.
- **Pelvic infection:** If infection is suspected, perform clinical examination; antibiotics need to be given, uterine evacuation and hospitalize if necessary.

Follow-up care of abortion cases

- **Mifepristone and misoprostol:** There is no need of routine follow-up. A follow-up visit may be arranged between 7 and 14 days, if needed.
- **Assesment for completion of abortion process,** analysis of clinical signs and symptoms, and bimanual examination is helpful. Ultrasonography may be done to confirm the diagnosis. It is useful to exclude ongoing intrauterine pregnancy, retained products of conception or an ectopic pregnancy.
- **Cases for further evaluation:** A woman may report with prolonged bleeding and cramping pain in the lower abdomen, and that no products of conception were obtained following termination of pregnancy (TOP). She needs investigations and management as appropriately. Ectopic pregnancy, retained products of conception or failure of the procedure need to be excluded. Ultrasonography is helpful in such cases.

CERVICAL PREPARATION BEFORE SURGICAL ABORTION

- It is done before surgical abortion for all women with pregnancies over 12–14 weeks.
- Osmotic dilators and pharmacologic agents are used for cervical preparation.
- Analgesics, such as ibuprofen and/or narcotics, oral anxiolytics may be needed to control the pain.

Procedure for Insertion of Osmotic Dilators

- Place a speculum in the vagina and wipe the cervix with betadine antiseptic solution.
- Administer **local anesthesia** to the cervical lip or a paracervical block then grasp the lip of the cervix with a tenaculum.
- Grasp the end of the **osmotic dilators with forceps** and insert it into the endocervical canal such that the tip extends just beyond the internal cervical os. Coating the osmotic dilator with lubricant jelly or with antiseptic solution can ease placement.
- Sequentially place the dilators adjacent to one another within the cervical os, so that they **fit snugly in the cervical** canal. Upper vagina is packed with a roller gauze to prevent the dislodgement of the dilators.

Additional Considerations for Misoprostol and Osmotic Dilator use for Cervical Preparation

Osmotic Dilators

- Maximum dilatation occurs between 6 and 12 hours after placement.
- As there is minimal risk of expulsion after placement of laminaria, women often leave the clinic and return for their procedure at a later scheduled time.

Misoprostol

- Women may experience some bleeding and cramping from the misoprostol.
- For observation, the woman is asked to wait for some time in the clinic.
- If the cervix does not dilate easily after one dose of misoprostol, the dose can be repeated.

DIFFERENT ROUTES OF MISOPROSTOL ADMINISTRATION

- **Oral:** Pills are swallowed.
- **Buccal:** Pills are placed between the cheek and gums and swallowed after 30 minutes.
- **Sublingual:** Pills are placed under the tongue and swallowed after 30 minutes.
- **Vaginal:** Pills are placed in the vaginal fornices (deepest portions of the vagina) and the woman is instructed to lie down for 30 minutes.

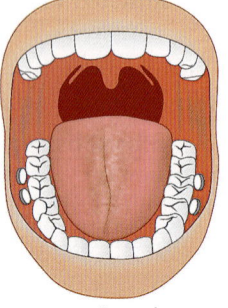 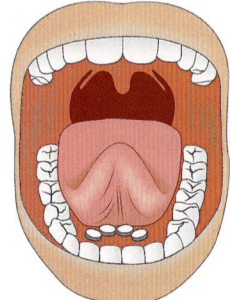

Buccal   Sublingual

Fig. 31.1: Buccal and sublingual routes of misoprostol administration.

TABLE 31.1: Selecting the cannula size for aspiration abortion.

Uterine size weeks since (LMP)	Suggested cannula size (mm)
4–6	4–7
7–9	5–10
9–12	8–12
12–14	10–14

(LMP: last menstrual period)

To reduce the risk of post-procedure infections, prophylactic antibiotics, preoperatively or perioperatively are recommended. Use of antibiotic depends on clinician's decision.

Manual vacuum apiration (MVA) or electrical vacuum aspiration (EVA): It is commonly done up to 12 weeks of pregnancy. It is done as an outpatient procedure. EVA/MVA is done using paracervical block. Intracervical 5 mL of 1–2% lignocine is injected at 2, 10 and/or 4, 8 o'clock. General and regional anesthesia may be used though it is not needed often. Aspiration of the conceptus done using manual vacuum aspiration cannula of appropriate size according to the weeks of pregnancy (Table 31.1).

The manual vacuum aspirator is connected to the cannula after creating a vaccum in the aspirator.
- Initiate the suction when the cannula tip is in the uterine cavity 1 cm below the fundus of uterus.
- Evacuate the contents of the uterus by gently and slowly rotating the cannula 180° in each direction. Blood and tissue will be visible through the cannula and in manual vacuum aspiration (MVA) syringe.

The cannula is gradually pulled down towards the OS. It is slowly rotated circumferentially to empty the entire surface of the uterine cavity. Endpoint of suction is noted when no more tissue is coming out or bubbles are started to come out. Curettage following evacuation is currently not recommended (WHO 2012).

MVA or EVA are safe and effective methods of surgical termination of pregnancy. The tissues need to be seen following rinsing them in a plastic container with clean water. Failure of the procedure may occur when pregnancy is ≤ 6 weeks and in bicornuate uterus.

Signs of Completion of Evacuation Process
- Red or pink froth appears and no more tissue is seen passing through the cannula and a gritty sensation is felt as the cannula passes along the surface of the evacuated uterus
- The uterus contracts (grips) around the cannula
- When the procedure is completed, remove the cannula and cervical tenaculum, wipe the cervix with a clean swab and assess the amount of uterine or cervical bleeding. Inspection of the products of conception (POC) is to be done.

EVACUATION OF THE UTERUS
- Wherever possible, complete the evacuation from the lowest section of the uterine cavity.
- Avoid probing deeply into the uterus, particularly with instruments in the horizontal position.
- Avoid reaching high into the uterus, where the perforation risk is greater. Instead, reinsert the cannula just inside the os and use suction to bring tissue down from the fundus to the internal os.
- Stop the procedure if signs of uterine perforation occur.
- Sudden loss of resistance, complaints of acute pain during the procedure, excess bleeding and/or detection some doubtful tissue (omentum) suggest perforation.
- Ultrasonography may be helpful to locate fetal parts if identification is otherwise difficult in some cases. All the fetal tissues are removed under ultrasonography guidance. Patient may need oxytocics for any additional bleeding.
  - 400–600 µg misoprostol sublingually, orally or buccally
  - 0.2 mg methergin orally or intramuscularly (IM)
  - High-dose oxytocin 20 units in 500 mL normal saline or Ringer's lactate solution, run at 30 drops per minute.

Inspection of the Tissues
After the evacuation procedure, the fetal tissues should be evaluated to ensure complete abortion specially in second trimester abortion. The extremities, trunk and the cranial bones need to be checked in products aspirated.

If the tissue inspection indicates that the abortion process is incomplete, ultrasonography is used to confirm complete evacuation.

To Perform Any Concurrent Procedures
When the aspiration procedure is completed, proceed with any concurrent procedures. IUD insertion or tubal ligation may be done as requested.

Recovery and Discharge from the Facility
- Reassure the woman that the procedure is finished and that it is done safely.
- Offer to address any emotional needs the woman might need immediately following the procedure.
- Monitor her for any complications and provide management as needed.
- Ensure that the woman has all necessary information and medications prior to leaving the facility.
- Document all outcomes of the treatment, including any adverse events.

POST-ABORTION CARE
- Prior to discharge from the healthcare facility
- Follow-up with a healthcare provider is advised for:
  - Assessing and managing any complications and
  - Post-abortion contraception.

Advice on Discharge From the Healthcare Facility
Client is provided a clear oral and written discharge instructions, including
- Sexual intercourse should occur only after the bleeding stops;

- Some amount of vaginal bleeding for 2 weeks after completed surgical or medical abortion is normal.

The woman should return to the clinic if she experiences:
- Increased intensity of cramping or abdominal pain
- Heavy vaginal bleeding

Provide contraceptive information and counseling to women who desire it:
- Assist her in choosing the most appropriate contraceptive method to meet her needs
- Provide the chosen contraceptive method. Ensure she knows how her selected method works, when to start it and how she can obtain future supplies
- Provide iron tablets for anemia
- Provide any pain medications, if needed

An IUD should not be inserted immediately after evacuation of a case of septic abortion.

Additional Follow-up with a Healthcare Provider
- Routine follow-up is not necessary following an uncomplicated surgical or medical abortion;
- Routine follow-up visit is recommended, only in cases with medical abortion using misoprostol alone to assess abortion completion;
- An optional follow-up visit 7–14 days after, may be organized to provide contraceptive counseling, for emotional support or to address any medical concerns.

Complications of Induced Abortion (MTP)
- Complications are more with increasing with gestational age.
- Common complications are: Hemorrhage, incomplete evacuation, and infections.
- Hemorrhage is more following: Medical (15%) compared to surgical procedure (2%). Rare complications are: Uterine perforation, lower genital tract lacerations, pelvic infections.

Complications of Medical Methods of Termination of Pregnancy and its Management

Excessive bleeding: Inj. Oxytocin infusion is continued to reduce the bleeding. The *major complications* are: Uterine perforation, cervical laceration, uterine bleeding, DIC or amniotic fluid embolism.

Complications due to abnormal placentation may cause perfuse bleeding. Placenta previa accreta (low lying placenta with morbid adhesions) may need blood transfusion or even hysterectomy. Prior cesarean delivery is not a contraindication for Dilation and Evacuation (D and E). Medical method of TOP may cause rupture of uterus (0.4–2.5%) in cases with prior one or more cesarean deliveries.

Management of Abortion-related Complications
- Unsafe abortions have more complications. Some of these women need immediate emergency attention for life-threatening conditions. They need admission for treatment.
- *Ongoing pregnancy:* Women with continuing signs of pregnancy or clinical signs of failed abortion, should be offered uterine evacuation.
- *Incomplete abortion:*
  - Common symptoms of incomplete abortion include vaginal bleeding and abdominal pain. It may be suspected when the POC aspirated during surgical abortion is not compatible with the estimated duration of pregnancy.
- Incomplete abortion may need repeat evacuation under anesthesia.

Recommended regimen for management of incomplete abortion with misoprostol.

Dose (μg)	Route
600 μg	Oral
400 μg	Sublingual
400–800 μg	Vaginal; may be used if vaginal bleeding is minimal

Other complications:
- Hemorrhage
- Infection
- Uterine perforation
- Anesthesia-related complications.

POST-ABORTION CONTRACEPTION

Generally, almost all methods of contraception can be initiated immediately following a surgical or medical abortion. With the start of any method of contraception, the woman's **medical eligibility** for that method should be verified.

Contraceptive Methods and Medical Eligibility after Abortion
- **Hormonal methods** (including pills, injections, implants, the patch and vaginal ring) may be started immediately after any abortion, including septic abortion.
- **IUDs** may be inserted immediately after first- or second-trimester abortion; however, the expulsion risk is slightly higher following second-trimester abortions than following first-trimester abortions. IUDs may be inserted after a medical abortion has been deemed complete.
- **Condom** use may start with the first act of sexual intercourse after abortion, including septic abortion.
- **Diaphragm or cervical cap** use may start with the first act of sexual intercourse after abortion, including septic abortion. It should be postponed for 6 weeks following abortion beyond 14 weeks' gestation.
- **Fertility-awareness-based methods** should be delayed until regular menstrual cycles return.
- **Female surgical sterilization** can be performed immediately after uncomplicated abortions. However, it should be delayed if abortion is complicated with infection, severe hemorrhage, trauma or acute hematometra.
- **Vasectomy** can be performed at any time.
- **Emergency contraception** women may use emergency contraceptive pills or an IUD within 5 days (120 hours)

Post-abortion medical eligibility recommendations for female contraception.

Method of contraception	Pregnancy duration		Post-abortion septic condition
	1st trimester	2nd trimester	
COC	1	1	1
CIC	1	1	1
Patch and vaginal ring	1	1	1
POP	1	1	1
DMPA, NET-EN	1	1	1
LNG/ETG implants	1	1	1
Copper-bearing IUD	1	2	4
LNG-releasing IUD	1	2	4
Condom	1	1	1
Spermicide	1	1	1
Diaphragm	1	1	1

(CIC: combined injectable contraceptive; COC: combined oral contraceptive; DMPA/NET-EN: progestogen-only injectables: depot medroxyprogesterone acetate/norethisterone enantate; IUD: intrauterine device; LNG/ETG: progestogen-only implants: levenorgestrel/etonorgestrel; POP: progesterone-only pill)

Definition of categories
1. A condition for which there is no restriction for the use of the contraceptive method.
2. A condition where the advantages of using the method generally outweigh the theoretical or proven risks.
3. A condition where the theoretical or proven risks usually outweigh the advantages of using the method. Use of method is not generally recommended unless other more appropriate methods are not available or not acceptable.
4. A condition that represents an unacceptable health risk if the contraceptive method is used.

Post-abortion condition	Surgical sterilization (Tubectomy)
Uncomplicated	A
Post-abortal sepsis or fever	D
Severe post-abortal hemorrhage	D
Severe trauma to the genital tract; cervical or vaginal tear at the time of abortion	D
Uterine perforation	S
Acute hematometra	D

Definition of Categories
A (accept): There is no medical reason to deny sterilization to a person with this condition.
C (caution): The procedure is normally conducted in a routine setting, but with extra preparation and precautions.
D (delay): The procedure is delayed until the condition is evaluated and/or corrected; alternative temporary methods of contraception should be provided.
S (special): The procedure should be undertaken in a setting with an experienced surgeon and staff, and equipment is needed to provide general anesthesia and other back-up medical support. For these conditions, the capacity to decide on the most appropriate procedure and anesthesia regimen is also needed. Alternative temporary methods of contraception should be provided, if referral is required or there is otherwise any delay.

of an act of unprotected sexual intercourse, to decrease pregnancy risk.
- **Withdrawal** use may start with the first act of sexual intercourse, after abortion, including septic abortion.

An effective contraceptive method should be initiated soon after abortion to reduce the risk of any unplanned pregnancy.

Suggested Reading

1. Based on Medical eligibility criteria for contraceptive use, 4th edition. Geneva: World Health Organization; 2009.
2. Cleland K, Creinin MD, Nucatola D, Nshom M, Trussell J. Significant adverse events and outcomes after medical abortion. Obstet. 2013;121(1):166–71.
3. Jackson E, Kapp N. Pain management for medical and surgical termination of pregnancy between 13 and 24 weeks of gestation: a systematic review; BJOG. 2020;127(11):1348-57.
4. FIGO's updated recommendations for misoprostol used alone in gynecology and obstetrics. International journal of gynecology and obstetrics: the official organ of the International Federation of Gynecology and Obstetrics. 2017;138(Suppl 2).
5. Maltzer DS, Maltzer MC, Wiebe ER, Halvorson-Boyd G, Boyd C. Pain management. In: Paul M, Lichtenberg ES, Borgatta L, Grimes DA, Stubblefield PG (Eds). A Clinician's Guide to Medical and Surgical Abortion. New York: Churchill Livingstone; 1999. pp. 73–90.
6. Konar H. Dutta's Textbook of Gynecology, 8th Edition, 2018. Jaypee Brothers and Medical Publishers, New Delhi; p. 398.

7. Shimoni N, Davis A, Ramos ME, Rosario L, Westhoff C. Timing of copper intrauterine device insertion after medical abortion: a randomized controlled trial. Obstet Gynecol. 2011;118:623–8.
8. Society of Family Planning/Contraception 89 (2014) 75–84. Cervical preparation for second trimester surgical abortion prior to 20 weeks gestation. SFP Guideline #2013-14, 2014.
9. Society of Family Planning Clinical Guidelines. Medical management of first-trimester abortion. Contraception. 2014; 89:148–61.
10. WHO Clinical practice handbook for safe abortion: https://apps.who.int/iris/bitstream/handle/10665/97415/9789241548717_eng.pdf;jsessionid=BF09C664A866D710A07EF28EA7FAEFEE?sequence=1.
11. WHO Medical eligibility criteria for contraceptive use, 5th ed. 2015.
12. WHO Reproductive Health Library: Cervical preparation for first trimester surgical abortion: RHL summary (last revised 4 March 2016). The WHO Reproductive Health Library; Geneva: World Health Organization.
13. World Health Organization (WHO). Health Worker Roles in Providing Safe Abortion Care and Post-Abortion Contraception. Geneva: WHO, Department of Reproductive Health and Research; 2015.
14. World Health Organization. Medical management of abortion. Geneva: World Health Organization; 2018.
15. World Health Organization. Safe abortion: technical and policy guidance for health systems. 2nd ed. Geneva: WHO, Department of Reproductive Health and Research; 2012.

Section 5: Gynecological Oncology

Section Outline

- Ch. 32. Carcinoma of the Endometrium (Early Stage Disease)
- Ch. 33. Surgical Management of Endometrial Carcinoma
- Ch. 34. Role of Pelvic and Para-aortic Lymph Node Dissection in the Surgical Management of Endometrial Cancer
- Ch. 35. Ovarian Tumor with Low Malignant Potential
- Ch. 36. Gestational Trophoblastic Disease
- Ch. 37. Human Chorionic Gonadotropin and the Management of Gestational Trophoblastic Disease
- Ch. 38 Fertility Preservation in Women
- Ch. 39. Fertility Preserving Options for Women with Ovarian Cancer
- Ch. 40. Fertility Preserving Options for Women with Cervical Cancer
- Ch. 41. Fertility Preserving Options for Women with Endometrial Cancer
- Ch. 42. Chemotherapy in Gynecological Cancers
- Ch. 43. Radiotherapy in Gynecological Cancers
- Ch. 44. Sentinel Lymph Node Mapping in Gynecologic Cancers

Chapter 32: Carcinoma of the Endometrium (Early Stage Disease)

CARCINOMA ENDOMETRIUM

FIGO EARLY STAGE DISEASE (2009)

Stage I*: Tumor confined to the corpus uteri
Stage IA*: No or invasion < 50% of the myometrium
Stage IB*: Invasion ≥ 50% of the myometrium (Fig. 32.1).
*Either grades I, II or III.
Positive peritoneal cytology has to be reported separately without changing the stage.
Stage II**: Tumor invades cervical stroma but does not extend beyond the uterus.
**Endocervical glandular involvement only is considered as stage I and no longer as stage II.

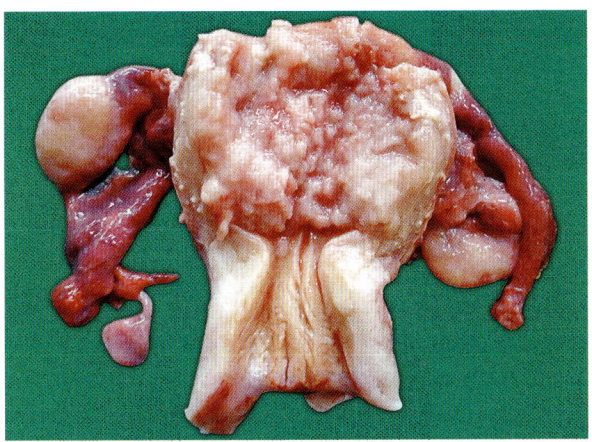

Fig. 32.1: Endometrial carcinoma diffuse type.

FIGO GRADING SYSTEM (1989)

Grade I: <5% of the tumors show a solid (nonsquamous or nonmorular) growth pattern.
Grade II: 6–50% of the tumors show a solid (nonsquamous or nonmorular) growth pattern.
Grade III: >50% of the tumors show a solid (nonsquamous or nonmorular) growth pattern.
Presence of any nuclear atypia increases the tumor grade by one.

Management Options

The current surgical management approach for a patient with endometrial cancer is: (a) Laparotomy, (b) peritoneal cytology, (c) total hysterectomy and bilateral salpingo-oophorectomy and (d) surgical staging. Majority of women with endometrial carcinoma have endometrioid type of adenocarcinoma (80%) on histology. In women with non-endometrioid case, surgical steps are extended to include: (a) Omentectomy, (b) appendectomy and (c) peritoneal biopsies.

The place of lymphadenectomy (pelvic and para-aortic) is an important issue to detect extrauterine spread of the disease. This is essential as to formulate the postoperative management. Incorporation of lymphadenectomy in all patients of endometrial carcinoma is not universally accepted. Two large prospective-randomized trials failed to show improved survival outcomes of the patients who underwent pelvic lymphadenectomy. Patients with endometrioid type histology, grades 1 or 2 disease, tumor diameter < 2 cm and superficial myometrial invasion did not have a lymphatic metastasis. There is no evidence of benefit in terms of overall survival or recurrence-free survival with pelvic lymphadenectomy in women with early endometrial cancer. Pelvic lymphadenectomy cannot be recommended as routine procedure for therapeutic purposes outside of clinical trials.

Therefore, it was necessary to identify the group of patients in whom lymphadenectomy likely to improve survival outcome instead of increasing the risk of surgical complications and consequent morbidity.

Treatment of endometrial cancer primarily is the surgery. The surgical procedures include: collection of peritoneal wash (or ascitic fluid) for malignant cell cytology, extrafascial hysterectomy, BSO, surgical staging and lymphadenectomy as recommended by FIGO revised staging (2018). Majority of the cases belong to Stage I disease.

Contraindications of surgery are few.
These are:
a. Younger age woman, desiring to preserve fertility
b. High surgical risk
c. Clinically unresectable disease
d. Associated comorbid conditions.

Extrafascial hysterectomy (type I) is commonly done. Radical hysterectomy (type III) is done in cases where cervical extension is present. Vaginal hysterectomy is also an accepted procedure in a selected case. Currently, minimally invasive surgery (MIS) is found to be safe, effective, feasible and is recommended. In early stage disease, laparoscopic or robot-assisted laparoscopic surgery is done in many centers.

The need to perform lymphadenectomy is based on the following factors:

- Histological type of the tumor
- Grade of the tumor
- Tumor size
- Depth of myometrial invasion as assessed during surgery
- Presence of extrauterine disease on exploration and biopsy.

Bilateral pelvic and para-aortic lymphadenectomy is performed in the presence of any of the following factors:
- Non-endometrioid type of endometrial cancer
- FIGO grade III tumor
- Tumor size > 2 cm
- Myometrial invasion >50%
- Evidence of extrauterine disease.

Differentiating features of type I and type II endometrial carcinoma		
Features	Type I	Type II
Clinical		
High-risk factors	Unopposed estrogen	Age
Histology	Endometrioid	Non-endometrioid
Stage	Early I/II	Advanced III/IV
Differentiation	Well-differentiated	Poorly differentiated
Molecular		
HER2/neu overexpression	No	Yes
P-53 overexpression	No	Yes
K-Ras overexpression	Yes	No

Q.1 What is the significance of peritoneal cytology in the management of endometrial carcinoma?

Ans. FIGO (2009) recommends positive peritoneal cytology to be reported separately without changing the stage. It is not included in direct-staging procedure.
- Positive peritoneal cytology generally indicates spread of the disease.
- On the other hand in the absence of any evidence of extrauterine spread of disease or without any evidence of poor prognostic factor, positive peritoneal cytology has no significant impact in terms of disease recurrence and/or survival outcome of the patient.
- Positive peritoneal cytology along with presence of other known poor prognostic factor(s) worsens the survival outcome of the patient.

Postoperative radiotherapy in stage 1 endometrial carcinoma reduces locoregional recurrence but has no effect on overall survival. Radiotherapy increases treatment-related morbidity. Postoperative radiotherapy is not recommended in patients with stage 1 endometrial carcinoma below 60 years and patients with grade 2 tumors with superficial invasion. However, patients with grade 3 tumors with a known propensity for deep myometrial invasion and lymph node metastasis may benefit from external beam radiotherapy.

Vaginal brachytherapy is better tolerated with high-dose rate (HDR) for women with endometrial cancer with high-risk of recurrence. Women with stage 1, grade 3 histology and invasion of lymphovascular space are the high-risk group. Women with these risk factors are benefitted with vaginal vault brachytherapy.

FIGO STAGE II

Stage II: Tumor invades cervical stroma, but does not extend beyond the uterus.

Incidence of lymph node metastasis in stage II endometrial carcinoma is about 36%. However, reliable diagnosis of cervical involvement is difficult as endocervical curettage, has high false-positive and false-negative rates. Ultrasonography, hysteroscopy or MRI may be helpful. Therefore, risk of spread outside the pelvis to the para-aortic nodes, adnexal and upper abdomen is high in stage II disease.

Management options for endometrial carcinoma stage II disease are:
- ***Radical hysterectomy, bilateral salpingo-oophorectomy, pelvic and para-aortic lymphadenectomy.***
  - ***Advantage:*** It provides accurate information as regard the spread of the disease.
  - ***Disadvantages:*** The women with endometrial carcinoma are often (i) elderly, (ii) obese and (iii) suffer from some medical disorders. They are often not suitable for such an extensive surgical procedure. Operative morbidities are high.
- ***Combined therapy***
  - ***Radiation therapy*** both external (pelvic) and intracavitary (cesium). This is followed after 6 weeks by ***total abdominal hysterectomy and bilateral salpingo-oophorectomy***. The results of the two above mentioned therapies are comparable.
  - ***Initial surgery:*** Exploratory laparotomy followed by extrafascial hysterectomy, bilateral salpingo-oophorectomy or modified radical hysterectomy with selected lymphadenectomy is done. This is ***followed by pelvic or extended field external and intravaginal radiation*** depending upon the spread of the disease. Results reported are excellent.

Suggested Reading

1. Benedetti Panici P, Basil S, Maneschi F, et al. Systematic pelvic lymphadenectomy vs no lymphadenectomy in early-stage endometrial carcinoma: randomized control trial. J Natl Cancer Inst. 2008;100(23):1707-16.

2. Creutzberg CL, van Putten WL, Warlam-Rodenhuis CC, et al. Outcome of high-risk stage 1C, grade 3, compared with stage 1 endometrial carcinoma patients: The postoperative radiation therapy in endometrial carcinoma trial. J Clin Oncol. 2004; 221234-41.

3. Kitchener H, Swart AM, Qian Q, et al. ASTEC study group. Efficacy of systematic pelvic lymphadenectomy in endometrial cancer (MRC ASTEC trial): A randomized study. Lancet. 2009;373:125-36.

4. Mariani A, Webb MJ, Keeney Gl, et al. Low-risk corpus cancer: Is lymphadenectomy or radiotherapy necessary? Am J Obstet Gynecol. 2000;182(6):1506-19.

5. Mariani A, Dowdy SC, Keeney GL, et al. Predictors or vaginal relapse in stage I endometrial cancer. Gynecol Oncol. 2005;97(3):820-27.

6. Mariani A, Webb MJ, Keeney GL, et al. Role of wide/radical hysterectomy and pelvic lymph node dissection in endometrial cancer with cervical involvement. Gynecol Oncol. 2001;83:72-80.

Surgical Management of Endometrial Carcinoma

Q.1 Discuss the place of vaginal hysterectomy in a case with endometrial carcinoma (EC).

Ans. Vaginal hysterectomy is an alternative option for the management of EC in some selected cases only. Such cases are:
- Stage I disease with well-differentiated tumor
- Without any extrauterine spread of disease. It is considered as the simplest and least morbid approach compared to abdominal hysterectomy. Treatment outcomes are similar to other methods of clinical stage I EC. This is specially helpful in obese and in patients with poor surgical risks.

Limitations of vaginal hysterectomy:
- Exploration of the intraperitoneal cavity is not possible.
- To procure peritoneal cytological washings, is not possible.
- May pose increased difficulty in oophorectomy procedure at times.
- Lymph node sampling to assess the spread of disease is not possible.

Q.2 What is the place of minimally invasive surgery in the management of endometrial cancer (EC)?

Ans. Minimally invasive surgery (MIS) in the management of EC is considered effective and is with comparable outcome to open surgery. Presently, it is considered as a standard care in the management of EC. It is useful for comprehensive surgical staging and appropriate risk stratification. This is again useful for correct treatment initiative.

MIS includes:
- Laparoscopically assisted vaginal hysterectomy (LAVH)
- Total laparoscopic hysterectomy (TLH)
- Robotic-assisted laparoscopic hysterectomy (RALH).

Surgical procedure is total hysterectomy, bilateral salpingo-oophorectomy with pelvic and para-aortic lymphadenectomy. This is the recognized mode of surgery.

Para-aortic node dissection up to the level of renal vein is recommended. MIS is used for transperitoneal and extraperitoneal assessment of nodes during hysterectomy. It may also be used at a later date to restage the disease when initial surgery was incomplete.

Robotic surgery has got additional benefits for obese women as it reduces the morbidity significantly. The overall benefits of LAVH/TLH or RALH are—reduced operative and postoperative complications, reduced hospital stay, improved recovery, fewer bowel adhesions and radiation-induced bowel injury. Robotic-assisted surgery has got all the benefits of laparoscopic surgery in terms of lymph node yield, shorter hospital stay, operative time and blood loss. However, it is pertinent that all gynecologic oncologists need to be trained with MIS to get the actual benefits.

Q.3 Discuss the place of nodal dissection in the management of EC.

Ans. *Surgical staging* is considered the most accurate way to determine the extent of disease spread. Selective use of nodal dissection was done to balance the benefit of detecting unrecognized disease against the cost, morbidity and the use of adjuvant therapy. The overall risks and benefits of lymphadenectomy are to weigh against the risks, cost and morbidity of adjuvant chemo and/or radiation therapy.

Intraoperative gross inspection of the uterus guides the surgeon for the need of nodal dissection. Visual inspection correlated with microscopic assessment in 85% of cases. However, myometrial invasion may be more extensive microscopically than is evident with the clinical inspection. Considering all the above facts, *routine nodal dissection is considered.*

There are two principal nodal basins that drain the uterus.

1. **Pelvic lymph nodes:** The lower and the middle portion of the uterus drain to the following pelvic nodes: External iliac, hypogastric, obturator and common iliac nodes.
2. **Para-aortic node:** The corpus and the fundus drain into the para-aortic nodes. As the nodes are bilateral, lymphadenectomy should be thorough and not sampling only. Isolated positive para-aortic nodes with negative pelvic nodes are uncommon and are found in only 2% cases.

However any suspicious pelvic or para-aortic lymph nodes, should be removed and histologically evaluated. Removal of grossly involved lymph nodes improves survival (Havrilesky 2005). **Women with serous or clear cell carcinoma** should undergo extensive surgical staging including infracolic omentectomy, peritoneal biopsies as in ovarian carcinoma.

Place of sentinel lymph node evaluation as done in vulvar, cervical and breast cancer is not yet standardized and is under evaluation for sensitivity and specificity. Laparoscopic surgery for pelvic and para-aortic lymphadenectomy in cases with stage I and IIa endometrial cancer, was found to be advantageous compared to laparotomy procedure. Overall survival rate and recurrence rate are similar to those with traditional laparotomy procedure.

Robot-assisted laparoscopic staging and surgery of endometrial cancer has been found to be feasible and safe. The procedure has less blood loss. However, women with extensive adhesive disease, morbid obesity, cardiopulmonary compromise are excluded from MIS. Morcellation is not performed and is avoided to prevent disease spread.

Patients with positive pelvic and/or para-aortic nodes are treated with complete node resection followed by adjuvant (radiation and/or chemotherapy) therapy. This resulted in superior (100% for pelvic and 75% for para-aortic) 5-year survival outcomes. In the absence of nodal disease, the recurrence risk is low and 5-year survival outcome is high either with no radiation or with vaginal cuff brachytherapy (VCB) only.

Suggested Reading

1. Abu-Rustum NR, Gomez JD, Alektiar KM, et al. The incidence of isolated para-aortic nodal metastasis in surgically staged endometrial cancer patients with negative pelvic lymph nodes. Gynecol Oncol. 2009;115(2):236-8.
2. ASTEC/EN.5 Study Group, Blake P, Swart AM, Orton J, Kitchener H, Whelan T, Lukka H, et al. Adjuvant external beam radiotherapy in the treatment of endometrial cancer (MRC ASTEC and NCIC CTG EN.5 randomised trials): pooled trial results, systematic review, and meta-analysis. Lancet. 2009;373:137–46.
3. ASTEC study group, Kitchener H, Swart AM, et al. Efficacy of systematic pelvic lymphadenectomy in endometrial cancer (MRC ASTEC trial): A randomized study. Lancet. 2009;373(9658):125-36.
4. Bakkum-Gamez JN, Gonzalez-Bosquet J, Laack NN, Mariani A, Dowdy SC. Current issues in the management of endometrial cancer. Mayo Clin Proc. 2008;83:97–112.
5. Creasman WT, Morrow CP, Bundy BN, et al. Surgical pathologic spread patterns of endometrial cancer. A Gynecologic Oncology Group Study. Cancer. 1987;60(8 Suppl):2035-41.
6. Creutzberg CL, van Putten WL, Koper PC, et al. Surgery and postoperative radiotherapy versus surgery alone for patients with stage 1 endometrial carcinoma: Multicenter randomized trial. PORTEC Study Group. Postoperative Radiation Therapy in Endometrial Carcinoma. Lancet. 2000;355(9213):1404-11.
7. Mariani A, Dowdy SC, Cliby WA, Gostout BS, Jones MB, Wilson TO, et al. Prospective assessment of lymphatic dissemination in endometrial cancer: A paradigm shift in surgical staging. Gynecol Oncol. 2008;109:11–8.
8. Onda T, Yoshikawa H, Mizutani K, et al. Treatment of node-positive endometrial cancer with complete node dissection, chemotherapy and radiation therapy. Br J Cancer. 1997;75(12):1836-41.
9. Seamon LG, Fowler JM, Cohn DE. Lymphadenectomy for endometrial cancer: The controversy. Gynecol Oncol. 2010;117(1):6-8.

Role of Pelvic and Para-aortic Lymph Node Dissection in the Surgical Management of Endometrial Cancer

Views and Counterviews

Surgical staging of endometrial cancer is essential for deciding the need and the type of postoperative management and adjuvant therapy. Rationality of bilateral pelvic and para-aortic lymph node dissection (in the management of endometrial cancer) needs to be standardized.

Surgical treatment of endometrial cancer includes total hysterectomy (extrafascial) and bilateral salpingo-oophorectomy.

Place of lymphadenectomy (pelvic and para-aortic) has the following objectives:
a. To document the extrauterine spread of disease
b. To determine the type and extent of postoperative therapy
c. To evaluate whether the procedure could be considered as a therapeutic modality
d. To evaluate treatment results in the woman following pelvic and para-aortic lymph adenectomy
e. Comparative evaluation of different therapeutic modalities in terms of disease-free interval and survival outcome
f. This will also help as a guide to avoid over- and under-treatment.

Predisposing factors for lymph node involvement are:
a. Primary tumor diameter measured after surgery
b. Histologic subtype
c. Depth of myometrial invasion
d. Tumor grade.

General Approach (Mayo Clinic-2009)

A low-risk woman can be managed with hysterectomy alone. This avoids the morbidity of lymphadenectomy.

'Low-risk' women are:
a. Myometrial invasion ≤ 50%
b. Endometrial cancer: histologic grade 1 or 2
c. Primary tumor diameter ≤ 2 cm
d. No macroscopic tumor beyond the uterine corpus
e. Endometrioid cancer and no myometrial invasion (independent of grade and primary tumor diameters).

Women with histology grade 3 and deep myometrial invasion are benefitted from external pelvic radiotherapy.

SURGICAL MANAGEMENT OF ENDOMETRIAL CANCER

- Peritoneal cytology
- Total hysterectomy
- Bilateral salpingo–oophorectomy
  Extended procedure includes: Bilateral pelvic and para-aortic lymph adenectomy (para-aortic dissection up to renal vessels).
- Omentectomy (nonendometrioid advanced cancer).

There is a lack of standardization as yet for the place of lymph node dissection in the management of endometrial cancer. **Lymph node evaluation varies from 'no evaluation' to 'sampling' to systematic pelvic and para-aortic lymphadenectomy**. As regards the extent of the procedure of lymphadenectomy, the upper limit should be the origin of the renal vessels to get its benefit for both diagnostic and therapeutic value. Routine dissections of lymphadenectomy up to the origin of inferior mesenteric artery misses nearly 45% cases with positive para-aortic lymph nodes. Postoperative radiotherapy in the node-positive cases is expected to improve the outcome in terms of therapy as well as to prevent the recurrence.

Suboptimal treatment is unlikely to improve survival outcome. On the other hand, it needs to be certain with more prospective randomized studies whether lymph node dissection ever in a high-risk woman would improve the outcome when judged in terms of prognosis, morbidity and the cost.

Risks: However, nodal dissection is not a complete risk-free procedure.

The known hazards are: Increased blood loss, increased operating time, vascular injury, injury to the genitofemoral nerve with subsequent development of paresthesia to the medial side of thighs, lymphocyte formation, ileus and lymphedema. The overall surgical complication of lymphadenectomy is above 20%. The major complication is about 6%.

Other Views (St. Mary's Hospital, Manchester, UK)

Endometrial cancer has the 5-year survival rate around 80%. The major area for improvement of survival rate is to manage the cases with more aggressive histological subtypes and the occult cases with extrauterine diseases (22%) and with lymph node metastasis (11%).

These observations raised the need of systematic pelvic and para-aortic lymph node dissection. However, till date, it is uncertain whether to use routine systemic lymphadenectomy in all cases or to be selective for few high-risk women.

A Study in the Treatment of Endometrial Cancer (ASTEC)

During laparotomy, full staging provides prognostic information and accurate knowledge of disease. There is little justification for routine removal of pelvic and para-aortic lymph nodes in women with disease that is confined to the uterus, on clinical examination, imaging and on histology.

ASTEC study with randomized 1400 women with endometrial cancer, did not show any significant difference in survival outcome between the lymphadenectomy and the control groups. However, it is expected that woman with high-risk nodal metastasis to be managed jointly by clinical oncologists and gynecological oncologists to develop guidelines to reduce inconsistencies of management results. PORTEC-3 trial is expected to reveal result of pelvic radiotherapy alone versus chemoradiation in the prevention of locoregional as well as distant disease. Women with no clinical or radiological suggestion of extrauterine disease, only 2% have metastasis to the para-aortic nodes. This increases to 17% with deep myometrial invasion.

MRI is superior to both computed tomography and ultrasound in the assessment of myometrial invasion. MRI is preferred imaging modality to indentify myometrial invasion as well as cervical extension. Therefore, imaging with MRI and preoperative endometrial biopsy can identify the women that are in the high-risk group with nodal metastasis.

Non-endometrioid tumors have the potential to early extrauterine dissemination and distant metastasis. Chemotherapy is usually given to these women postoperatively although the disease-free interval and the overall survival rate are no different. Women with endometrial carcinoma should have full surgical staging by a gynecological oncologist. Benefit of routine lymphadenectomy is not supported by evidence.

The role of sentinel lymph node (SLN) mapping in the staging of endometrial carcinoma is currently being done (*See* Ch 43). This procedure is expected to identify positive lymph nodes and to reduce the need of full lymphadenectomy. This procedure has high sensitivity and a high negative predictive value.

Suggested Reading

1. ASTEC/EN.5 Study Group, Blake P, Swart AM, Orton J, Kitchener H, Whelan T, Lukka H, et al. Adjuvant external beam radiotherapy in the treatment of endometrial cancer (MRC ASTEC and NCIC CTG EN.5 randomised trials): pooled trial results, systematic review, and metaanalysis. Lancet. 2009;373:137–46.
2. ASTEC Study Group, Kitchener H, Swart AM, Qian Q, Amos C, Parmar MK. Efficacy of systematic pelvic lymphadenectomy in endometrial cancer (MRC ASTEC trial): a randomised study. Lancet. 2009;373:125–36.
3. Bakkum-Gamez JN, Gonzalez-Bosquet J, Laack NN, Mariani A, Dowdy SC. Current issues in the management of endometrial cancer. Mayo Clin Proc. 2008;83:97–112.
4. Benedetti Panici P, Basile S, Maneschi F, Alberto Lissoni A, Signorelli M, Scambia G, et al. Systematic pelvic lymphadenectomy vs no lymphadenectomy in early-stage endometrial carcinoma: Randomized clinical trial. J Natl Cancer Inst. 2008;100:1707–16.
5. Creutzberg CL, van PuttenWL J, Koper PCM, et -al: PROTECT study group Surgery and post operative radiotherapy versus surgery alone for patients with stage -1 endometrial carcinoma: multicenter randomised trial. Lancet. 2000;335:1404-11.
6. Mariani A, Dowdy SC, Cliby WA, Gostout BS, Jones MB, Wilson TO, et al. Prospective assessment of lymphatic dissemination in endometrial cancer: A paradigm shift in surgical staging. Gynecol Oncol. 2008;109:11–8.
7. Mariani A, Webb MJ, Keeney GL, Haddock MG, Aletti G, Podratz KC. Stage IIIC endometrioid corpus cancer includes distinct subgroups. Gynecol Oncol. 2002;87:112–7.

Chapter 35: Ovarian Tumor with Low Malignant Potential

Ovarian tumors of low malignant potential (LMP) are also known as **borderline ovarian tumors**. Ovarian tumors with LMP are characterized by histological features that are intermediate between a clearly benign tumor and a frankly invasive carcinoma. These tumors do not belong to any of the hereditary breast ovarian cancer syndromes. These tumors were first described by Taylor. Overall prevalence of borderline tumors or ovarian tumors of low malignant potential is 10–15%.

The characteristic histological features of LMP tumors are:
- Nuclear atypia
- Epithelial stratification
- Cellular pleomorphism
- Cellular mitotic activity
- Microscopic papillary projections
- No stromal invasion
- However, up to 10% of LMP tumors exhibit areas of microinvasion measuring <3 mm in diameter

RISK FACTORS

It is often suggested that LMP tumors represent a disease of distinct entity. LMP tumors may progress to invasive disease. In such a situation, the tumor is of low-grade invasive phenotype rather than that of the high-grade type. Most studies combine LMP tumors and invasive cancers together for epidemiological factors. Younger women are more likely to develop LMP tumors when compared with older women. Risk factors evaluation have been observed to have different correlation. Lactation is found to be protective whereas oral contraceptive is not **protective**. LMP tumors are not considered to be the result of any hereditary breast-ovarian cancer (*BRCA* gene mutations) syndrome.

LMP TUMORS AND THE HISTOLOGICAL TYPES

LMP Tumors of the ovary
- **Serous type**
  - Most common (50%)
  - Bilateral in 30% of cases
- **Extraovarian site implants are also observed**
  These may be:
  - Noninvasive
  - Invasive
- **Mucinous type 46%**
  - Interstitial (85%)
  - Endocervical/Mullerian types (15%)
- **Others**
  - Endometrioid, clear cell, Brenner or mixed types (4%)
  - LMP tumors of mucinous types may cause pseudomyxoma peritonei

DIAGNOSIS

Diagnosis of borderline tumors is problematic as there is no means to determine preoperatively. These tumors are mostly asymptomatic and the diagnosis is mainly incidental. The **clinical features are**: pelvic pain, dyspepsia, abdominal fullness, bloating and pelvic pressure symptoms. Several tumor markers have been studied. Values of tumor markers like CA125, CA19-9, CEA, CA15-3 are often raised. However, tumor markers are not specific. Values of tumor markers may be normal or marginally elevated in some cases. Like other cases of benign and invasive ovarian tumors, ultrasonography can provide useful information as regards the tumor size, dimensions, solid areas, septa, presence of ascites or papillary projections. MRI is helpful to detect the presence of peritoneal (extraovarian) implants or omental caking.

MANAGEMENT

All women should be considered for laparotomy, as in a case with ovarian cancer. Surgical staging (FIGO) and maximal cytoreductive surgery is the plan.

Laparoscopic surgery may be an option for a selective case (Figs. 35.1 and 35.2).

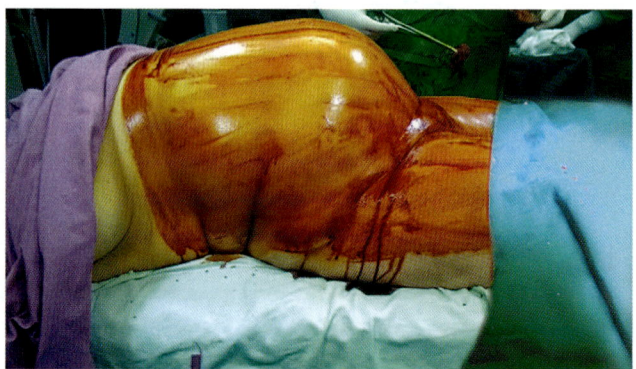

Fig. 35.1: 65 years old parous lady, diagnosed with huge ovarian tumor, is for laparotomy.

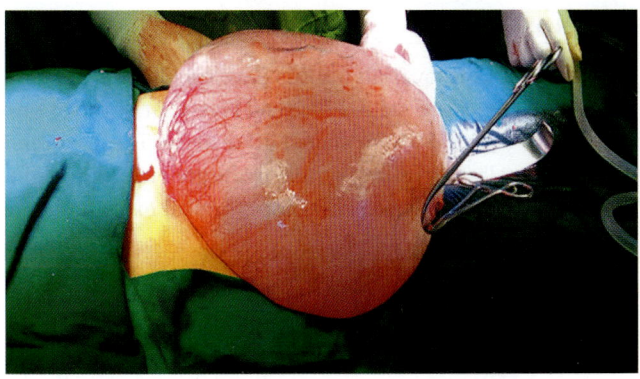

Fig. 35.2: Laparotomy done. A huge ovarian mass is seen. Histology confirmed ovarian tumor with low malignant potential.

Standard Procedure of Laparotomy includes

- Through exploration of the abdominal cavity as in a case with invasive tumor (FIGO)
- Collection of peritoneal washings for malignant cell cytology
- Total abdominal hysterectomy
- Bilateral salpingo-oophorectomy and infracolic omentectomy
- Appendicectomy in a case with mucinous tumor.

Ovarian tumor tissues should be subjected to frozen section biopsy where facilities are available. Diagnosis may sometimes be difficult as the accuracy of frozen section biopsy in the diagnosis of LMP tumors is relatively low. About one third of cases with ovarian tumors reported as borderline on frozen section, are later on reclassified as invasive tumors.

The actual plan for surgery for an individual woman varies depending upon the following factors:
a. Age of the woman
b. Desire of fertility
c. Stage of the disease
d. Peritoneal implants
e. Histological features.

Frozen section evaluation is helpful for planning the surgery. However, it is almost impossible to know with certainty whether a patient has a benign tumor, LMP tumor or an invasive ovarian cancer until final histologic slides have been revised. Biopsies of the peritoneum and omentum have limited values unless tissues appear clearly abnormal.

Procedure of routine pelvic and para-aortic nodes dissection may not be done unless the tumor is finally invasive.

Plan of Surgery

Women with LMP tumor diagnosed intraoperatively may be considered for actual surgery as mentioned below:
- **Older women with no desire to fertility preservation**
    - Ovarian cancer surgical staging throughly and maximum cytoreduction surgery including appendicectomy (mucinous tumor).
- **Younger women with the need of fertility preservation**
    - Fertility-sparing surgery with preservation of the uterus and contralateral ovary.

This is a reasonable approach even if the final histological diagnosis shows invasive stage I cancer.

The main difficulties in the management of LMP tumors are:
a. In majority of cases, the diagnosis is not suspected intraoperatively.
b. No frozen section is requested.
c. Frozen section report may not correctly diagnose the disease.

The clinician is to work with the final and confirmed pathology report. Comprehensive surgical restaging is not necessarily required if the tumor appears to a single ovary. Cases where cystectomy has been performed, the risk of residual disease is a possibility.

Till date there is no consensus as regards the need of restaging and completion of surgery. Survival outcome did not differ for women with LMP tumor, who have undergone restaging compared with those who have not.

The determining factors for restaging are:
a. Micropapillary projections
b. Invasive implants
c. DNA aneuploidy
d. When no fertility preservation is needed.

Women with invasive disease have higher risk of recurrence (31%) compared with those with noninvasive implants (21%) over 5 years.

The need of relaparotomy is less for women who have undergone full staging laparotomy as per FIGO-2018. Assessment of the contralateral ovary, tube, omentum and the peritoneal surfaces, during primary surgery, should be a routine.

Place of Fertility-sparing Surgery

Fertility-sparing surgery is considered for women with younger age, following appropriate discussion with different treatment options. It may be an acceptable treatment option for young women with early stage disease especially who are desirous of babies. However, women need to be counseled adequately as regards the risk of recurrence.

Fertility-sparing surgery includes:
a. Complete staging (FIGO)
b. Preservation of the uterus
c. Preservation of one ovary or a part of it

Options of surgery for the pathological ovary may be:
a. Ovarian cystectomy
b. Unilateral salpingo-oophorectomy
c. With or without infracolic omentectomy

It has been observed that relapse rates are higher after cystectomy (12–58%) compared to salpingo-oophorectomy (0–20%) and that of following radical surgery (2.5–5.7%).

Delayed recurrences have been observed hence, long-term follow-up of these women need to be stressed. The prognosis of a recurrent disease is excellent following relaparotomy and complete surgery. The fertility outcome of women with LMP tumors is satisfactory. No adverse effect of pregnancies on the disease or vice versa has been observed. Spontaneous conception has been observed up to 65% of cases. Most centers advise to limit the number of stimulation cycles as minimum possible. The place of relaparotomy and removal of the remaining ovary and the uterus following completion of child bearing is debatable. Many prefer not to go for radical surgery as long as there is no recurrence. Recurrent disease is easily resectable and the prognosis is excellent. However, complete definitive surgery may be done if the woman chooses to have it because of her psychological stress.

Laparotomy Versus Laparoscopic Surgery

Presently laparoscopic surgery has been used in oncology more and more. However, difficulties faced are: cyst rupture, understaging of the disease, port-site metastasis, risk of recurrence and lower survival outcome. LMP ovarian tumors and the invasive tumors are preferably treated by midline laparotomy until supported by evidence.

Place of Adjuvant Therapy

Adjuvant chemotherapy has not been recommended in cases with LMP ovarian tumors. There are no clinical trials to support the benefits. Recurrent LMP ovarian tumor, not amenable to surgical resection, may be considered. Majority of such cases are undiagnosed invasive diseases (30%).

Follow-up of Cases with LMP Ovarian Tumors

Ovarian tumors with LMP run the risk of recurrence. It varies between 0–58% depending upon the histological type and the stage of the disease. Recurrence may occur after few years or even decades after initial surgery. Majority of the cases with recurrence are observed with invasive disease (8–73%). Clinical examination and ultrasonography are helpful for the detection of recurrence. ***Many centers follow-up the women every 3 months for the first 2 years, every 6 months for the next 2 years and annually thereafter.***

PROGNOSIS

Women with LMP ovarian tumors have excellent prognosis. More than 80% have stage I disease. Five-year survival rate range from 96% to 99% for stage I–III disease. These women have an overall survival rate similar to the general population. For the recurrent disease, complete surgical excision is the most effective therapy.

CONCLUSION

LMP ovarian tumors belong to a distinct entity of ovarian tumors. LMP tumors characterized histologically by cellular proliferation, nuclear atypia, nuclear mitosis without any stromal invasion. The cornerstone of management is surgical staging as in FIGO and maximal cytoreduction surgery. Fertility-sparing surgery can be performed in young women and it does not affect the overall survival. These women need long-term follow-up as recurrences have been observed (15%) even after years of diagnosis. Usually, recurrences occur in the contralateral ovary. Recurrent diseases are curable by relaparotomy and resection. Chemotherapy is usually not needed except for the invasive disease.

Suggested Reading

1. Cadron I, Amant F, Van Gorp T, Neven P, Leunen K, Vergote I. The management of borderline tumours of the ovary. Curr Opin Oncol. 2006;18:488–93.
2. Camatte S, Morice P, Atallah D, Thoury A, Pautier P, Lhomme C, et al. Clinical outcome after laparoscopic pure management of borderline ovarian tumors: Results of a series of 34 patients. Ann Oncol. 2004;15:605–9.
3. Morice P, Camatte S, El Hassan J, Pautier P, Duvillard P, Castaigne D. Clinical outcomes and fertility after conservative treatment of ovarian borderline tumors. Fertil Steril. 2001;75:92–6.
4. Morice P. Borderline tumours of the ovary and fertility. Eur J Cancer. 2006;42:149–58.
5. Vandenput I, Amant F, Vergote I. Peritoneal recurrences might be less common in advanced stage serous borderline ovarian tumors that were treated by laparotomy. Gynecol Oncol. 2005;98:523–5.

Chapter 36: Gestational Trophoblastic Disease

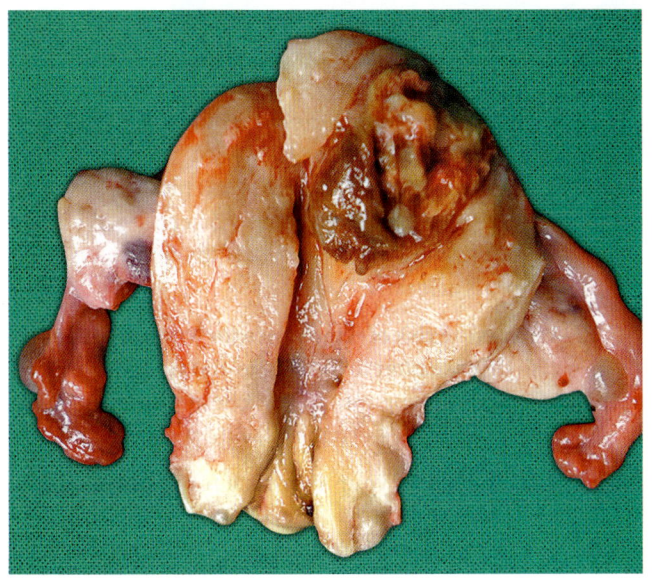

Fig. 36.1: Choriocarcinoma invading myometrium.

Q.1 Regarding gestational trophoblastic neoplasia (GTN):
  a. Nearly 20–30% of patients with partial mole develop GTN following evacuation
  b. Metastatic tumor without established primary site with raised human chorionic gonadotropin (hCG) is diagnosed
  c. Decline in hCG level by >10% following chemotherapy indicates response
  d. Risk of recurrence is nearly 13% despite use of chemotherapy.

Ans. a. F b. T
    c. T d. T

Q.2 What is meant by gestational trophoblastic disease (GTD)?

Ans. GTD comprises a spectrum of neoplastic conditions derived from the placenta. GTN refers especially to those GTD cases with potential for tissue invasion and metastasis (Fig. 36.1).

Q.3 How the diagnosis of GTN could be made following evacuation of hydatidiform mole?

Ans.
- Four or more values of plateaued hCG (±10%) over at least 3 weeks (days 1, 7, 14 and 21)
- Three or more values of rise in hCG (≥ 10%) over at least 2 weeks (days 1, 7 and 14)
- Histologic diagnosis of choriocarcinoma, invasive mole or placental site trophoblastic tumor (PSTT)
- Metastatic tumor without established primary site with raised hCG.

Q.4 What percentage of women develop GTN following evacuation of a hydatidiform mole?

Ans. About 6–30% of patients develop GTN following evacuation of complete mole whereas, nearly 2–8% of patients develop GTN following evacuation of partial mole.

Q.5 How do you evaluate a case of GTN?

Ans.
- Complete general physical and pelvic examination
- Baseline hematologic parameters
- Baseline renal and hepatic functions
- Baseline hCG values
- Chest radiograph or computed tomography (CT) chest
- Brain magnetic resonance imaging (MRI) or CT scan (Fig. 36.2A)
- CT or MRI scan of abdomen (Fig. 36.2B) and pelvis.

Q.6 What is 'phantom' (false-positive) hCG? How this problem could be overcome?

Ans. Many patients after receiving chemotherapy or after surgery present with low level of hCG (100–300 mIU/mL). This is due to interference with hCG immunometrics and sandwich assays caused by nonspecific heterophile antibodies in patient's serum. False-positive hCG assays will have markedly different values using different assay techniques. Heterophile antibodies are not excreted in the urine. Therefore, when serum hCG is detected in such a patient, a urine sample should be tested for hCG. Urinary hCG values would not be detected in a case with phantom GTN. This will avoid unnecessary chemotherapy for such a patient.

Q.7 What is 'real' low level hCG?

Ans. Persistent low levels of hCG in patients with GTN (<500 mIU/mL) may be observed without any evidence of lesion. This is known as 'quiescent GTN' where hCG is not hyperglycosylated. These patients need

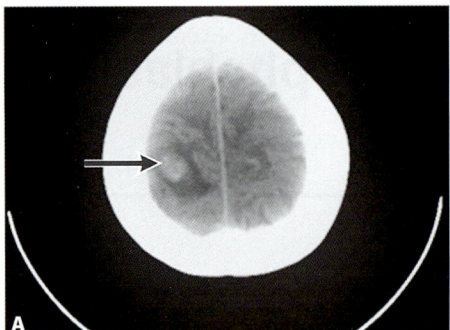 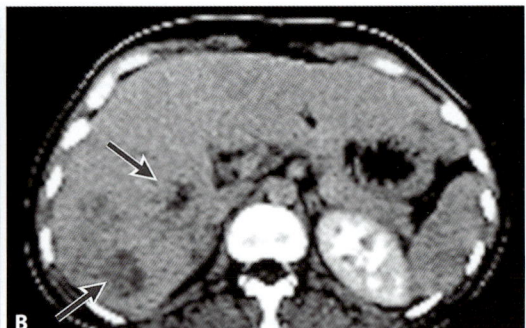

Figs 36.2A and B: Patient with choriocarcinoma, CT view showing: (A) Brain metastasis, (B) Multiple metastases in the liver.

follow-up for long time. Risk of recurrence for such a patient is about 10%. Usually these patients respond well to chemotherapy in the event of recurrence.

Q.8 What factors have got prognostic importance for GTN?

Ans. Initially, World Health Organization (WHO) clinical classification (1980) and International Federation of Gynecology and Obstetrics (FIGO) anatomic staging were considered. In 2000, FIGO revised its staging for GTN with uniformity for comparative evaluation and treatment in all the centers worldwide.

Adoption of current FIGO revised (2000) scoring system (*See* Dutta's Textbook of Gynecology, 8th Edition, p. 306) has categorized patients into low-risk (score: 0–6) and high-risk (score ≥ 7) groups. Low-risk group patients are treated initially single agent regimen. Patients with metastatic disease (score ≥ 7) are treated with multiagent chemotherapy.

Q.9 What hCG value should be considered for risk scoring?

Ans. It is important to note that the hCG level obtained immediately before starting treatment for GTN should be considered for ***risk scoring***. The hCG level obtained at the time of evacuation is not to be used for this purpose. Current FIGO staging will help uniformity of patient evaluation and comparison of treatment results.

Q.10 How do you follow-up the women during and after chemotherapy for GTN?

Ans. Serum hCG level is monitored weekly during and after the chemotherapy:
- ***Response:*** Decline in hCG level by >10% following one cycle therapy.
- ***Plateau:*** Change ± 10% in hCG following one cycle therapy.
- ***Resistance:*** Rise > 10% in hCG following one cycle or plateau for two cycles of chemotherapy.
- ***Remission:*** Normal hCG values weekly for 3 consecutive weeks.
- ***Maintenance*** chemotherapy should be given for at least three more cycles after normalization of serum hCG values.

Q.11 How do you maintain the surveillance for remission after chemotherapy for GTN?

Ans.
- hCG values every 2 weeks for 3 months
- hCG values every month for 1 year
- hCG values every 6–12 months for lifelong (3–5 years at least).

Q.12 What is the risk of recurrence for women with high-risk disease after achieving initial remission?

Ans. In spite of using multiagent chemotherapy aggressively, nearly 13% of patients will develop recurrence.

Q.13 What would be your approach for management of such cases?

Ans. Even with intensive chemotherapy, patients may have recurrence following initial remission especially the women with high-risk disease.

Management options for such women are:
- Patient needs to be evaluated for metastasis.
- Patient may be considered for alternative (EMA-CO, EMA-EP or MAC/CHAMOCA) chemotherapy regimens (*See* Dutta's Textbook of Gynecology, 8th Edition, p. 308).
- Patient may be considered for additional surgery (to extirpate drug resistant tissues, e.g. thoracotomy for lung wedge resection) or radiotherapy (for brain metastasis).

Twin pregnancy: Coexistent molar pregnancy and a normal fetus: Coexistent molar pregnancy with a normal fetus is relatively rare (1 in 22,000 to 1 in 1,00,000 pregnancies). Mrs R, a 34-year-old lady; P-0, G-4, A-3, L-0, conceived following IVF-ET. USG revealed the diagnosis (Figs. 36.3A to C). Pregnancy ended in miscarriage at 18 weeks gestation due to the complication of excessive hemorrhage. Medical complications of such a twin pregnancy including hyperthyroidism, PIH and hemorrhage are increased. These patients have an increased risk of developing post molar GTN and metastatic disease. Invasive prenatal testing for fetal karyotyping is needed to confirm the diagnosis of complete mole with a coexisting normal twin and to exclude partial molar pregnancy. Perinatal outcome is often poor.

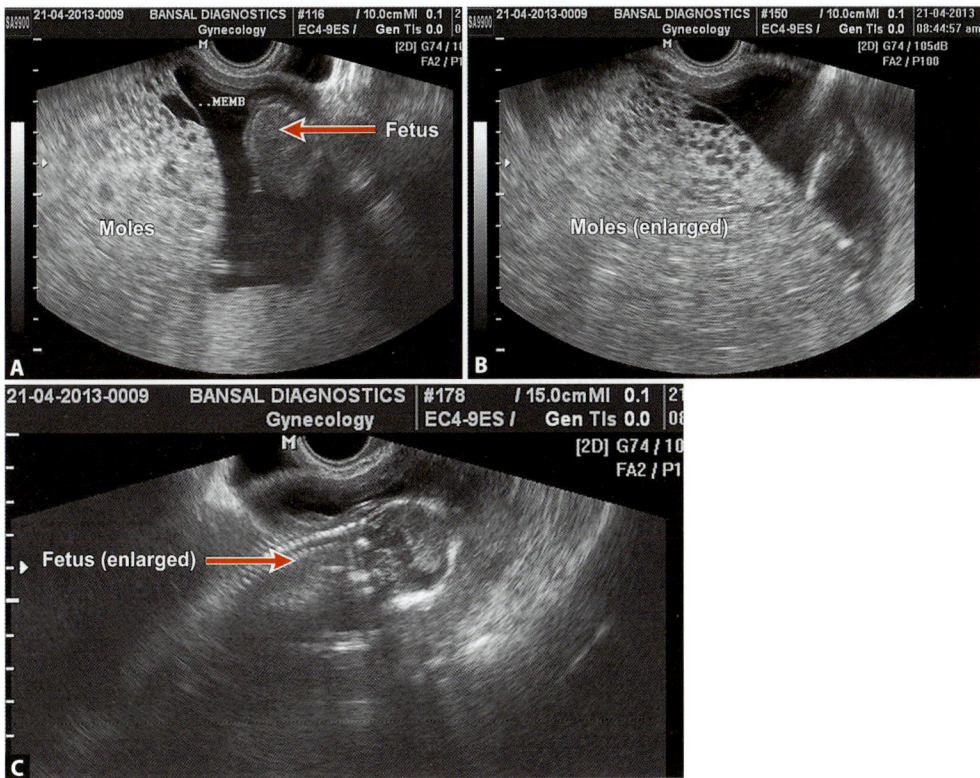

Figs. 36.3A to C: Twin pregnancy: Coexistent molar pregnancy and a normal fetus.

Q.14 What is the reproductive outcome of a woman with GTN following remission of the disease?

Ans. Such a woman can have normal pregnancy and successful outcome in majority (79%). Risk of premature ovarian failure has been reported. However, risks of fetal congenital malformation are not increased but of stillbirths may be high.

Q.15 What are the long-term health consequences of women treated for GTN?

Ans.
- Increased risk of second malignancy, especially following the use of multiagent chemotherapy with etoposide. Risks of developing myeloid leukemia and colon cancer are there.
- Early onset of menopause and premature ovarian failure have been observed.

FOLLOW UP OF CASES AFTER TREATMENT OF GESTATIONAL TROPHOBLASTIC DISEASES

- Following medical abortion (medical termination of pregnancy) women should do a urinary pregnancy test 3 weeks after the procedure to ensure that it is negative.
- For women with complete molar pregnancy if hCG has reverted to normal within 56 days following evacuation then follow up will be for 6 months from the date of uterine evacuation.
- If hCG has not reverted to normal within 56 days of pregnancy event, then follow up will be 6 months from normalization of the hCG level.
- Follow up for partial molar pregnancy is concluded once hCG has returned to normal on two samples, at least 4 weeks apart.
- Placental site trophoblastic tumor (PSTT) and epithelioid trophoblastic tumor (ETT) are the recognized variants of GTN. They are treated with surgery because they are less sensitive to chemotherapy.
- **Plan of pregnancy following treatment of molar (complete or partial) pregnancy:** Women who received chemotherapy are advised not to conceive for 1 year after the completion of treatment.
- Women who have a pregnancy following prior molar pregnancy where no treatment for GTN was needed, there is no need to send post-pregnancy sample for hCG.
- Use of oxytocin infusion prior to evacuation is not recommended. Preparation of the cervix immediately prior to uterine evacuation is safe.
- Overall prognosis for woman treated with GTN is good. Cure rate is close to 100%.
- Use of exogenous estrogens and other fertility drugs are safe for women undergoing ART after a molar pregnancy.
- **Assay technology for hCG:** Definitive diagnosis of molar pregnancy is made by histological examination. Very rarely, some women may have familial raised hCG (levels ranging between 10 IU/L and 200 IU/L) levels. These women have menstrual cycles and can conceive. Other conditions where elevated low levels of hCG observed are: malignant germ cell tumors, any epithelial cancers (bladder, breast, lungs,

gastric and colorectal cancers). It may also be due to the presence of pituitary hCG.

The hCG glycoprotein can be present in many forms, in both the serum and urine. **The different forms are:** intact hCG, free hCG β-subunit, nicked hCG and hCG β-core fragment. Molar pregnancy and the GTN can produce all these variants of hCG. The commonly used hCG assay technology, do not measure all the hCG fragments. For follow up of cases with GTDs assay technology for all the forms hCG is needed.

- GTN can develop after miscarriage, therapeutic abortion or rarely after a term pregnancy. The prognosis for a woman with GTN after a non-molar pregnancy may be worse owing to delay in diagnosis or the advanced stage of the disease.
- **Twin pregnancy**: There are increased risks of perinatal morbidity, mortality and the outcome of GTN. Prenatal invasive testing for fetal karyotyping should be done to confirm the diagnosis of complete moles with a co-existing normal twin or it is a partial molar pregnancy. **There is high risk of early fetal loss (40%) and preterm delivery (36%).**
- Anti-D prophylaxis is not required for complete molar pregnancies. There is poor vascularisation of the chorionic villi and absence of the D antigen in the trophoblast cells. However, it is required for partial molar pregnancies. If the diagnosis of complete molar pregnancy cannot be established within 72 hours, anti-D prophylaxis can be administered for practical reasons.

Follow up of GTDs: In women with GTN following chemotherapy, there is increased risk of premature menopause.

Contraceptive measures following treatment of GTD (*See* Ch 28).

Suggested Reading

1. Angelopoulos G, Palmer JE, Hancock BW, Tidy JA. Healthy women with persistently elevated hCG levels: a case series of fourteen women. J Reprod Med. 2012;57:249–53.
2. Benachi A, Garritsen HS, Howard CM, Bennett P, Fisk NM. Lack of expression of Rh-D in human trophoblast cell. Am J Obstet Gynecol. 1998;178:294–9.
3. Coyle C, Short D, Jackson L, Sebire NJ, Kaur B, Harvey R, et al. What is the optimal duration of human chorionic gonadotrophin surveillance following evacuation of a molar pregnancy? A retrospective analysis on over 20,000 consecutive patients. Gynecol Oncol. 2018;148:254–7.
4. Earp KE, Hancock BW, Short D, Harvey RA, Fisher RA, Drew D, et al. Do we need post-pregnancy screening with human chorionic gonadotrophin after previous hydatidiform mole to identify patients with recurrent gestational disease. Eur J Obstet Gynecol Reprod Biol. 2019;234:117–9.
5. FIGO Oncology Committee. FIGO staging for gestational trophoblastic neoplasia 2000. FIGO Oncology Committee. Int J Gynecol Obstet. 2000;77:285–7.
6. Ghorani E, Kaur B, Fisher RA, Short D, Joneborg U, Carlson JW, et al. Pembrolizumab is effective for drug-resistant gestational trophoblastic neoplasia. Lancet 2017;390:2343–5.
7. Kaur B, Short D, Fisher RA, Savage PM, Seckl MJ, Sebire NJ. Atypical placental site nodule (APSN) and association with malignant gestational trophoblastic disease; a clinicopathologic study of 21 cases. Int J Gynecol Pathol. 2015;34:152–8.
8. Ngan HYS, Seckl MJ, Berkowitz RS, Xiang Y, Golfier F, Sekharan PK, et al. Update on the diagnosis and management of gestational trophoblastic disease. Int J Gynecol Obstet. 2018;143 (Suppl 2):79–85.
9. Russell JC, Niemann I, Sebire NJ, Kaur B, Fisher RA, Short D, et al. Outcomes in Twin Pregnancies with Complete Hydatidiform Mole and Normal Co-Twin: A Retrospective National Cohort Study in 153 New Cases. 20th Biennial World Congress on Gestational Trophoblastic Diseases, 20–23 October 2019, Toronto, Canada.
10. Schmid P, Nagai Y, Agarwal R, Hancock B, Savage PM, Sebire NJ, et al. Prognostic markers and long-term outcome of placental-site trophoblastic tumours: a retrospective observational study. Lancet. 2009;374:48–55.
11. Seckl MJ, Gillmore R, Foskett MA, Sebire NJ, Rees H, Newlands ES. Routine terminations of pregnancies–should we screen for gestational trophoblastic neoplasia? Lancet. 2004;364:705–7.
12. The Faculty of Sexual & Reproductive Healthcare. Contraception After Pregnancy. FSRH Guideline Executive Summary. London: FSRH; 2017.

Chapter 37: Human Chorionic Gonadotropin and the Management of Gestational Trophoblastic Disease

The level of beta-human chorionic gonadotropin (hCG) correlates well with volume of proliferating trophoblastic tissues. Estimation of this hormone is essential as it is an important biomarker. Levels of serum β-hCG is used for diagnosis, scoring the risk factors, response of therapy following chemotherapy or surgery and also for follow-up of women with gestational trophoblastic neoplasia (GTN). GTN is a significant cause of morbidity, loss of fertility and rarely mortality in young women.

Gestational trophoblastic disease (GTD) covers both the benign and the malignant conditions of the neoplastic trophoblastic conditions.
A. **Benign conditions are:** Complete hydatidiform moles (CHM) and the partial hydatidiform moles (PHM)
B. **Malignant conditions are:** Gestational trophoblastic neoplasia (GTN). GTN includes:
   i. Invasive moles (IM),
   ii. Choriocarcinoma (CC), and
   iii. Placental site trophoblastic tumors (PSTT).

All the forms of the neoplastic conditions of the trophoblasts secrete hCG which is an important biomarker for the disease. All the forms of GTD need close follow-up. Follow-up is done by serial estimation of serum β-hCG. Overall risk of malignancy in cases with CHM is 15% and that of PHM is 0.5%.

The prevalence of GTD is higher in the Asian countries compared with Europe and the US.

Human Chorionic Gonadotropin

Human chorionic gonadotropin is a glycoprotein produced mainly by the syncytiotrophoblast cells of the placenta. It has two subunits.
1. Alfa-subunit, which is common to α-subunit of hCG, TSH and LH.
2. The β subunit which is specific to trophoblast-secreted hCG. Furthermore, it is known that β-hCG exists in at least two-intact forms:
   A. **Regular β-hCG** which is produced by the syncytiotrophoblasts throughout the normal pregnancy. Its physiological function is to maintain pregnancy with the secretion of progesterone.
   B. **hCG-H** is a variant of hCG having double-sized oligosaccharide side chains. It is produced by the invasive cytotrophoblasts. Its presence is specific to the implantation phases of normal pregnancy. It has autocrine function. It promotes the growth, proliferation and invasion of the trophoblasts. It is detected in cases with GTN (invasive mole, choriocarcinoma, and PSTT). In GTN, there are few other fragmented components of β-hCG. These are: free β-subunit, β-core, nicked free-β, and C-terminal fragments.

Estimation of β-hCG level is essential for the management of GTD. Decision to start or stop chemotherapy, or to go for surgical management (e.g. hysterectomy) is based on the levels of serum β-hCG. It is essential that the assays used in oncological hCG analysis to be used for the purpose of managing cases of GTD. It is different from the usual hCG estimation what is done in pregnancy. It is more reliable and accurate. The increasing sensitivity of hCG assays and identification of β-hCG variants have helped in the understanding for the management of cases with GTD.

1. **False-negative result:** Unless an assay can detect all forms of hCG, it may result in failure to make the correct diagnosis of GTN. This may cause failure or inadequate treatment for a patient with GTN. It is important that assays used for hCG monitoring during pregnancy are not adequate for management of GTD.
2. **False-positive result:** It is due to cross-reactivity of the assay with circulating heterophile antibodies. This can be eliminated by measuring urine hCG levels. Heterophile antibodies are too large to be excreted through the glomerular filtration.
3. **Presistently elevated low-levels of β-hCG** without clinical or radiological evidence of active GTD. This is observed, though rarely, in few patients of GTD. This may be due to the increasing assay sensitivity. On rare occasions, women with GTN who had been treated with adequate chemotherapy or following hysterectomy, failed to show hCG normalization. It is important to identify the cause of the persistence or elevated low level of hCG. Otherwise, women with GTN, those who need further treatment, will be missed. On the other hand, unnecessary treatment would be given to the women who do not need it.

Reasons for Persistence or Low-level Elevation of hCG
1. Presence of heterophile antibodies to cause false-positive result.

2. **Quiescent state of GTN**: It is observed in patients with previous GTD that had been treated. A small percentage of these patients may subsequently develop active disease and require treatment. Estimation of serum **elevated levels of hCG-H** is to be done. This is essential to determine which cases are having the activation of the disease and need further chemotherapy.
3. **Pituitary-derived hCG:** This may be observed in a postmenopausal woman or a woman with premature ovarian failure. It could be differentiated by measuring changes in the serum LH/FSH levels.
4. **Nongestational neoplasia:** Germ cell and epithelial tumors with some trophoblast differentiation may produce hCG. Thorough investigation is needed to exclude this.
5. **Physiological elevation:** Some women may have an elevated baseline hCG.

Significance of Elevated hCG

Elevated hCG-H levels indicate development of GTN in majority of cases. Elevation of **hCG-H level** occurs much earlier than the rise in conventional hCG levels. Therefore, routine hCG-H estimation is helpful for early detection of GTN. This is helpful in early initiation of treatment or change of therapy when one drug is found in a case of GTN.

Free fragments of β-hCG: It is observed that free fragments of hCG are produced in PSTT. Levels are often raised. Differentiation between PSTT and choriocarcinoma is difficult. Free fragments of β-hCG are very sensitive and are used to differentiate PSTT from choriocarcinoma.

MANAGEMENT OF GTD

It is recommended that for monitoring of GTD, all the forms of β-hCG should be assayed. hCG detection tests done in normal pregnancy are not reliable for monitoring the cases of GTN.

Histological diagnosis of GTN is not always needed. Placental site trophoblastic tumor (PSTT) has different histological presentations. Syncytiotrophoblasts cells are generally absent. But the intermediate trophoblast cells are abundant. β-hCG secretion is low and secretion of human placental lactogen (hPL) is high. hPL is monitored for follow-up.

GTN is diagnosed when there is persistence or rising values of serum β-hCG following evacuation of molar pregnancy. Usually, serum levels of β-hCG normalize by 9 weeks following evacuation.

Chemotherapy is the mainstay in the treatment of cases with GTN. Type of chemotherapy, whether single agent or multidrug therapy, depends on the FIGO prognostic score. Successful treatment of GTN is considered only with the normalization of serum. β-hCG levels and not with the complete response of tumor with imaging studies (USG, CT or MRI). PSTT usually do not respond to any chemotherapy. Hysterectomy is the preferred treatment.

Currently anti-hCG-H antibody is being tried to block tumorigenesis and to prevent development of choriocarcinoma.

Anti-hCG-H vaccine is under trial to promote endogenous antibody formation. This vaccine when given to a woman with hydatidiform mole, is expected to prevent its malignant transformation.

β-hCG is synthesized by the syncytiotrophoblasts. Synthesis continues throughout the pregnancy (smaller amount in latter months). It is detected in the serum in all the types of patients with GTD. Its main physiological function is to secrete progesterone to maintain pregnancy.

hCG-H is produced by the (i) Invasive cytotrophoblasts of normal pregnancy during the implantation phase, and (ii) by the tissues of GTN.

Suggested Reading

1. Cole La, Butler SA, Khanlian SA, et al. Gestational trophoblastic disease: Hyperglycosylated hCG as a reliable marker of active neoplasia. Gynecol Oncol. 2006;102:151-9.
2. Mitchell H, Seckl M. Discrepancies between commercially available immunoassays in the detection of tumor derive hCG. Mol Cell Endocrinol. 2007;262:310-3.
3. Palmieri C, Dhillon T, Fisher RA, et al. Management and outcome of healthy women with a persistently elevated β-hCG. Gynecol Oncol. 2007;106:35-43.

38 Chapter — Fertility Preservation in Women

Q.1 What is the clinical relevance of this subject in context of current gynecologic practice?

Ans. Gynecologic malignancies are commonly diagnosed in elderly and postmenopausal women. However, no age is immune to any malignancy. When such a malignancy is diagnosed in woman with younger age, fertility conservation is a major concern. Standard treatment of such malignancies ends in sterility. There are now few options for fertility conservation for such women who are diagnosed with a gynecologic malignancy before they are married or child bearing is completed or even in adolescence.

Q.2 What is the prevalence of such gynecologic malignancies?

Ans.
- Ovarian cancer
  - For women < 20 years — 0.7–1.4 per 100,000 women
  - For women 20–49 years — 1.6–16.6 per 100,000 women
- For cervical cancer
  - For women 20–49 years — 1.5–14.9 per 100,000 women
- Endometrial cancer

FERTILITY PRESERVATION IN WOMEN

Fertility preservation (FP) is the process of preservation of an individual's oocytes, sperm or gonadal tissue with the prospective that the same may be used in future when one needs to have his/her biological children.

Indications of Fertility Preservation

- Patients with cancer who are waiting for different methods of treatment, e.g., surgery, chemotherapy, radiotherapy including proton therapy or combination of therapy.
- Patients with cancer who had undergone surgical treatment (radical hysterectomy and ovarian conservation) for cervical cancer and are waiting subsequent treatment of chemotherapy or radiotherapy (*See* Ch 40).

FP can help individuals as there is improved survival rates of childhood, adolescent and adult cancers. The late effects of cancer treatment is the loss of fertility.

Total body irradiation or radiotherapy over a field covering the ovaries or testes or use of chemotherapy (alkylating agents), all have risk of gonadotoxicity. Irradiation of the ovaries ≥ 10 GY is associated with premature ovarian failure.

Cryopreservation of oocyte or sperm: Cryopreservation is the process of cooling of cells and tissues to subzero temperatures. This stops all cellular biological activity so that they can be preserved for future use. The human metaphase II oocytes is a large cell. It is fragile as it has large cytosolic water content and chromosomal rearrangements. Oocyte freezing was used earlier. It was known as slow freezing technique. This method caused cellular damage, formation of ice crystal and/or excessive cellular dehydration. Currently slow freezing technique has been replaced by vitrification. Vitrification is a process of cryopreservation using high concentration of cryoprotectant. Uniform presence of cryoprotectant in the ooplasm and rapid cooling avoid the formation of ice crystal. The process of vitrification has improved the viability of cryopreserved cells significantly. In order to achieve the ice-free, glass like solidification of cells, high cryoprotectant concentrations and very rapid cooing rate are used. Cryotop vitrification technique, was used for cryopreservation of oocytes and embryos. The Cryotec vitrification method has resulted in almost 100% survival rate followed by excellent fertilization, blastocyst development, pregnancy and birth after embryo transfer (ET).

Ovarian tissue cryopreservation (OTC): Whole or part of ovary is taken out laparoscopically. This is processed for cryopreservation for the purpose of auto-transplantation in future. This tissue is transplanted back to the patient either in pelvic cavity (orthotopically) or outside in the forearm or rectus muscle (heterotopically). Oocyte retrieval and embryo development have been done following heterotopic transplantation of ovarian tissue. Successful pregnancies after replacement of cryopreserved human ovarian tissue have been reported. Ovarian activity starts within 4 months of transplantation. Its biological function is maintained for a variable period of time (upto several years).

Testicular tissue cryopreservation (TTC): In vitro maturation (IVM) is useful to generate sperm cells.

In vitro maturation (IVM) of oocytes is a technique that avoids ovarian stimulation. IVM of cryopreserved oocytes, involves retrieval of immature oocytes from the ovaries after minimal or no gonadotropin stimulation. Maturation of these retrieved immature oocytes is done in the laboratory subsequently.

Livebirths have been reported following vitrification of metaphase II (M II) oocytes after human chorionic gonadotropin (hCG) primed IVM cycles. IVM is helpful for patients with cancers. IVM does not need ovarian stimulation.

Ovarian transposition and use of GnRH agonists: Ovaries along with the fallopian tubes may be transposed (laparoscopically) to the abdominal wall or below the kidneys to avoid the radiation effect. Ovarian transposition or oophoropexy is done for fertility preservation in women that they need pelvic radiation for nonovarian cancers. Overall efficacy is around 50%.

GnRH agonists have been used to suppress ovarian activity to minimize the gonadotoxic effects of chemotherapy. It is found useful in women with breast cancer when FP is needed.

Suggested Reading

1. Anderson RA, Wallace WHB, Telfer EE. Ovarian tissue cryopreservation for fertility preservation: clinical and research perspectives. Hum Reprod Open. 2017;2017:hox001.
2. Cohen Y, St-Onge-St-Hilaire A, Tannus S, Younes G, Dahan MH, Buckett W, et al. Decreased pregnancy and live birth rates after vitrification of in vitro matured oocytes. J Assist Reprod Genet. 2018;35(9):1683-9.
3. Donnez J, Dolmans MM, Demylle D, Jadoul P, Pirard C, Squifflet J, et al. Livebirth after orthotopic transplantation of cryopreserved ovarian tissue. Lancet. 2004;364:1405-10.
4. ESHRE Female Fertility Preservation Guideline Development Group. Female Fertility Preservation. Guideline of the European Society of Human Reproduction and Embryology (ESHRE). Review Report Grimberg: ESHRE; 2020.
5. ESHRE Working Group on Oocyte Cryopreservation in Europe; Shenfield F, de Mouzon J, Scaravelli G, Kupka M, Ferraretti AP, et al. Oocyte and ovarian tissue cryopreservation in European countries: statutory background, practice, storage and use. Hum Reprod Open. 2017;2017:hox003.
6. Goldfarb SB, Kamer SA, Oppong BA, Eaton A, Patil S, Junqueira MJ, et al. Fertility preservation for the young breast cancer patient. Ann Surg Oncol. 2016;23:1530-6.
7. Grynberg M, Mayeur Le Bras A, Hesters L, Gallot V, Frydman N. First birth achieved after fertility preservation using vitrification of in vitro matured oocytes in a woman with breast cancer. Ann Oncol. 2020;31:541-2.
8. Sauvat F, Binart N, Poirot C, Sarnacki S. Preserving fertility in prepubertal children. Hormone Res. 2009;71 (Suppl 1):82-6.

Chapter 39: Fertility Preserving Options for Women with Ovarian Cancer

Q.1 What is the significance of fertility conservation in malignant ovarian tumors?

Ans. Ovarian malignancy is most lethal and 5-year survival rate of ovarian malignancy in spite of all modalities of treatment remained the same for last four decades. Most patients are in advanced stage except few (39%) that are diagnosed in stage IA. Presently, there is delay in women's child bearing. Therefore, it is important to have the fertility conservation options that are safe and available.

Q.2 What are different options for fertility conservation in a young woman with ovarian malignancy?

Ans. Options available are:
- **Surgery:** Conservation of the uninvolved ovary while doing surgery to the pathological one.
- **Medical**
  - Assisted reproductive technology
  - Surrogacy.

Q.3 How the woman with gynecologic malignancy should be counseled for available fertility conservation options?

Ans.
- Oncologist should keep in mind that the desire to have a biological child is strong in most couples.
- Before cancer therapy, oncologists should address the possibility of infertility in women with reproductive age.
- Options for third-party reproduction should be given.
- Oncologists should discuss issues of limitations, as regard to nonavailability of accurate data to predict for any individual.

Q.4 What are the different options available for fertility preservation with the help of ARTs?

Ans. Options available are:
- **Before treatment:** Embryo cryopreservation following harvesting eggs, IVF and embryo freezing. This procedure is standardized now.
- **Oocyte cryopreservation:** Harvesting and freezing unfertilized eggs. This procedure is still investigational.
- **Ovarian tissue cryopreservation:** Freezing healthy ovarian tissues and reimplantation later on. This procedure is investigational.
- **Gonadal shielding during radiotherapy:** It is done to reduce the radiation dose and damage to the gonads. This procedure is standardized.
- **Ovarian transposition (oophoropexy):** It is the surgical repositioning of the ovary(ies) away from the field of radiation. This procedure is standardized.
- **Ovarian suppression with GnRH** (agonist/antagonist) for conservation of ovarian tissue during therapy.
- **Conservative ovarian surgery** like ovarian cystectomy or preserving healthy contralateral ovary.

Q.5 What are the criteria for selecting a woman with ovarian malignancy for fertility conserving surgery?

Ans. These are the selected women who may be considered following counseling only:
- Epithelial ovarian cancers with stage IA and may be stage IB
- Borderline tumor of the ovary
- Malignant ovarian germ cell tumor (stage I)
- Sex cord stromal tumors (stage I).

Surgery in stage I, grade I and possibly grade 2 ovarian cancer does not significantly compromise survival and allows future fertility.

However, it is important that removal of the preserved ovary may be considered after pregnancy(ies) is over, to reduce the risk of recurrence.

Q.6 How the staging of ovarian cancer is made?

Ans. Ovarian cancer is staged following surgical and pathological procedures. These include laparotomy and findings on exploration and histopathological reports. Surgical (exploratory laparotomy) procedures include:
- Peritoneal fluid cytology
- Multiple peritoneal biopsy
- Biopsy of any suspicions area
- Retroperitoneal lymph node sampling
- Pelvic and para-aortic node sampling
- Infracolic omentectomy.

It is important that tumor should be removed intact without any cyst rupture or intraperitoneal spread of the disease.

Q.7 How to assess the involvement of the contralateral ovary?

Ans. Contralateral ovary may be involved even it looks clinically normal. Confirmation of involvement may be done only following biopsy that may be with wedge-resection or tissue biopsy only. However, such methods are unreliable. Risks of microscopic involvement for a normal looking contralateral ovary is 2.5% only. It is virtually absent when the stage of the disease is IA.

Q.8 What should be the surgical approach in a young woman with unilateral and stage I (grade 1) ovarian cancer?

Ans. Unilateral salpingo-oophorectomy with preservation of the contralateral healthy ovary and the uterus is now considered the appropriate surgical treatment.

Q.9 What is the effect of adjuvant chemotherapy on fertility outcome after conservative surgery?

Ans. Actual situation is unclear and it is different with different chemotherapeutic agents.
- Alkylating agents (cyclophosphamide) may cause menstrual abnormalities and even premature ovarian failure (high risk).
- Methotrexate, 5-FU and vincristine cause less ovarian dysfunction (low risk).
- Taxanes, oxaliplatin are of unknown risks.
- Pubertal ovary has been found to be more resistant to the adverse effects of chemotherapy. However, successful pregnancy has been reported even following combined chemotherapy.

Q.10 What are the important issues that the oncologists should know and accordingly counsel the patients?

Ans.
- Oncologists should be familiar with the fertility sparing management options for a young woman with ovarian malignancy.
- Women must be counseled with the options available, limitations, eligibility criteria and importantly the risks and the benefits of such a procedure.
- Multidisciplinary team approach (oncologists, reproductive endocrinologists and perinatologists) should be there.
- It is difficult to predict outcome for anyone individual woman as there is nonavailability of accurate data that are based on large number of controlled studies.

Suggested Reading

1. Ayhan A, Celik H, Taskiran C, et al. Oncologic and reproductive outcome after fertility-saving surgery in ovarian cancer. Eur J Gynecol Oncol. 2003;24(3-4):223-32.
2. Heintz AP, Odicino F, Maisonneuve P, et al. Carcinoma of the ovary. FIGO 26th Annual Report on the Results of Treatment in Gynecological Cancer. Int J Gynaecol Obstet. 2006;95(1): S161-92.
3. Meirow D, Levron J, Eldar-Geva T, et al. Pregnancy after transplantation of cryopreserved ovarian tissue in a patient after chemotherapy. N Engl Jr Med. 2005;353(3):318-21.

Fertility Preserving Options for Women with Cervical Cancer

Cervical cancer is treated in majority by hysterectomy (simple or radical and/or pelvic radiation). Unfortunately, this treatment results in sterility. The surgical options available for fertility conservation are:
- Excisional procedures on the cervix—(a) cervical amputation, (b) conization.
- Other extensive procedures are—(a) radical abdominal trachelectomy (RAT), (b) radical vaginal trachelectomy (RVT).

Q.1 Who are the women that may be considered for excisional procedures?

Ans.
- Women with stage IA1 (< 3 mm stromal invasion, microinvasive carcinoma)
- Without any lymphovascular space involvement (LVSI)
- There should be negative endocervical curettings and the cone margin (following excision) should be free of disease.

Q.2 What is the place of ovarian transposition for a woman with cervical cancer?

Ans. It is done to reduce the risk of radiation injury to the ovaries, in the event that the woman needs radiation therapy following treatment of cervical cancer.

Q.3 How and at what place ovarian transposition could be done?

Ans. Ovarian transposition could be done either laparoscopically (commonly) or by laparotomy.
Ovaries are transposed to a position away from the pelvis, in the paracolic gutters below the lower pole of the kidneys.

Q.4 What are the suggested eligibility criteria for ovarian transposition?

Ans.
- Any gynecologic malignancy that needs pelvic radiation therapy where ovarian function is to be preserved.
- Patient's age < 40 years seeking fertility conservation.
- Cancer confined to the cervix only.
- No evidence of LVSI.
- Extent of tumor spread has been assessed and excluded by pelvic magnetic resonance imaging (MRI).

Q.5 What is radical vaginal trachelectomy (RVT)?

Ans. RVT was originally performed by Daniel Dargent in 1987. RVT has two-step procedure:
1. A laparoscopic pelvic (with or without para-aortic) lymphadenectomy is done.
2. Trachelectomy is done via vaginal route.

Principal steps of vaginal trachelectomy are:
- A rim of 1–2 cm of vagina is delineated and a vaginal incision is made.
- Posterior colpotomy is performed.
- Paravesical and pararectal spaces are developed.
- Uterosacral ligaments are transected.
- The bladder pillars are transected mobilizing the ureters.
- Descending cervical branch of the uterine artery is ligated.
- The cervix is amputated keeping 1 cm of cervix attached to the body of the uterus.
- A permanent cerclage is placed at the remaining cervical stroma.
- The vaginal margin is sutured to cervical stroma without occluding the new external os.

The cervical tissue is sent for frozen section biopsy for examination of the resected margin. RVT is abandoned and a radical hysterectomy is done if the resected margin is found positive.

Q.6 What are the eligibility criteria for RVT?

Ans.
- Histologically confirmed cervical cancer—squamous cell carcinoma, adenosquamous carcinoma or adenocarcinoma. Neuroendocrine tumors of cervix are not considered for RVT.
- Women desirous to preserve fertility and ready for regular follow-up.
- Stage of the disease: FIGO stages IA1 (without LVSI), IA2 or IB1.

- Size of the lesions < 2 cm.
- No evidence of distant metastasis on preoperative assessment using MRI.
- Adequate cervical length (≥2 cm).
- No evidence of lymph node metastasis.

Q.7 What is the outcome of RVT?

Ans. Pregnancy has been documented after RVT. However, risks of miscarriage and preterm labor are there. Recurrence risks (3.1%) have also been observed.

Suggested Reading

1. Schlaerth JB, Spirtos NM, Schlaerth AC. Radical trachelectomy and pelvic lymphadenectomy with uterine preservation in the treatment of cervical cancer. Am J Obstet Gynecol. 2003;188(1):29-34.
2. Shepherd JH, Mould T, Oram DH. Radial trachelectomy in early stage carcinoma of the cervix: outcome as judged by recurrence and fertility rates. BJOG. 2001;108(8):882-5.

Chapter 41: Fertility Preserving Options for Women with Endometrial Cancer

Up to 35% of endometrial cancers are diagnosed in premenopausal women. Endometrial cancers are diagnosed even in women younger than 25 years of age, less common though. **High-risk factors to develop endometrial cancer are:** (a) Hyperestrogenism, (b) anovulation, (c) obesity, (d) dyslipidemia, (e) diabetes mellitus (carbohydrate intolerance) and (f) women with polycystic ovarian syndrome (PCOS).

Standard treatment of early stage endometrial cancer (*See* Ch 32) is total abdominal hysterectomy, bilateral salpingo-oophorectomy (BSO), pelvic and para-aortic lymph node sampling. Few patients may need adjuvant therapy either radiotherapy and/or chemotherapy.

Q.1 Who are the women to be considered for fertility conservation options?

Ans. Women with:
- Stage I, grade I endometrioid adenocarcinoma limited to the endometrium
- Without any evidence of lymph vascular space involvement (LVSI)
- Without any evidence of extrauterine spread of the disease based on CT imaging
- No evidence of myometrial invasion based on MRI
- No evidence of a suspicious adnexal mass on CT or USG.

Q.2 What are the different parameters that should be reviewed as pretreatment evaluation of the woman?

Ans.
- Detailed history and physical examination and to look for any signs and symptoms of advanced or metastatic disease.
- Dilatation and curettage of the endometrium should be done.
- Hysteroscopy and endometrial sampling is considered for women who are considered for hysterectomy. It is extremely operator dependent.
- Contrast-enhanced MRI is most reliable, accurate and is comprehensive for assessment of women with endometrial carcinoma to assess myometrial invasion. MRI is superior to TVS and CT in assessing myometrial invasion.

Q.3 What are the fertility sparing treatment options available for endometrial carcinoma?

Ans. Preventive measures to be taken are:
- To stop any unopposed estrogens
- Other risk factors are to be taken care of: (i) weight reduction, (ii) glycemic control, etc.
- **Progestin therapy:** Medroxyprogesterone acetate (MPA) or LNG-IUD. MPA is given continuously 40 mg (orally) per oral a day or higher is recommended for 6–9 months.

Q.4 How do you follow-up these women?

Ans.
- Office endometrial sampling is done at an interval of 10–12 weeks or sooner if necessary. Dilatation and curettage may be performed if endometrial sampling results are not informative.
- Women are followed up depending upon their response with endometrial histology.
  - ♦ **Complete regression:** Therapy may be continued or stopped and advised for fertility improvement therapy.
  - ♦ **Persistence of disease:** Therapy may be continued and repeat evaluation is to be done. Persistent disease may need hysterectomy.
  - ♦ **Progression of the disease:** Recommended for hysterectomy.

Indications of hysterectomy:
- Poor compliance of the women with medication and/or follow-up.
- Evidence of progression of the disease.
- Child bearing is completed.

Q.5 What is the outcome of fertility conservative management of a woman with endometrial carcinoma?

Ans. Experience of managing such patients are less as the total number of patients managed are less as yet. Pregnancy has been documented and live birth rate is 47%.

Suggested Reading

1. Gotlieb W, Beiner ME, Shalmon B, et al. Outcome of fertility-sparing treatment with progestins in young patients with endometrial cancer. Obstet Gynecol. 2003;102(4):718-25.
2. Niwa K, Tagami K, Lian Z, et al. Outcome of fertility-preserving treatment in young women with endometrial carcinomas. BJOG. 2005;112(3):317-20.

Chapter 42: Chemotherapy in Gynecological Cancers

ANTIMETABOLITES

Methotrexate (MTX) is an antimetabolite. It blocks the cell metabolism by competing with naturally occurring purines or pyrimidines. Methotrexate blocks the reduction of dihydrofolate to tetrahydrofolate (the active form of folic acid). It binds tightly to the enzyme dihydrofolate reductase.

As a result, the synthesis of the thymidylate synthase and ultimately purine synthesis are blocked.

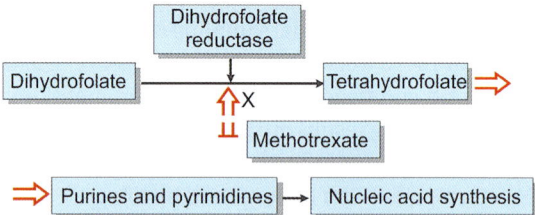

Ultimately, MTX causes arrest of DNA, RNA and protein synthesis. The drug affects predominantly the S phase of the cell cycle. The effects of methotrexate can be overcome by folinic acid (citrovorum factor). Methotrexate may be given by oral, IV, IM or by intrathecal route.

MTX has several side effects. Citrovorum factor (leucovorin) is given as a 'rescue' to overcome the severe toxic side effects, following very high doses. It should be given 24 hours after methotrexate is given.

Main side effects: Myelosuppression, mucositis, renal toxicity, CNS dysfunction and hepatotoxicity.

Leucovorin in folinic acid has the function similar to folic acid. It is readily converted to tetrahydrofolic acid. It does not need dihydrofolate reductase for conversion. Therefore, function of leucovorin is not affected by MTX.

Dose: Leucovorin is given 0.1 mg/kg. It may be given orally or IM.

MTX is predominantly excreted through the kidneys. Dose should be reduced in women with renal dysfunction.

Gemcitabine is an antimetabolite. It binds to DNA to form a wrong base pair. It stops DNA synthesis. It affects the S phase of the cell cycle. It is given as an infusion over a period of half an hour. Dose varies between 600 and 1250 mg/m^2. It is given once a week for 2–3 weeks.

Toxicities: Myelosuppression, neutropenia, GI toxicity (nausea, vomiting, mucositis), malaise, fever and chills, rarely pulmonary toxicity.

Alkylating Agents

The positively charged alkyl groups bind to the negatively charged DNA to form adducts. This binding leads to DNA breaks or cross-linking. Ultimately, there is block of DNA synthesis. Alkylating agents affect the rapidly dividing cells like the bone marrow.

Alkylating agents commonly used are: Cyclophosphamide, ifosfamide.

Cyclophosphamide is given orally or IV. IV: 500 to 750 mg/m^2 over 30 min, every 3 weeks.

Toxicities: Bone marrow depression (BMD), hemorrhagic cystitis, nausea, vomiting, alopecia, leukopenia, thrombocytopenia, and amenorrhea. Hemorrhagic cystitis is due to severe urothelial damage due to the metabolite acrolein. Development of leukemia is a long-term complication.

Ifosfamide has all the above mentioned side effects. The additional complications are: Neurotoxicity (CNS) and renal toxicity.

Hemorrhagic cystitis can be prevented by:
1. Adequate hydration before the drug administration
2. Mesna (2-mercaptoethane sulfonate) is given IV as it binds with acrolein metabolite of alkylating agents. It detoxifies acrolein in the bladder.

Plant derivatives and taxanes: These are cell cycle specific agents. Taxanes cause disturbances of normal assembly, disassembly and stabilization of intracellular microtubules. It stops cell division during mitosis.

Drugs: Vinca alkaloids, topoisomerase inhibitors, paclitaxel, docitaxel.

Topoisomerase Inhibitors

Functions of topoisomerase (TOPO) enzymes are to unwind and rewind DNA to help DNA replication. Inhibitors of TOPO isomerase interefere with this function and block DNA synthesis. There are two types of inhibitors. Camptothecin (Topotecan) inhibit TOPO I and Podophyllotoxins (etoposide) inhibit TOPO II.

Topotecan (TOPO 1 inhibitor) is an alkaloid extract of camptothecin. It binds TOPO I-DNA complex resulting in break of double-strand DNA. It is commonly used in recurrent cases of ovarian and cervical cancer.

Toxicities: Myelosuppression, neutropenia and GI toxicity (nausea, vomiting, diarrhea, abdominal pain) are common.

Others: Headache, arthralgia, myalgia, fever, and alopecia.

Etoposide: It is cycle-specific as it acts in the late S and G_2 phase of the cell cycle. It forms TOPO II-DNA complex. It thus blocks DNA unwinding and causes break of double-strand DNA.

Etoposide is commonly used IV, as a part of combination therapy. The 'E' of EMA-CO regimen is used in GTN (100 mg/m^2) and the **"E"** of BEP regimen is used in ovarian germ cell cancers. The dose of etoposide varies from 75 to 100 mg/m^2.

Carboplatin: Similar to alkylating agents, it causes DNA adducts and inhibits DNA synthesis.

It is commonly used in epithelial ovarian cancer.

The used IV dose of carboplatin is calculated to a target "area under the curve" (AUC) from 5 to 7, based on the glomerular filtration rate (GFR). The Calvert equation is most often used.

{Carboplatin total dose (mg) = target AUC x [GFR + 25]}

In clinical practice, creatinine clearance (CrCl) is usually done instead of GFR.

It is given as infusion over 30–60 minutes. It is repeated at every 3–4 weeks.

Toxicities: Myelosuppression, thrombocytopenia, GI toxicities (nausea, vomiting), HSR, and less commonly peripheral neuropathy.

Antiangiogenesis Agents

Angiogenesis is a process of new blood vessel formation. The blood vessels are remodeled for transport of oxygen and nutrient transport to tissues. The process is regulated by various pro- and antiangiogenic factors. Malignant process dysregulates the normal balance and initiates abnormal angiogenesis through the lymphatic and vascular system.

Antiangiogenic agents are targeted to inhibit angiogenesis. Antiangiogenic agents prevent the binding of vascular endothelial growth factor (VEGF) to VEGF receptor as a primary step.

Bevacizumab: It is a monoclonal antibody that binds to VEGF to prevent VEGF binding with its receptor. Bevacizumab is used in cases with recurrent or metastatic cervical cancer as well as in recurrent epithelial ovarian cancer.

Dose: 15 mg/kg IV every 3 weeks. It may be given with other cytotoxic drug.

Toxicities: Minimal; Rise in blood pressure may lead to hypertensive crisis, intestinal perforation has been reported.

Others are: Delayed wound healing, proteinuria.

VEGF Trap is a recombinant "fusion protein", works by fusing two specific portions of the VEGF receptor and the "Fc" region of IgG molecule. The receptor portions have high affinity binding of VEGF.

Sunitinib: It is an oral agent. It inhibits several receptor tyrosine kinases (RTKs) and also blocks the angiogenic growth factors. Receptor tyrosine kinases (RTKs) are proteins present in the plasma membrane of cells and act as receptors. Drugs in this group are: pazopanib, sorafenib.

Dose: 50 mg daily.

Mammalian Target of Rapamycin Inhibitors

Mammalian target of rapamycin (mTOR) is a protein kinase. It regulates membrane trafficking, transcription, translation and maintains cytoskeleton. mTOR increases production of VEGR.

Rapamycin inhibits mTOR. Temsirolimus, everolimus are currently being studied in gynecological cancers.

Poly (ADP-ribose) Polymerase (PARP) Inhibitors

During cell division, both the double and single-stranded DNA break several times. The double-stranded breaks are repaired by BRCA proteins. PARP repairs the single-strand breaks. In normal functioning cells, PARP will repair the break even if it is not repaired by BRCA. About 10 percent of women with ovarian cancer have mutations of *BRCA1* or *BRCA2* gene. This leads to loss of homologous DNA repair. Replications of cancer cells are very fast compared with normal cells. Normal cells without any mutated *BRCA1* or *BRCA2*, can repair DNA breaks. This allows them to survive PARP inhibition. Thus only cancer cells with *BRCA* defects are almost entirely dependent on PARP repair. When PARP repair is blocked, damaged cancer cells cannot be repaired and these cells die eventually. On the contrary, normal cells are unaffected.

Olaparib is a PARP inhibitor. It is currently approved by FDA. Women with ovarian cancer, known to be *BRCA1* and *BRCA2* mutation carriers, are treated with PARP inhibitors when they are resistance to platinum drugs. It is also used in patients without mutations.

Dose: 400 mg twice daily.

Side effects: Nausea, vomiting, fatigue.

Doxorubicin Hydrochloride Liposome

Doxorubicin is an antitumor antibiotic. The liposomal encapsulation of doxorubicin improves the pharmacokinetic and toxicity profile. It has less cardiac toxicity. Though nausea and vomiting may be present.

Dose: 30–60 mg/m² given IV as infusion over 30–60 minutes. Course is repeated at an interval of 4 weeks.

However, increased rate of stomatitis and palmar-plantar erythrodysesthesia (PPE) are reported. PPE is noted with the complaints of tingling sensation on the sole, palm, swelling, development of erythematous plaques, desquamation with skin cracking and pain.

GROWTH FACTORS TO COMBAT CHEMOTHERAPY-INDUCED SIDE EFFECTS

Synthetic Erythropoietin

Epoetin alfa and darbepoetin alfa are the synthetic erythropoietin. These are used as hematopoietic drugs to stimulate the development of red blood cells and granulocytes. They have the same biologic effects of endogenous erythropoietin. Common indication of use is chemotherapy-induced anemia. It should not be used when the hemoglobin level is high as it may cause tumor progression.

Epoetin alfa is usually used as 40,000 units SC weekly.

Side effects: Diarrhea, nausea, or hypertension.

Granulocyte Colony-stimulating Factors (G-CSF)

G-CSF (Filgrastim, pegfilgrastim) are produced by recombinant DNA technology. These cytokines bind to hematopoietic cells to activate proliferation, differentiation and stimulation of granulocyte progenitor cells. These are used to prevent development of febrile neutropenia (ANC <1500).

Filgrastim is given SC, 5 μg/kg/day. It is given 24 hours after the completion of chemotherapy. Pegfilgrastim is similar to filgrastim. Polyethylene glycol (PEG) unit of pegfilgrastim prolongs its duration in the body.

Dose: 6 mg, SC injection once per Chemotherapy Cycle.

DRUG DOSE CALCULATION

Commonly, chemotherapy doses are calculated based on patient's body surface area (BSA). It is expressed as mg per meter squared (mg/m²).

BSA is better indicator of metabolic mass than the body weight as it is less affected by abnormal adipose mass. However, height is a fixed variable, patient's weights are to be taken prior to each course of therapy, as it may fluctuate significantly. BSA provides a better measures of potential toxicity than body weight. BSA closely reflects the cardiac output and blood flow than the body weight. For drugs excreted through renal route, dose is calculated on the basis of glomerular filtrartion rate (Calvert Formula). Drugs metabolized in liver need monitoring of liver function. Drug dose needs modification for a woman with hepatic dysfunction. Normal adult BSA for women approximates 1.7 m².

ANTIEMETIC DRUGS USED DURING CHEMOTHERAPY

Drugs 5HT3 (SRA)	Dose	Time
Ondansetron	Oral : 24 mg IV : 8 mg	Before therapy
Granisetron	Oral : 2 mg IV : 1 mg	Before chemotherapy
Dexamethasone (Decadron)	Oral : 12 mg	Before chemotherapy
	Oral : 8 mg	Daily: Oral—8 mg (Days 2–4)

5HT3: 5-hydroxytryptamine-3
SRA: Serotonin receptor antagonists

CHEMOTHERAPEUTIC DRUGS AND RISKS OF VOMITING (HESKETH 2008)

High risks: > 90%: Cisplatin, cyclophosphamide, dactinomycin.

Moderate risks: > 30–90%: Carboplatin, ifosfamide, doxorubicin.

Low/Minimal risks: < 30%: Paclitaxel, docetaxel, gemcitabine, MTX, etoposide, topotecan, bleomycin, vinblastin and bevacizumab.

EVOLUTION OF CHEMOTHERAPY RESPONSE*

Response	Criteria
Complete response (CR)	Disappearance of all "target" lesions
Partial response (PR)	A decrease of ≥ 30% in the sum of greatest diameters of l target lesions
Progressive disease (PD)	An increase in ≥ 20% in the sum of greatest diameters of target lesions or identification of one or more new lesions
Stable disease (SD)	Neither sufficient shrinkage to qualify for PR nor sufficient increase to qualify for PD

*Eisenhauer EA- 2009

CHEMOTHERAPEUTIC DRUGS AND TISSUE INJURY FOLLOWING EXTRAVASATION

Tissue injuries	Drugs
Vesicants are drugs that can cause skin ulceration, tissue necrosis and sloughing	Doxorubicin, actinomycin D, paclitaxel
Exfoliants cause skin exfoliation	Cisplatin, topotecan, docetaxel
Irritants cause skin irritation	Carboplatin, etoposide
Inflammants cause inflammation of the skin	Methotrexate
Neutral drugs: Bleomycin, cyclophosphamide, gemcitabine, ifosfamide	

CHEMOTHERAPEUTIC DRUGS, INDICATIONS OF USE AND THE TOXICITY

Drugs	Uses	Toxicity
Paclitaxel	Recurrent epithelial ovarian cancer, endometrial cancer, GTN	Neurotoxicity (peripheral), BMD, alopecia, bradycardia, arrhythmia, HSR
Docetaxel	Recurrent ovarian epithelial cancer	BMD, alopecia, HSR, peripheral neuropathy
Vincristine	GTN	Neurotoxicity, alopecia
Etoposide	Germ cell Sex cord stromal tumor (SCST) Recurrent epithelial ovarian cancer	BMD, alopecia Secondary cancers
Topotecan	Recurrent epithelial ovarian cancer, cervical cancer	BMD, nausea, vomiting, alopecia, fever, malaise

Suggested Reading

1. Bafaloukos D, Linardou H, Aravantinos G, Papadimitriou C, Bamias A, Fountzilas G, et al. A randomized phase II study of carboplatin plus pegylated liposomal doxorubicin versus carboplatin plus paclitaxel in platinum sensitive ovarian cancer patients: A Hellenic Cooperative Oncology Group study. BMC Med. 2010;8:3.
2. Monk BJ, Pujade-Lauraine E, Burger RA. Integrating bevacizumab into the management of epithelial ovarian cancer: The controversy of front-line versus recurrent disease. Ann Oncol. 2013;24 (Suppl 10):x53–x58.
3. Pujade-Lauraine E, Wagner U, Aavall-Lundqvist E, Gebski V, Heywood M, Vasey PA, et al. Pegylated liposomal doxorubicin and carboplatin compared with paclitaxel and carboplatin for patients with platinum-sensitive ovarian cancer in late relapse. J Clin Oncol. 2010;28:3323–29.
4. Tewari KS, Sill MW, Long HJ 3rd, Penson RT, Huang H, Ramondetta LM, et al. Improved survival with bevacizumab in advanced cervical cancer. N Engl J Med. 2014;370:734–43.

Radiotherapy in Gynecological Cancers

EXTERNAL BEAM RADIATION THERAPY (EBRT)

Linear accelerator *(linac)* is a radiation-producing unit. Linac can produce both photon and electron beams. Photons are used in External Beam Radiation Therapy (EBRT). Photon therapy mode is used for deep-seated tumors. Electron therapy mode is used for superficial lesions. The accelerated electron beam is directed to hit a metal target (lead scattering foil) to generate photons. The unit used to describe the energy of a photon beam is MV (million volts).

BRACHYTHERAPY

Brachytherapy provides treatment at a short distance. It is used for small tumor volumes (<4 cm). Brachytherapy may be intracavitary or interstitial. Interstitial brachytherapy needs placement of needles directly in the cancer tissues.

Newer technology includes: Image-guided Adapted Brachytherapy (IGABT). There are two modes for the delivery of brachytherapy. These are: intracavitary and interstitial.

New technologies in external beam radiation therapy (EBRT) include: Intensity-modulated radiation therapy (IMRT) and volumetric modulated arc therapy (VMAT). These newer methods help to get greater precision to the target volume with the use of computer software and at the same time reduce the radiation dose to organs at risk (OAR).

Low-dose Rate (LDR) Versus High-dose Rate (HDR) Brachytherapy

LDR brachytherapy is delivered over the period of few days and requires the patient hospitalization. For several reasons, HDR has become more popular. HDR treatment time is reduced to minutes. LDR is defined as dose rates from 0.4 Gy to 2 Gy/hr. High-dose rates are higher than 12 Gy/hr. Intracavitary implant for cervical cancer: LDR technique, a dose of 30 to 40 Gy delivery takes several days. Whereas with HDR, the same dose is delivered in 3–5 weekly fractions. The dose per fraction is 5–7 Gy and is given in 10–20 minutes. The HDR has the following advantages:
a. Short hospital stay
b. Reduces patient immobility
c. Reduces thromboembolic problems.

Multileaf Collimator (MLC) is helpful to shape the radiation beam which also permits OAR shielding. Reducing toxicity to OAR in gynecology is important. The OAR includes: the rectum, bladder, small bowels, kidney and bone marrow.

PLACE OF RADIOTHERAPY IN GYNECOLOGICAL MALIGNANCY

1. As a neoadjuvant—before operation
2. As an adjuvant—post-operation
3. As the primary and definitive treatment of advanced carcinoma (endometrial cancer)
4. Concomitantly with chemotherapy.

Preoperative Radiotherapy

Indications: Cases with locally advanced cancers (carcinoma cervix).

Benefits

a. It reduces the tumor volume so that subsequent surgical resection is complete.
b. It reduces tumor dissemination at the time of surgery.
c. Improves the outcome when compared to surgery alone.

Limitations

a. It is not commonly used these days.
b. Patients are not properly staged, whereas primary surgery can stage the disease properly.
c. Primary surgery gives the histological diagnosis also.

Postoperative Radiotherapy

Indication

1. It is used when disease has been staged and the histological features are known.
   This is helpful to assess the dose schedule.
2. Radiotherapy may be EBRT or brachytherapy or both (postoperative; vaginal vault radiation, in cases with endometrial carcinoma).
3. High-risk group of women with endometrial carcinoma:
   a. Age > 60 years
   b. Histologically grade – III disease
   c. Invasion of outer half of myometrium
   d. Invasion of lymphovascular space.

Benefits

1. Postoperative radiotherapy is helpful to assess the dose schedule.
2. EBRT when used with the application of IMRT or VMAT, can improve the outcome and, at the same time, can reduce

the long-term morbidity. Case selection should be made with the multidisciplinary team following a tumor-based meeting.
3. Vaginal vault brachytherapy (VBT) significantly reduces the risk of local relapse. It has less morbidity.
4. IMRT with improved conformality can decrease the bowel and bladder toxicity during pelvic radiation therapy.
   - **Stereotactic body radiation therapy (SBRT)** uses hypofractionated regimen of five or less fractions (10–20 Gy per fraction). Combined image-guided radiation therapy (IGRT) and safe SBRT can overcome some of the technical problems. The common technical problems are: patient organ motion, changes in tumor size and shape during a treatment course.

Conformal radiation technique (CRT) maximizes tumor damaged and minimizes injury to the OAR. This needs patient's tumor imaging with CT, MRI or PET. This imaging report along with patient's pathology and operative report helps in defining 3-D target (tumor and the area of tumor spread) and normal tissue volumes. These are needed for a radiation oncologist to delineate the anatomic areas that will receive the tumoricidal dose. In this process, practice of simulation with patient positioning, immobilization, shielding the normal tissues are all done.

Four volumes are considered important and are defined as:
1. Gross tumor volume (GTV)—which covers any gross disease.
2. A clinical target volume (CTV)—that covers areas at risk for microscopic tumor spread.
3. Planning the target volume (PTV).
4. A volume that defines the normal organs at risk (OAR).

CERVICAL CANCER

Radiotherapy for Cervical Cancer

Radiotherapy in cervical cancer may be used as:
1. **Definitive treatment**: In cases with advanced disease.
2. **Adjuvant therapy** for high or intermediate risk cases. It is used postoperatively. Adjuvant radiotherapy is used with or without chemotherapy.
   Cases for adjuvant postoperative radiotherapy with or without chemotherapy are:
   i. Tumors > 2 cm in size
   ii. Stromal invasion > 50%
   iii. Lymphovascular space involvement
   iv. Parametrium involvement
   v. Involvement of lymph nodes.

Definitive Treatment with Radiation

Cases for primary radiation therapy:
a. Locally advanced cervical cancer in an older woman
b. Women unfit for radical surgery (associated comorbidity).

Place of Neoadjuvant Chemotherapy

a. Neoadjuvant chemotherapy followed by surgery is an option for patients with carcinoma cervix.
b. Women with carcinoma cervix with bulky tumors (>4 cm) are considered for neoadjuvant chemoradiation (platinum-based) therapy to reduce the tumor volume. Platinum-based chemotherapy is radiosensitizer. Dose-dense neoadjuvant chemotherapy with carboplatin and paclitaxel is found to be superior.
c. Neoadjuvant chemoradiation (platinum/taxanes-based) therapy, increases local disease control and decreases distant metastasis or development of secondary neoplasia (Table 43.1).
d. Addition of a taxane to cisplatin group of drugs may improve the outcome for adenocarcimona cases as these cases appear to be more radioresistant. Combination therapy can maximize tumericidal effects and minimize toxicities and complications.

TABLE 43.1: Risk of developing secondary cancer following radiation therapy.

Risks	Tissues
High	Bone marrow, female breast, thyroid
Moderate	Bladder, stomach, colon, ovary
Low	Bone, muscle, cervix, uterus, rectum

Brachytherapy for Cervical Cancer

There are two modes for delivery of brachytherapy for cervical cancer:
a. Intracavitary, and
b. Interstitial.

Currently gynecologic brachytherapy has moved from radium to cesium to modern-day cobalt and iridium sources.
- Remote control after loaders are used for safety of the staff.
- High-dose rate (HDR) delivery is now the standard care. Pulse dose rate (PDR) delivery are used in some centers.
- HDR therapy takes about 5–10 minutes and is usually given in 2–5 weekly doses or fractions.
- PDR is given as a single or two treatments (pulsed method over only 10 to 30 minutes of each hour) and requires the presence of a physicist or a physics support staff.
- Conventional brachytherapy is based on Manchester rules. Fixed points: Point A and point B are considered. Orthogonal X-ray images are used for calculating the treatment doses. This method assumes that all tumors are the same. The doses prescribed to the fixed points are irrespective of tumor size or shape. This therapy works well with small volume tumors. Recurrences are high where the tumors are large. However, X-ray images cannot identify OAR. Point estimations are made for doses to these organs. With this, toxicity to bowel and bladder is reduced in about 5–20% of cases. Traditional approach is to insert a central

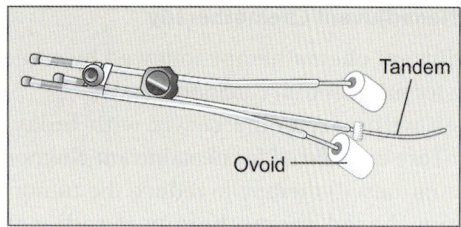

Fig. 43.1: Tandem and ovoid applicator.

tube (tandem) into the uterus through the cervical OS and to place a pair of ovoids (colpostats) into the posterior fornix (tandem and ovoid applicator) (Fig. 43.1). Presently ovoids are replaced by a ring which surrounds the cervix. This technique is known as **ring and tandem applicator**. Perforating the ring, it allows the needles to be introduced to provide interstitial boost. Computerized planning may allow modifications to the plan, to adapt the tumors with symmetrical parametrial spread.

Most advanced radiation oncology centers are shifting more towards **image-guided brachytherapy (IGBT)**. Computed tomography or preferably magnetic resonance imaging (MRI) are used to view the applicators to localize the tumor more correctly and also the OAR. It is proved that 3D image-based planning is superior in the assessment of gross tumor volume (GTV), clinical target volume (CTV) and in the delineation of CTV. IGBT allows dose calculation and prescription of radiation to these defined target volumes that are at risk of microscopic tumor spread.

Intensity-modulated radiotherapy (IMRT) has reduced the morbidity following radiation therapy. Patients with large and unresectable tumors, primary radiotherapy with concomitant cisplatin chemotherapy is an option worth considering. Both radiation and cisplatin cause single and double-stranded DNA breaks and base damage. Taxanes also enhance the effects of radiation by causing microtubule damage and blocking cell division. Newly targeted chemotherapeutic agents like poly (ADP-ribose) polymerase (PARP) inhibitors in combination with radiation give a synergistic effect.

Dose volume histogram (DVH) is made for assessing the entire dose distribution to the cancer (tumoricidal dose) and surrounding normal tissues (minimal dose). The dose distributions are reviewed by the radiation oncologists and radiation physicist for final approval.

Once brachytherapy instruments are in place, the radioactive sources are inserted. This remote after loading approach is commonly done at present.

Radiation effects and cell death: These are two main pathways of cell death:
a. **Mitotic catastrophe:** Mitotic catastrophe is the main mechanism for cell death. In this process, the cells with damaged DNA, enter the process of mitosis prematurely before DNA is repaired. These cells die in their attempt to complete next two to three mitotic divisions.
b. **Apoptosis:** Apoptosis is due to the intracellular stress following radiation-induced irreparable double-strand breaks.

Cells' response to radiation: Four phases of cellular response are observed. It is commonly expressed by 4 "R's"
a. **Cellular repair** is observed following sublethal damage. Sublethal damage repair (SLDR) occurs when radiation dose is split into two or more fractions with a gap of few hours in between the fractions. Cells have the time to repair the damage and their survival rate increases. With this **repopulation** of cells, it is possible to restore the cell pool.
b. **Reassortment** is the phase following SLDR. The proliferating cells are in the different phases of the cell cycle. Cells in phases of mitosis (M) and (G2) are sensitive to radiation compared to the G1 and S phases. The ultimate result of radiation is the death of some cells in phases of M and G2.
c. **Repopulation,** however in the reassortment phase, the surviving cells restart their progression by mitotic divisions to cause cellular repopulation.
d. **Reoxygenation:** The tumor cells situated within 100 microns of the capillaries are oxygenated but the cells lying beyond distance of 100 microns are hypoxic. Following radiation therapy, the oxygenated cells are killed and the tumor shrinks. Due to the shrinkage of tumor volume, the hypoxic cells come closer to the capillaries to become oxygenated.

Tissue Response to Radiation Therapy

Situations where radiation therapy is less tolerated:
1. Tissue hypoxia is an important factor for poor tumor response and survival outcome.
2. Response is poor when the volume of tissue is large for irradiation.
3. The dose of radiation is high.
4. The dose per fraction is large.
5. Patient's age is advanced.

Suggested Reading

1. Duenas Gonzalez A, Zarba JJ, Alcedo JC, et al. A phase III study comparing concurrent gemicitabine (Gem) plus cisplatin (Cis) and radiation followed by adjuvant Gem plus Cis versus concurrent Cis and radiation in patients with stage IIB to IVA carcinoma of the cervix. Abstract No. CRA5507, Presented at the 45th Annual Meeting of the American Society of Clinical Oncology. 1-2 June 2009.
2. Heron De, Gerszten K, Selvaraj RNm, et al. Concentional 3D conformal versus intensity-modulated radiotherapy for the adjuvant treatment of gynecologic malignancies: A comparative dosimetric study of dose-volume histograms. Gynecol Oncol. 2003;91(1):39.
3. Wong FC, Tung SY, Leung TW, et al. Treatment results of high-dose rate remote afterloading brachytherapy for cervical cancer and retrospective comparison of two regimens. Int J Radiat Oncol Biol Phys. 2003;55(5):1254.

Sentinel Lymph Node Mapping in Gynecologic Cancers

One study (Rossi-2017) reported a bilateral SLN dissection. Detection rate was 58%. The rate of false negative sentinel lymph node (SLN) mapping was less than 3% [National Comprehensive Cancer Network (NCCN)].

NCCN guidelines now support SLN mapping as an alternative lymph node assessment strategy. Use of indocyanine green (ICG) dye is found superior for bilateral SLN identification compared to isosulphan blue. SLN mapping is an accurate method of lymph node assessment. This is used as an alternative to performing full lymphadenectomy.

SLN mapping includes cervical injection of indocyanine green dye. This enhances the fluorometric imaging to maximize SLN detection.

The sole objective of SLM is to get the information about the metastatic spread of the disease to the lymph nodes. This has the benefit of avoiding the morbidity of full lymphadenectomy.

With this approach, the rate of lymphadenectomy can be reduced by 50% in patients with type 1 tumors. About 15 to 50% of patients develop some degree of lymphedema following the procedure. This more so in women who undergo radiotherapy thereafter.

The surgical staging of endometrial cancer is based on the pattern of spread.
- **Type I:** Initially spreads by direct extension.
    - Endometrium → Myometrium → Adjacent structures (lymphnodes, cervix, parametria) → Distant metastasis to lung, liver, usually occur late.
- **Surgical management of women with Type 1 tumors:** To include pelvic lymphadenectomy with or without para-aortic lymphadenectomy as most patients will have negative lymph nodes. This strategy reduces overtreatment.
- **Type II tumors:** Spread similar to type 1 tumors and also through the peritoneal cavity to distant sites (as in a case with ovarian cancer). This is more in cases with serous adenocarcinomas. Therefore all patients with type II tumors should be included for pelvic and para-aortic lymphadenectomy.
- **Cases with type II tumors** are found to have occult omental spread between 5% and 25% of cases.
- **Pelvic lymphadenectomy** includes removal of: internal iliac, external iliac, common iliac and the obturator nodes as to dissect the SLN.
- **Para-aortic lymphadenectomy** should extend atleast to the level of inferior mesenteric artery. Ideally, it should be up to the level of renal vessels.
- **Omentectomy:** It should be done in cases with type II tumors.

Hereditary nonpolyposis colorectal cancer, an autosomal dominant inherited cancer is caused by mutations of DNA mismatch repair (MMR) genes. Individuals with Lynch syndrome have an increased risk of secondary malignancies. These are: (A) Colon cancer (50%), (B) Bladder cancer (10%), (C) Upper urinary tract cancer (10%). In a young woman with endometrial cancer, seeking fertility sparing surgery, endometrial curettage specimen should be sent for DNA MMR testing.

Lymphadenectomy in Ovarian Cancer

Lymph node metastasis with advanced ovarian cancer occurs in about 60% of cases. Studies have not established that lymphadenectomy is associated with distinct clinical benefit. On the contrary lymphadenectomy is associated with increased postoperative morbidities. Lymphodenectomy is associated with more operative time, more blood loss and postoperative morbidity. Also, there is more need of blood transfusion, increased morbidity and readmission.

Therefore lymphadenectomy in all cases of advanced ovarian cancer is not a routine procedure. In cases with mucinous ovarian histology, lymph nodes are less commonly involved.

Moreover lymph node metastasis in cases with sex cord stromal tumor is uncommon. Similarly germ cell tumors like dysgerminoma are more sensitive to chemotherapy even if these lymphnodes are involved.

Bilateral SLN mapping provides information about the lymph node status without subjecting patients to the morbidity of full lymphadenectomy.

Suggested Reading

1. Rossi EC, Kowalski LD, Scalici J, Cantrell L, Schuler K, Hanna RK, et al. A comparison of sentinel lymph node biopsy to lymphadenectomy for endometrial cancer staging (FIRES trial): a multicentre, prospective, cohort study. Lancet Oncol. 2017;18(3):384-92.

Section 6: Operative Gynecology

Section Outline

- Ch. 45. Abdominal Incisions
- Ch. 46. Tubal Ectopic Pregnancy
- Ch. 47. Cervical Insufficiency (Incompetence)
- Ch. 48. Surgical Management of Heavy Menstrual Bleeding
- Ch. 49. Surgical Site Infection
- Ch. 50. Endoscopy in Gynecology (Laparoscopic Surgery)
- Ch. 51. Prevention of Urinary Tract Injuries in Gynecological Laparoscopic Surgery
- Ch. 52. Management of Urinary Tract Injuries Following Laparoscopic Surgery
- Ch. 53. Place of Prophylactic Salpingectomy or Salpingo-oophorectomy in Current Gynecologic Practice
- Ch. 54. Surgical Management of Polycystic Ovarian Disease
- Ch. 55. Bariatric Surgery in Gynecology and Obstetrics
- Ch. 56. Robotic Surgery in Gynecology
- Ch. 57. Interventional Radiology in Obstetrics and Gynecology

Chapter 45: Abdominal Incisions

Most gynecological surgeons perform abdominal operations, making either a vertical or a transverse incision. Abdominal incisions in gynecological surgery can be made with a scalpel or with electrosurgery. Prophylactic antibiotics should be given within one hour of surgical incision and is completed after 48 hours of surgery. Wound infections are mainly related to patient and surgical factors. In selecting an incision, surgeon need to consider the underlying pathology, possibility of adhesions or malignancy.

VERTICAL INCISION

i. **Midline or**
ii. **Paramedian.**

Advantages of a Vertical (Midline/Paramedian) Incision

- Quick entry in the abdominal cavity
- Minimal blood loss
- May be extended upward when needed
- No important nerve or blood vessels are damaged
- Excellent exposure of operation field.
- *Principal steps:*
  - ♦ **Incision**: Skin incised vertically in the midline. It usually starts at a point below the level of the umbilicus (may be extended upward depending on the need) and ends 2–3 cm above the symphysis pubis. When it needs extension, incision is arched on the left of the umbilicus to avoid transection of the ligament of teres and the remnant of the umbilical vein. Moreover, arching the incision laterally provides more fascial tissue support to secure good closure.
  - ♦ **Subcutaneous fascial layers**
    - Camper's fascia and
    - Scarpa's fascia are incised
  - ♦ **Rectus sheath** incised in the midline and it is extended first cephalad and then caudally
  - ♦ **Rectus muscle** bellies are bluntly separated in the midline and retracted laterally.
  - ♦ **Peritoneal layer** is identified. It is grasped with two hemostatic forceps in the upper part to avoid injury to the bladder. The interposed peritorneum is palpated and visually examined to exclude any intervening viscera. It is then cut. An index finger is introduced and is swiped around the undersurface of the peritoneum to feel any adherent bowel loops or omentum.

The incision can be extended cephalad and caudally as needed. Fascia transversalis remains superficial to the peritoneum. The urachus (remnant of the allantois) is seen as a white fibrous cord.

Limitations of Vertical Incision

a. Wound dehiscence
b. Burst abdomen
c. Wound hematomas
d. Hernia formation.

Complications are more in cases associated with chronic lung disease, cough, vomiting or ileus.

PFANNENSTIEL INCISION (FIG. 45.1)

It is a suprapubic transverse incision most commonly used in obstetrics and gynecology. It has excellent cosmetic value.

It follows the **Langer lines** of the skin. Karl Langer (1861), described such lines. In the trunk, these lines are horizontal. Incision is made horizontal on the abdomen to cut the skin, parallel to these lines. This wound heal nicely with a fine scar, whereas a wound following a vertical incision on the abdomen, heal with a broad scar.

Advantages	Disadvantages
• Excellent cosmetic value	• Exposure is limited
• Maximum wound safety	• Injury to iliohypogastric and ilioinguinal nerves may occur
• Less postoperative pain	• It cannot be extended cephalad when needed
• Less need of analgesia	• It should preferably not to be used for cases with gynecological malignancy, large pelvic mass or when performing relaparotomy for postoperative complications (hemorrhage)
• Less of risk of developing incisional hernia	

Other Incisions

Suprapubic transverse incision of about 8–10 cm is made 2–3 cm above the symphysis pubis. It is made slightly arched with convexity downward. The vessels cut in the incision are superficial epigastric, superficial external pudendal and the superficial circumflex iliac vessels. These vessels may be coagulated.

Rectus sheath is incised transversely. Anterior rectus sheath composed of two layers—aponeurosis of external oblique

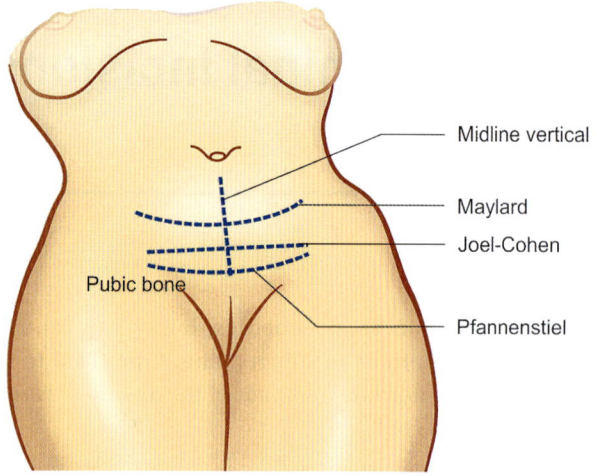

Fig. 45.1: Types of abdominal incision.

muscle and a fused aponeurotic layer of internal oblique, and transversus abdominis muscles. The iliohypogastric, ilioinguinal nerves run between these two fascial layers. The inferior epigastric vessels typically lie outside the lateral border of the rectus abdominis muscle. These vessels are injured when the incision is extended laterally. Unless these vessels are indentified, clamped and ligated or coagulated, massive hemorrhage may remain undetected. Lateral extension of the incision, also cause injury to the iliohypogastric and ilioinguinal nerves. The upper edge of fascial (rectus sheath) incision is grasped with a lens tissue forceps one or either side of the midline. It is kept retracted upward and is separated for the rectus abdominis muscle by sharp and blunt dissection. The perforating vessels are coagulated during dissection. Lower edge of the fascial incision is similarly held and separated from the rectus abdominis muscle. The pyramidalis muscle lies superficial to the rectus abdominis, and remain separated at the midline.

Peritoneum: Peritoneum incised vertically. Steps are same as described above.

Cherney incision: Skin incision is similar to Pfannenstiel incision. It is also similar to Maylard's muscle dividing incision (see below). Rectus sheath is opened. The tendinous part of the rectus abdominis and pyramidalis muscles are transected 1–2 cm above their insertion on the symphysis pubis. These muscles are then lifted upward to get access to the peritoneum. The inferior epigastric vessels are seen on the lateral aspect of the rectus muscle.

> **Advantages**
> a. Space of operating field is increased.
> b. Access to the space of Retzius is easy.
> c. Exposure to the pelvic side walls is also adequate.

Pfannenstiel incision can be converted to Cherney incision when needed.

Index finger is insinuated beneath the rectus muscle tendons when the tendons are divided. The insinuate fingers are also guard the bladder from injury during tendon division (Fig. 45.2).

During closure, the cut ends of the tendons are fixed to the under surface of the rectus sheath. Delayed absorbable suture material. 1-0 (Vicryl) is used with interrupted stitches. Stitching to symphysis pubis is not done to avoid the risk of osteitis pubis or osteomyelitis.

Risk of injury to the femoral and genitofemoral nerves are increased with the use of self-retaining retractors.

Maylard incision (1907): It is a true transverse muscle cutting incision (Fig. 45.3). It gives good pelvic exposure, specially for radical pelvic surgery. Initial steps are similar to that Pfannenstiel incision. Maylard's incision differs from Pfannenstiel incision in the following respects:

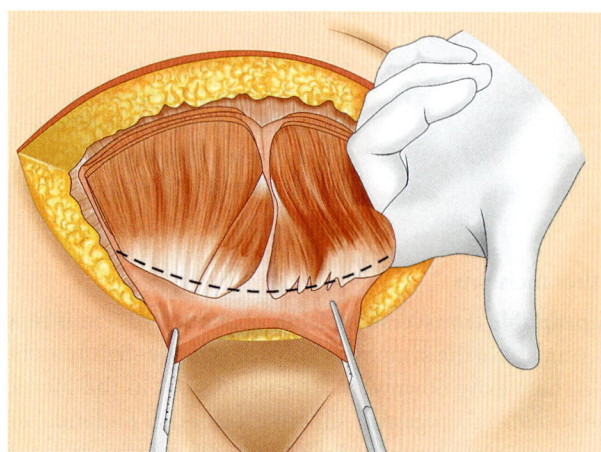

Fig. 45.2: Tendon transection.

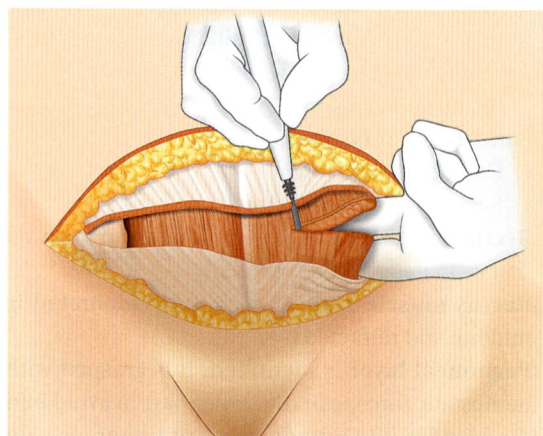

Fig. 45.3: Muscle transection incision. It gives extensive exposure and access within the pelvis.

A. Rectus abdominis muscle is not separated from the rectus sheath.
B. The bellies of the rectus abdominis muscles are transected to create more spaces during surgery within the pelvis. The inferior epigastric vessels lie posterolateral to the rectus abdominis muscles. These vessels are identified and ligated and transected bilaterally. The rectus abdominis muscles are to be dissected from the underlying fascia transversalis and peritoneum. Electrosurgical cutting blades are often used during dissection. Surgeon's fingers are insinuated beneath the rectus of the muscle. The peritoneum is incised transversely. Maylard's incision is avoided in cases where superior epigastric vessels have already been interrupted.

Wound closure: The rectus sheath is closed with a continuous stitch. Vicryl (delayed absorbable) suture material 1-0 is used. The divided muscle bellies do not need to be sutured together. Closing the fascial layer approximates the transected muscle fibers.

This incision is less commonly used as it is technically difficult.

Common difficulties of Maylard incision
a. Risks of injury to the inferior epigastric vessels
b. Postoperative pain is more and more need of analgesia
c. Longer-operating time
d. Increased postoperative febrile morbidity
e. More abdominal wall weakness

Joel-Cohen incision (1954) was initially introduced for abdominal hysterectomy. It is currently used widely for cesarean section. A straight transverse incision is made on the skin, at the level of 3 cm below the joining the anterior superior iliac spines. It is made slightly higher than the Pfannenstiel incision. The subcutaneous tissues and the rectus sheath are opened in the midline. It is extended laterally with blunt finger dissection. Rectus muscles are separated vertically with blunt dissection along with the peritoneum.

Paramedian incision: It has the advantage extending the incision on the same side of the pelvis when needed. There is no other difference from that of a midline incision.

Oblique incision: Gridiron (muscle splitting) incision of McBurney is commonly used for appendicectomy. It is a downward and inward incision at the McBurney's point. The incision is deepened through the skin and subcutaneous fat to the abdominal muscles. The muscle fibers are split along the direction of the fibers. The peritoneum may be opened up for as in appendectomy; otherwise, it may be reflected away from the abdominal wall. This allows extraperitoneal approach for drainage of abscess.

Advantages of Joel-Cohen incision
a. Less operating time
b. Less postoperative morbidity
c. Less need of postoperative analgesia
d. Less blood loss
e. Lower risk of wound infection and
f. Lesser hospital stay

Advantages and Disadvantages of Transverse Incision

Advantages	Disadvantages
• Cosmetically superior	• More time consuming
• Less postoperative pain	• More bleeding, more injury to vessels and nerves
• No restriction of respiratory excursions as the pain is less	• Difficulty in exploration of the upper abdominal viscera
• Early mobility	• Technically difficult

Advantages and Disadvantages of Vertical Incision

Advantages	Disadvantages
• Exposure adequate	• Poor cosmetic acceptance
• Can be extended as needed	• Risk of hernia formation
• Less bleeding	• Less respiratory excursion in the postoperative period due to pain
• Less injury to the nerves	• Risk of burst abdomen
• Entry into the abdominal cavity is quick	• More postoperative pain
• Technically easy to perform	• Need of more postoperative analgesia

Commonly used abdominal incisions for most gynecological procedures are either a transverse or a vertical incision. While deciding the type of incision, the surgeon must consider the underlying pathology, its size, morbidity, possibility of adhesions or malignancy and the need of exploring other organs (upper abdomen).

Suggested Reading

1. Joel-Cohen S. Abdominal and Vaginal Hysterectomy: New Techniques Based on Time and Motion Studies, 2nd edn. London: Heinemann, 1977.
2. Morrow CP, Curtin JP. Incisions and wound healing. In: Gynaecologic Cancer Surgery. New York: Churchill Livingstone, 1996. p. 152.
3. Raghavan R, Arya P, Arya P, China S. Abdominal incisions and sutures in obstetrics and gynaecology. The Obstetrician and Gynaecologist. 2014;16:13-8.
4. Rock JA, Jones III HW. TeLinde's Operative Gynecology. 10th edn. revised. Philadelphia: Lippincott Williams and Wilkins, 2011. p. 285–307.

Chapter 46: Tubal Ectopic Pregnancy

Q.1 Regarding ectopic pregnancy:
a. Laparoscopy should be done in all cases to confirm the diagnosis
b. Laparoscopic salpingotomy increases the chance of subsequent intrauterine pregnancy
c. Pregnancy of unknown location is a type of abdominal pregnancy
d. Persistent ectopic and recurrent ectopic pregnancy are the same.

Ans. a. F b. F
c. F d. F

Q.2 Tubal ectopic pregnancy can be managed by:
a. Laparotomy once the patient is hemodynamically stable
b. Laparoscopy when there is tubal rupture
c. Medical method in all cases with unruptured state
d. Observation alone occasionally.

Ans. a. F b. F
c. F d. T

Women who are rhesus negative and nonimmune should be given anti-D immunoglobulin 50 mg IM who have an ectopic pregnancy.

MANAGEMENT ISSUES

When a patient with tubal ectopic pregnancy is hemodynamically unstable, it is mostly due to the rupture of tube resulting in massive intraperitoneal hemorrhage. Patient may be in hypovolemic shock. Hemoperitoneum can be diagnosed with transvaginal ultrasonography. Laparotomy should be done in such a patient as an emergent procedure with simultaneous resuscitation. It is indicated as the most expedient method to prevent further blood loss.

Laparoscopic surgery is preferable in the patient who is hemodynamically stable. This method has the advantage of shorter operation time, less intraoperative blood loss, shorter hospital stays and lesser need for analgesic drugs.

However, subsequent intrauterine pregnancy rate is similar in both the procedures, the risk of repeated ectopic pregnancy is lower in following laparoscopic procedure.

The actual surgical procedure on the tube includes salpingectomy or salpingotomy. The chance of subsequent intrauterine pregnancy appears to be the same following any of the procedure provided the contralateral tube is healthy.

When the laparoscopic conservative (salpingotomy) and radical treatment (salpingectomy) are compared, the chances of subsequent intrauterine pregnancy rates are similar but the risks of ectopic pregnancy rates are higher in the salpingotomy group. In the presence of contralateral tubal disease, conservative tubal surgery (salpingotomy) is appropriate. This is done for the chance of future intrauterine pregnancy though the risk of ectopic pregnancy is increased. Therefore, the women must be counseled about the risk. Once understood, laparoscopic salpingotomy is the primary method of treatment when the contralateral tube is diseased and the women desire for future fertility. Otherwise, if salpingectomy is done, women need in vitro fertilization.

Irrespective of the type of surgery (laparotomy or laparoscopy), it is essential to follow-up the women when salpingotomy is done. Few patients need treatment for persistent trophoblastic activity (4–8%).

Medical Management of Tubal Ectopic Pregnancy

Estimation of serum human chorionic gonadotropin (hCG) and transvaginal ultrasonography can make the diagnosis of ectopic pregnancy confidently. Many women may not need the help of laparoscopy. However, the main reason for the use of laparoscopy is not only for the diagnosis but also for the purpose of therapy. Therefore, medical therapy has got its place for selected woman.

Overall selection criteria of a patient for medical therapy includes:
- Unruptured tubal ectopic pregnancy (Fig. 46.1)
- Patient hemodynamically stable
- Serum hCG <3,000 IU/L
- Absence of fetal cardiac activity.

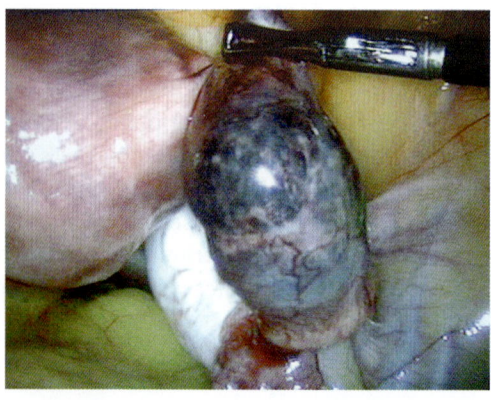

Fig. 46.1: Laparoscopy view of unruptured tubal ectopic pregnancy (right).

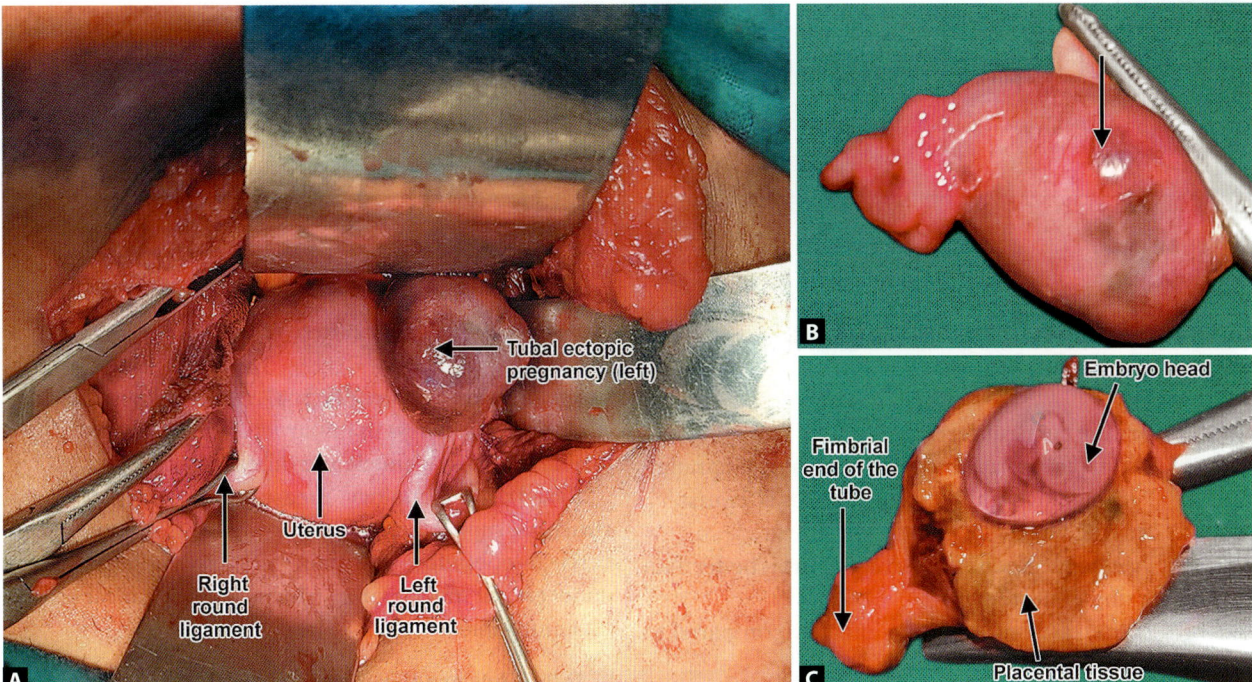

Figs. 46.2A to C: Emergency laparotomy for tubal ectopic pregnancy: (A) Unruptured tubal ectopic pregnancy is seen on the left (see arrow). Uterine fundus and the round ligaments are also seen; (B) Salpingectomy has been done; (C) The tube has been cut opened to show the embryo.

A variety of medical treatments are as effective as that of surgical treatment. Intramuscular methotrexate is commonly used. A single dose of 50 mg/m² is recommended. Serum hCG levels are checked on D4 and D7. There should be a fall in the level of serum hCG by more than 15%. Otherwise the women need further doses. About 14% of women require more than one dose. Another about 10% women will need surgical therapy in spite of medical therapy. Therefore, they should be counseled about the need of further therapy, follow-up and also the adverse effects of drug.

The adverse effects of the drug (methotrexate) are: (1) abdominal pain (75%), (2) stomatitis, (3) gastrointestinal upset, (4) conjunctivitis, (5) tubal rupture (7%).

Women should be advised to avoid sexual intercourse during the period of treatment. Similarly, forceful clinical pelvic examination should be avoided.

Pregnancy of unknown location is a situation when serum hCG level is positive but no pregnancy is visible neither within nor outside the uterus on transvaginal ultrasonography. See Clinics in Obstetrics, Section 2, Chapter 18.

The level of serum hCG at which any viable intrauterine pregnancy will be visualized by transvaginal scan (TVS) is considered as the discriminatory zone. When serum hCG levels are <1,000 IU/L, no pregnancy is visible so as to define it as a pregnancy of unknown location. Levels of serum hCG between 1,000 IU/L and 2,000 IU/L have also been used as discriminatory levels.

Usually, 40–70% of such pregnancies resolve spontaneously with expectant management. Remainder of such cases were diagnosed subsequently as ectopic pregnancy (15–30%) and the rest were intrauterine that ended in miscarriage. However, these cases need follow-up with serum hCG levels until the levels are ≤ 20 IU/L. Woman needs to be counseled accordingly. About 20–30% women may need intervention.

Expectant Management for Unruptured Tubal Ectopic Pregnancy

The criteria for expectant management:
- Patient hemodynamically stable
- Woman without any symptoms
- Ultrasound diagnosis of unruptured tubal ectopic pregnancy
- Size of adnexal mass < 5 cm
- Initial value of serum hCG <1000 IU/L
- Follow-up hCG levels are falling (>15% in 24 hours)
- No evidence of rupture or blood in the POD.

PERSISTENT TROPHOBLASTS OR PERSISTENT ECTOPIC PREGNANCY

Persistent trophoblasts activity is observed in women treated with salpingotomy rather than following salpingectomy. This results in failure of serum hCG levels to fall as expected following initial treatment. Overall 10% women suffer from persistent trophoblastic activity. A single dose of methotrexate 50 mg/m² has been found to be effective.

Suggested Reading

1. Hajenius PJ, Mol F, Mol BW, et al. Interventions for tubal ectopic pregnancy. Cochrane Database Syst Rev. 2007;1:CD000324.

Chapter 47: Cervical Insufficiency (Incompetence)

SINGLE BEST ANSWER (SBA) AND MULTIPLE CHOICE QUESTIONS (MCQs)

Q.1 Regarding cervical cerclage:
a. Use of perioperative tocolytics should be a routine
b. Perioperative antibiotic prophylaxis is a must
c. It should be under general anesthetic
d. Placement of two purse-string suture is better than a single suture
e. Shirodkar suture is more effective compared to McDonald's.

Ans.
a. F   b. F
c. F   d. F
e. F

MANAGEMENT OPTIONS

No significant different results are obtained when tocolytic drugs are used or not during the perioperative phase. Similarly, there are no studies of perioperative antibiotic use in women undergoing cervical cerclage operation. Choice of anesthesia should be at the discretion of the anesthetic for any individual patient. Either of general or a regional anesthesia can be used. There is no study to support the placement of two sutures over one suture.

No significant differences of results in terms of fetal survival or major postoperative morbidity, had been observed between the two techniques (Shirodkar versus McDonald).

Midtrimester recurrent fetal loss and spontaneous preterm birth may be due to cervical incompetence (insufficiency). This is due to impaired anatomy and/or function of the cervix (internal os).

Etiological factors may be—uterine anomalies, cervical trauma (forceful dilatation of the internal os), conization, trachelectomy or vaginal operative delivery (forceps) through undilated cervix.

History suggestive of cervical incompetence are:
- Recurrent midtrimester fetal loss
- Painless cervical shortening and dilatation
- Painless expulsion of the products of conception
- Painless rupture of membranes.

Measures to prevent recurrent fetal loss due to cervical incompetence.

Cervical incompetence (Figs. 47.1A and B) may be due to:
- Intrinsic weakness in the structure of the cervix
- Premature effacement and dilatation of the cervix.

Based on the etiology, measures are taken to provide a structural support to the weak cervix. This support, given by cerclage operation, maintains the cervical length and the endocervical mucous plug which is a mechanical barrier to ascending infection.

Q.2 What are the different types of cervical cerclage operations?

Ans.
- History indicated cerclage
- Ultrasound indicated cerclage
- Rescue (emergency) cerclage.

History indicated cerclage: Cerclage is done based on woman's obstetric and gynecological history (discussed above). History indicated suture is performed prophylactically in an asymptomatic woman.

History indicated cerclage may be helpful to woman with previous two or more second trimester loss and/or preterm births.

Ultrasound indicated cerclage: Ultrasound indicated cerclage is done in cases with shortening of cervical length as seen on transvaginal sonography (TVS). This procedure is done electively (asymptomatic women).

Rescue (emergency) cerclage: Cervical cerclage is done in a case with premature cervical dilation and/or with herniation of fetal membranes in the vagina. Emergency cerclage usually done on the basis of patients' symptoms like vaginal discharge, bleeding or due to sensation of pelvic pressure. Often there are evidences of cervical effacements, dilatation and shortening of the cervix when the woman is examined by a speculum or by ultrasonography.

Q.3 What is the appropriate time for an elective cerclage procedure?

Ans. It is done electively at 14–16 weeks of gestation but may be done up to 24 weeks of gestation.

Q.4 What are the different routes and methods of cervical cerclage operation?

Ans. *Transvaginal (common)*
- *McDonald's operation:* A purse-string suture is placed at the cervicovaginal junction without dissecting the bladder.
- *Shirodkar's operation:* Here, the similar type of purse-string suture is placed at the upper level of the cervix (level of internal os) after mobilization of the bladder.
- *Wurm's operation:* Sutures are placed crosswise (from above-down and side-to-side) at or below the level of cervicovaginal junction. Purpose is to support the cervix and to retain the mucus plug.

Transabdominal: This procedure is performed via laparotomy or laparoscopy. Suture is placed at the level of cervicoisthmic junction (internal os). The mersilene tape is placed at the level of the isthmus, between the uterine wall and the uterine vessels.

Q.5 What are the indicaions of transabdominal procedure?

Ans. 1. Cervix is hypoplastic
2. Cervix is torn and no adequate length is obtained to pass the suture virginally
3. Prior vaginal cerclage has failed.

Disadvantages of transabdominal procedure:
- Increased complications (injury to uterine vessels, ureter, bladder and hemorrhage), during the operation.
- Subsequent laparotomy for delivery or for removal of the tape when needed in pregnancy.

Q.6 What are the contraindications of cervical cerclage operation?

Ans.
- Presence of intrauterine infection (chorioamnionitis)
- Ruptured membranes (PPROM) before or during the operation
- Cervical dilatation > 4 cm
- Fetal compromise (malformation or death)
- Vaginal bleeding.

History indicated cerclage operation should be performed for women with recurrent (three or more) previous second trimester losses and/or preterm births. Three randomized controlled trials (RCTs) comparing history indicated cerclage with expectant management, showed no significant difference between the two groups in forms of fetal and neonatal outcome (Fig. 47.1B).

Women with a singleton pregnancy and no history of spontaneous midtrimester loss or preterm birth should not be considered for cervical cerclage operation, even if incidentally they are found to have short cervix (cervical length ≤ 25 mm) on ultrasonography (Fig. 47.2).

Meta-analysis of four RCTs of cerclage versus expectant management in women with short cervix, reported no evidence of benefits of cerclage operation in women, who had no other risk factors for spontaneous preterm birth.

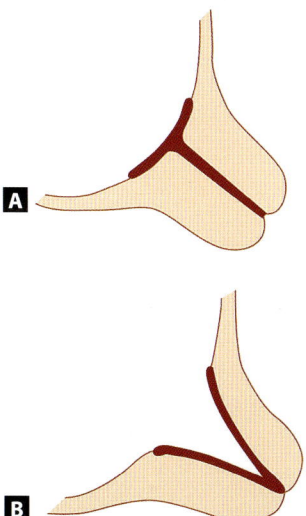

Figs. 47.1A and B: Schematic presentation of the cervix: (A) Normal cervix-closed internal os, the cervical canal appear T shaped; (B) Incompetent cervix-showing V shaped.

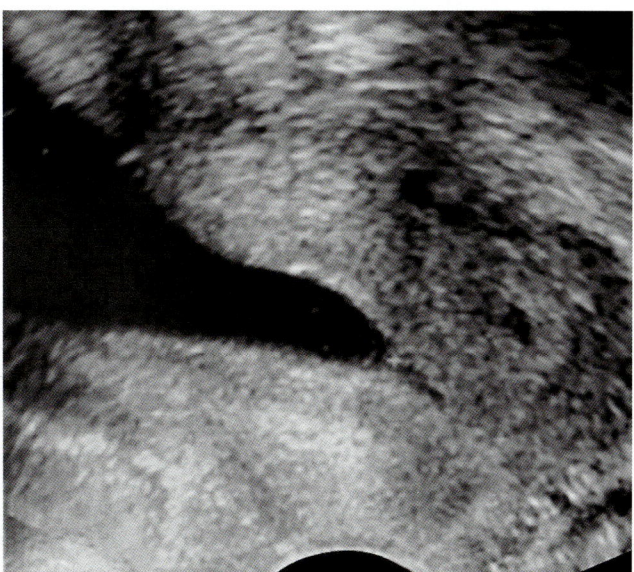

Fig. 47.2: USG of the cervix showing funneling of the cervical canal. The amniotic sac is seen herniated within the cervical canal.

The criteria to be fulfilled for performing cervical cerclage operation for a woman with singleton pregnancy are:
- History of spontaneous (≥ 2) midtrimester loss or preterm birth
- TVS surveillance revealed, cervical length ≤ 25 mm
- Funneling of the cervix (dilatation of the internal os) on TVS.

Women, found to have cervical length of ≤ 25 mm detected during serial sonographic examinations between 10+ and 21+ weeks of gestation, with history of spontaneous preterm birth/midtrimester loss, have reduced preterm birth and perinatal death with cervical cerclage.

Therefore, women with a history of spontaneous second trimester loss or preterm delivery may be offered serial sonographic surveillance to detect cervical shortening. Women having cervical shortening, are benefited from ultrasound indicated cervical cerclage compared to a woman who has a long cervix.

Investigations to be done prior to insertion of cervical cerclage: First trimester ultrasound scan and screening for aneuploidy before insertion of cervical cerclage is recommended. This practice helps to ensure fetal viability and the absence of major or lethal fetal abnormality. It is a good practice to ensure an anomaly scan before a rescue cerclage.

Q.7 Regarding cervical cerclage:
   a. Progesterone supplementation following cerclage operation should be a routine
   b. Transvaginal cervical cerclage should be removed after 38 completed weeks of pregnancy
   c. Women with transabdominal cerclage, suture may be left in place if delivered by cesarean section
   d. Fetal fibronectin testing during the postcerclage period is very useful.

Ans. a. F   b. F
       c. T   d. F

A transcervical cerclage should be removed usually after 36 weeks of pregnancy. When the woman is in established preterm labor, the suture is to be removed immediately to avoid trauma to the cervix irrespective to the period of gestation. Fetal fibronectin testing in such a woman is not much informative because of its increased false-positive result. Women with transabdominal suture require delivery by cesarean section. In such a situation the suture may be left in place if further future pregnancy is desired. Routine use of progesterone supplementation following cerclage operation is restricted to clinical trials only. This is helpful in women with high risk of preterm delivery only.

Suggested Reading

1. Berghella V, Odibo AO, To MS, Rust OA, Althuisius SM. Cerclage for short cervix on ultrasonography: Meta-analysis of trial using individual patient-level data. Obstet Gynecol. 2005;106(1):181-9.
2. Final report of the Medical Research Council/RCOG multicenter randomized trial of cervical cerclage. Br J Obstet Gynecol. 1993;100(6):516-23.
3. McDonad IA. Suture of the cervix for inevitable miscarriage. J Obstet Gynecol Br Emp. 1957;64(3):346-50.
4. Royal College of Obstetricians and Gynecologists: Clinical Governance. London: RCOG. 2006.
5. Shirodkar VN. A new method of operative treatment for habitual abortion in the second trimester of pregnancy. Antiseptic. 1955;52:299-300.

Surgical Management of Heavy Menstrual Bleeding

Heavy menstrual bleeding (HMB) is defined as excessive menstrual bloodloss, which interferes with a woman's physical, social, emotional and/or material quality of life occurring alone or in combination with other symptoms (NICE-2007).

International Federation of Gynecology and Obstetrics (FIGO) **defines heavy menstrual bleeding (HMB)** as the women's perspective of increased menstrual blood loss regardless of regularity, frequency or duration. Treatment for HMB is offered to a woman on the basis of reported deterioration or intolerance of menstrual bleeding. An objective proof of excessive blood loss has been considered a requirement. **Abnormal uterine bleeding (AUB)** according to the **FIGO is coined by the acronym 'PALM-COEIN'.**

Other different terminologies **'Dysfunctional uterine bleeding (DUB)'** which was accepted as a state of abnormal uterine bleeding without any clinically detectable organic, systemic and iatrogenic cause (pelvic pathology, e.g. tumor, inflammation or pregnancy is excluded).

Currently DUB is accepted as a state of abnormal uterine bleeding following anovulation due to dysfunction of hypothalamo-pituitary-ovarian axis (endocrine origin). The causes of anovulatory bleeding may occur either alone or in various combinations in a woman with AUB.

Management issues for women with AUB need careful history taking, thorough examination (general, systemic and pelvic) and appropriate investigations. Treatment is initiated thereafter.

INVESTIGATIONS

Blood: Full blood count, blood biochemistry, endocrine assays, thyroid function tests, hysteroscopy, endometrial biopsy, to exclude endometrial hyperplasia, malignancy especially in women with age > 45 years. **Ultrasonography scan** is the initial investigation to exclude any organic pelvic pathology. Hysteroscopy, laparoscopy to be organized depending upon the abnormalities as detected on ultrasonography.

MANAGEMENT

Management options for AUB vary widely.
- **Management is decided upon the following factors:**
    - Age of the woman
    - Desire for child-bearing
    - Severity of bleeding
    - Pathology as revealed on investigations.
- **Associated with any other pathology**
  Broadly the treatment protocol is divided into:
    - Medical and /or
    - Surgical methods.

Considering the importance of age and the pathology, the treatment protocol is classified as:
- Pubertal and adolescent menorrhagia (<20 years)
- Reproductive period (20–40 years)
- Premenopausal (>40 years)
- Postmenopausal
- Presence of associated pathology (pain)
- Impact on quality of life.

Management Options

Medical	Surgical
■ **Non-hormonal** 　■ Prostaglandin synthetase inhibitors (Mefenamic acid) 　■ Antifibrinolytic agents (Tranexamic acid) ■ **Hormones** 　■ Norethisterone acetate 　■ Medroxyprogesterone acetate 　■ Progesterone-releasing IUCD (LNG-IUS) 　■ Combined oral pills 　■ GnRH analogs	■ **Uterine curettage** ■ **Endometrial ablation/resection** 　■ First generation (hysteroscopic) 　■ Second generation (non-hysteroscopic) ■ **Myomectomy** ■ **Hysterectomy**
NICE recommends combined oral contraceptive pills, tranexamic acid, LNG-IUS as the first-line medical treatment	

Woman with AUB have the opportunity of wide range of options to accept. Informed decision about the treatment modalities can reduce the risk of major operations (hysterectomy). The incidence of hysterectomy has been reduced steadily with the introduction of LNG-IUS and endometrial ablation.

Women, those do not respond to medical treatment or where medical treatment is unacceptable, can have the surgical methods of treatment including endometrial ablation.

Endometrial Ablation

It is a procedure that is used to control AUB by destroying the functioning active endometrium (glands and stroma) located in the endomyometrial junction and up to 5 mm of the myometrium. The indications for endometrial ablation are:

> **Indications for endometrial ablation**
> - Women with failed medical treatment for AUB
> - Women completed their family
> - Women who do not wish to preserve menstrual reproductive function
> - Size of the uterus is either normal or <10 weeks pregnancy size
> - Uterine fibroid, if present <3 cm
> - Women requesting for preservation of the uterus

Endometrial ablation techniques both the first and second generation have been thoroughly evaluated and are evidence based (NICE). Second generation techniques are safer, simple to learn and use.

Endometrial Destruction Techniques

First generation: Ablation of endometrium is done through a hysteroscope. Whole of endometrium is ablated and 5 mm of adjacent myometrium is also ablated along with. Glycine is the distension medium used when monopolar diathermy is used.

Commonly used First-generation Methods of Endometrial Destruction

Transcervical resection of endometrium (TCRE)

Operative hysteroscope is used with a 3 mm electrosurgical loop. Distension medium is glycine when monopolar blend current at 80–100 W is used for resection. However, normal saline can be used as the distension medium when bipolar energy source resectoscopes are used. Complications are more and learning curve is also long. It is the preferred method when hysteroscopic myomectomy is required along with ablation.

Rollerball endometrial ablation

A rollerball electrode is used for ablation of the endometrium instead of a resectoscope. Principally, it is similar to TCRE. The ablation of the endomyometrium is done up to a depth of 5 mm. Complications are relatively less compared to TCRE. The procedure may be repeated when needed.

Laser ablation of endometrium

It is rarely performed. ND:YAG laser energy to endometrium is used. The power use ranges from 50 W to 80 W. This procedure is expensive, time-consuming and needs arrangement of safety in the theater.

Second-generation Methods of Endometrial Destruction

Different devices are available to ablate the endometrium.
A. Thermal balloon ablation system is commonly used. It consists of a catheter and a silicon balloon filled with circulating hot liquid at a high pressure. *Thermochoice III and Cavaterm* (endometrial ablation systems) both use 5% dextrose at temperature of 87°C and pressure of 160–180 mm Hg. Other devices use hot saline at 85°C with pressure of 200 mm Hg (Monotreat balloon). *Thermablate* (endometrial ablation system, EAS) uses glycerine at 173°C, with a pressure at 220 mm Hg.

The time required for endometrial ablation for these systems is 2–10 minutes.

The mechanism for endometrial ablation is based on the effects of combined high temperature and high pressure. This causes coagulation of the endovascular and endomyometrial vessels resulting in immediate damage and subsequent development of permanent fibrosis.

> **Contraindications of second-generation endometrial ablation methods**
> - Uterine size >10–12 weeks of pregnancy size
> - Submucous fibroids >3 cm
> - Women with prior classical cesarean delivery
> - Women with prior history of transmural myomectomy
> - Any suspicion of uterine perforation
> - Uterus acutely anteverted or retroverted
> - Presence of intrauterine adhesions

This procedure is not done under the direct version of a hysteroscope. However, it is better to have evaluation of the endometrial cavity with prior hysteroscopy.

B. Bipolar radiofrequency endometrial ablation, i.e., commonly used in the UK. Novasure delivers radiofrequency energy up to 50 Ohm, to ablate the endometrium. The electrode array of the device conforms to the uterine contour. The average treatment time is 90 seconds but may go up to 120 seconds. The endometrium is desiccated up to the adjacent myometrium.

C. Hydrothermal balloon ablation is done with circulating heated normal saline at 90°C. Cervix is to be kept closed to prevent leakage of hot saline and to prevent vaginal burns. The method is done under direct hysteroscopic vision.

Mechanism of Action for Endometrial Ablation Method

When the endometrium is ablated or resected out with its full thickness along with superficial myometrium (5 mm), all the basal endometrial glands are removed. Endometrial regeneration usually occurs from the basal endometrial glands. Regeneration of endometrium is not possible once the full thickness of endometrium along the basal glands is removed. This makes these procedures effective to control HMB with minimum or no failure rates.

Place of Pretreatment Endometrial Preparation

Use of danazol or progestogens or GnRH analogs pretreatment is helpful to reduce the time of endometrium ablation. For the second-generation procedure to pretreatment may not be done.

Precautions: Endometrial pathology (atypia, malignancy) needs to be excluded prior to therapy.

Pregnancy after Endometrial Ablation and Place of Contraception

Pregnancy following endometrial ablation has been reported (0.7%). It is advisable to use some form of contraception following endometrial ablation (EA). Essure system may be inserted 3 months before and left for 3 months after the procedure. Simultaneous endometrial ablation and Essure sterilization is not recommended.

Pregnancy complications: Miscarriage, ectopic pregnancy, preterm birth, FGR, abnormal placentation, placenta accreta, uterine rupture, cesarean delivery and PPH.

Results of Various Endometrial Ablation Procedures

TCRE takes longer time, compared to rollerball ablation. Rollerball may be used alone or in combination with TCRE to treat the area of fundus and cornual regions. For the first-generation method, the overall development of amenorrhea varies between in 33% and 55% and need of hysterectomy was between 15% and 30%. For the second-generation methods, development of amenorrhea was 40–60% and the need of hysterectomy was 10–12%. Rates of failure and the need of re-operation are about 20%.

Fluid deficit of 1.5 liters warns to stop the procedure. **Use of saline as the distension media with bipolar resection equipment can reduce the problem.**

Complications of TCRE
Intraoperative/Postoperative complications
■ Fluid over load (Glycine overload)
■ Hemorrhage
■ Uterine perforation
■ Hyponatremia
■ Hyperammonemia
■ Congestive cardiac failure
■ Hemolysis
■ Coma
■ Cerebral edema
■ Death

Long-term postoperative complications	
■ Infection	■ Pregnancy-related complications are also there (discussed above)
■ Endometriosis	
■ Pyometra	■ **Post-ablation syndrome** may occur: pain during menstruation due to uterine scarring, synechiae formation, or hematometra formation. This may ultimately end in hysterectomy
■ Pelvic inflammatory disease (PID)	
■ Pelvic abscess	
■ Pyrexia	
■ Hematometra formation	

Surgical treatment for a woman with uterine fibroid principally includes myomectomy or hysterectomy. Uterine artery embolization (UAE) have also been done as an alternative. Myomectomy is the option for a woman where fertility needs to be preserved.

FIGO classification (Fig. 48.1) and **STEPW** (**s**ize, **t**opography, **e**xtension, **p**enetration and **w**all) classification (Lasmar, 2005) (Table 48.1) are helpful for planning treatment.

Myomectomy could be done

Abdominal Route
a. Open (laparotomy)
b. Laparoscopic
c. Laparoscopic-assisted robotic surgery.

Blood loss during myomectomy could be reduced significantly using GnRH analogs, vasopressors or using tourniquets. Ulipristal acetate can also reduce the size and vascularity of the myomas, morcellation procedures allow removal of a large tumor mass to be taken out through a 12 mm port, though dissemination of unsuspected malignancy during morcellation has been the concern. The European Society of Gynecological Endoscopy and American Association of Gynecologic Laparoscopists have given the guidelines based on the risk of malignancy that is 1:2000.

TABLE 48.1: Lasmar/STEPW fibroid classification.

	Size (cm)	Topography	Extension of the base	Penetration	Lateral wall	Total
0	<2	Low	<1/3	0	+1	
1	>2 to 5	Middle	1/3–2/3	<50%		
2	>5	Upper	>2/3	>50%		
Score	+	+	+	+	+	=

Score	Group	Complexity and therapeutic options
0–4	I	Low-complexity hysteroscopic myomectomy
5–6	II	High-complexity hysteroscopic myomectomy. Consider GnRH use. Consider two-step procedure
7–9	III	Consider alternatives to hysteroscopic techniques

(GnRH: gonadotropin-releasing hormone; STEPW: size, topography, extension, penetration and wall)

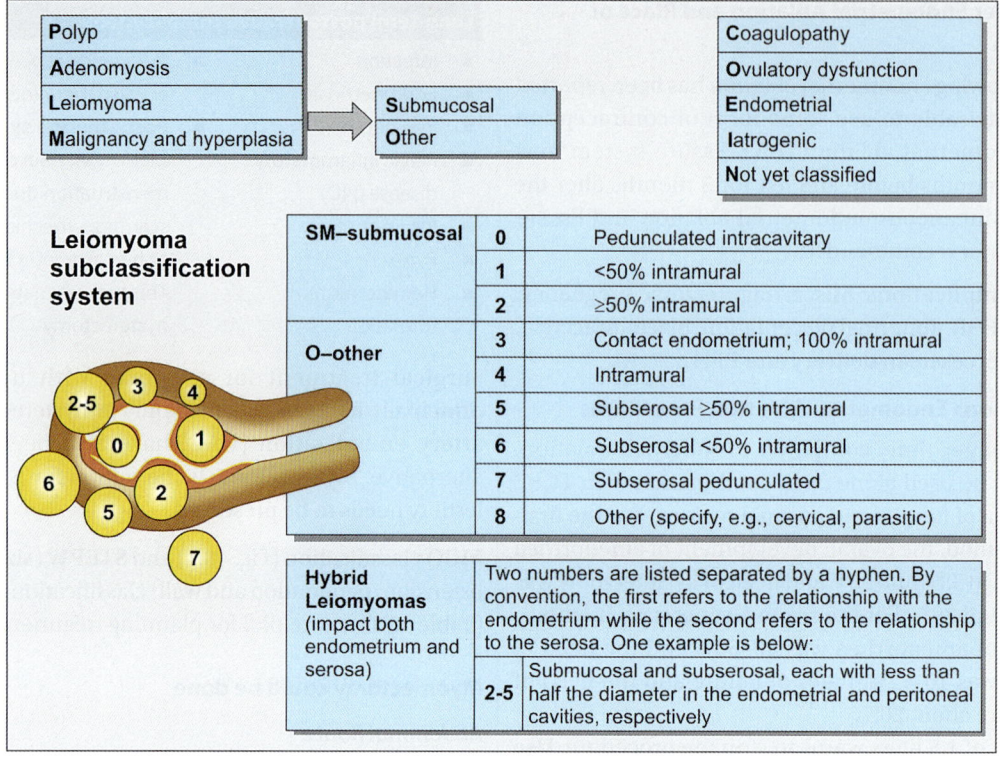

Fig. 48.1: Classification system including leiomyoma and the subclassification system.
Source: FIGO Classification System (PALM-COEIN), IJGO, 2011.

Morcellation is avoided in the following situations:
a. Postmenopausal women
b. Premenopausal women with larger and solitary lesions
c. Women with fibroids that do not respond to treatment with GnRH analogs.

Morcellation without dispersion of fragmented tissues can be done using intraperitoneal isolation bag (contained morcellation).

Hysteroscopic myomectomy: It is the choice of operation for the submucosal or the intracavitary myomas. Resectoscope is commonly used. Fibroids belonging to FIGO type 0, 1 and 2 are commonly resected out. However, one has to be careful against the perforation of the uterus. Intraoperative ultrasound can be useful to assess the wall thickness. Resection may be performed under laparoscopic guidance or by two-stage procedure at interval of 4–6 weeks. This is especially done in Lasmar group II or III tumors.

Hysterectomy: It is the common surgical procedure. Hysterectomy is the only definitive form of treatment for HMB.

Route of hysterectomy depends upon the pelvic or extrapelvic pathology, previous surgeries, associated comorbidities, the choice of the patient and the expertise of the surgeon.

Abdominal or vaginal hysterectomy are commonly done. **Nondescent vaginal hysterectomy** (NDVH) is popular and also being done. Results of NDVH are comparable to laparoscopic-assisted vaginal hysterectomy (LAVH). Laparoscopic hysterectomy is currently being done and it is categorized as:

a. **Laparoscopic-assisted vaginal hysterectomy** where the round ligaments and the infundibulopelvic ligaments are done laparoscopically and the rest of the procedure is done vaginally.
b. **Laparoscopic hysterectomy:** All the steps up to the ligation of the uterine vessels, removal of the cervix are done laparoscopically. Colpotomy cup is used to complete the surgery. Colpotomy cup is placed in the vaginal fornix. This helps the dissection of the Mackenrodt's ligament and to displace the ureters laterally. This colpotomy cup allows maintenance of the uterosacral ligaments attached to the vaginal vault. This prevents vault prolapse, at the end of the procedure the uterus is delivered through the vagina. The vaginal vault is closed laparoscopically.

CHAPTER 48: Surgical Management of Heavy Menstrual Bleeding

c. **Laparoscopic-assisted supracervical hysterectomy**:

A. Outline of the surgical procedures	B. Advantages
i. Vagina is not opened	i. Procedure is simple.
ii. Less risk of infection	ii. Patient may be discharged by 24 hours.
iii. No dissection of the uterosacral complex	iii. She can resume her activities by 2 weeks.
iv. No dissection of bladder is needed	iv. Complications are less.
v. Uterine arteries are ligated	
vi. Uterus is removed making colpotomy incision through the vagina or by morcellation	

d. **Robot-assisted hysterectomy**: Robot-assisted procedures have the following advantages:
   i. 3D vision
   ii. Intuitive movements
   iii. Allows complex maneuvers (with seven degrees of hand movements)
   iv. High accuracy
   v. No or less surgeon fatigue
   vi. Learning curve is easy compared to laparoscopy.

Disadvantages are: (a) No haptic feedback; (b) expensive.

Hysterectomy is the only definitive management procedure for cure of HMB. Patient's satisfaction is higher (90%) with hysterectomy compared with endometrial ablation procedures.

Suggested Reading

1. Clark TJ, Samuels N, Malick S, et al. Bipolar radiofrequency compared with thermal balloon endometrial ablation in the office: a randomized controlled trial. Obstet Gynecol 2011; 117:1228.
2. Cooper KG, Parkin DE, Garratt AM, et al. A randomised comparison of medical and hysteroscopic management in women consulting a gynaecologist for treatment of heavy menstrual loss. Br J Obstet Gynaecol. 1997;104:1360-6.
3. Daniels JP, Middleton LJ, Champaneria R, et al. Second generation endometrial ablation techniques for heavy menstrual bleeding: network meta-analysis. BMJ 2012;344:e2564.
4. Daniels JP. The long-term outcomes of endometrial ablation in the treatment of heavy menstrual bleeding. Curr Opin Obstet Gynecol. 2013;25:320-6.
5. Jack SA, Cooper KG, Seymour J, et al. A randomised controlled trial of microwave endometrial ablation without endometrial preparation in the outpatient setting: patient acceptability, treatment outcome and costs. BJOG. 2005;112:1109-16.
6. Lasmar RB, Barrozo PR, Dias R, Oliveira MA. Submucous myomas: a new presurgical classification to evaluate the viability of hysteroscopic surgical treatment—preliminary report. J Minim Invasive Gynecol. 2005;12:308-11.
7. Lethaby A, Shepperd S, Cooke I, et al. Endometrial resection and ablation versus hysterectomy for heavy menstrual bleeding. Cochrane Database Syst Rev. 2000;(2):CD000329.
8. Munro MG, Critchley HO, Broder MS, et al. FIGO Working Group on Menstrual Disorders. FIGO classification system (PALM-COEIN) for causes of abnormal uterine bleeding in nongravid women of reproductive age. Int J Gynaecol Obstet. 2011;113:3-13.
9. National Institute for Health and Care Excellence. Heavy Menstrual Bleeding. CG44. London: NICE; 2007.
10. Pritts EA, Vanness DJ, Berek JS, et al. The prevalence of occult leiomyosarcoma at surgery for presumed uterine fibroids: a meta-analysis. Gynecol Surg. 2015;12:165-77.
11. Roberts TE, Tsourapas A, Middleton LJ, et al. Hysterectomy, endometrial ablation, and levonorgestrel releasing intrauterine system (Mirena) for treatment of heavy menstrual bleeding: cost effectiveness analysis. BMJ. 2011;342:d2202.

Chapter 49: Surgical Site Infection

Postoperative surgical site infections (SSIs) are the important cause of patient mortality and prolonged hospital stay. This increases hospital cost. Some patients have increased risk factors for SSI.

SSI is defined as an infection of the superficial or deep skin tissues of an organ or space, occurring up to 30 days after surgery (if no implant was left behind) or within a year if an implant was left in place.

TABLE 49.1: Risk factors for surgical site infection (SSI).

- Intraoperative contamination
- Malnutrition
- Pre-existing anemia
- Older age
- Excess operative blood loss > 1500 mL
- Prolonged operative time (> 3.5 hours)
- Placement of foreign body (drain, catheter)
- Obesity
- Smoking
- Prior chemotherapy
- Prior radiation
- Prior operations
- Immunocompromised individual
- Preoperative HbA1C >7% or
- Capillary blood glucose >200 mg/dL
- Presence of systemic disease

In obstetrics:
- Rupture of membranes
  - Prolonged
  - Premature
- Chorioamnionitis
- Prolonged labor
- Prolonged surgery
- Repeated vaginal examinations
- Emergency operations
- Non-use of antibiotic prophylaxis

CLINICAL ISSUES AND PREVENTION OF SSI (MODIFIABLE OR NON-MODIFIABLE FACTORS)

Patient factors associated with SSI are discussed in Table 48.1. **Risk factors may be modifiable or non-modifiable.** Modifiable risk factors could be improved with lifestyle changes. These are: controlling the glycemic status (diabetes), cessation of smoking, improvement of anemia, improvement of other associated comorbid conditions (obesity).

Preoperative factors: Patients, who are the positive carriers of Methicillin-resistant *Staphylococcus aureus* (MRSA) from anterior nares, are with increased risk of SSI. These patients need decolonization of the bacteria using mupirocin (NICE). To reduce SSI, screening for MRSA status and decontamination of women, is needed before operation.

There are several recommendations (NICE, ACOG, ACS, CDC, SIS, WHO) for prevention of SSI.

Use of prophylactic antibiotics: Single dose of a broad spectrum antibiotic recommended within 120 minutes of incision (WHO). Otherwise prophylactic antibiotic may be started IV with the start of anesthesia (NICE). For carriers of MRSA, screening and prophylaxis has been recommended. Nasal mupirocin 2% ointment in combination with chlorhexidine body wash before surgery reduces the risk of SSI.

	Common microbials involved in SSI in obstetrics and gynecology		
	Gram-positive aerobes	**Gram-negative aerobes**	**Anaerobes**
	Staphylococcus aureus	Klebsiella spp	Clostridium (Clostridioides) spp
	Enterococcus spp	Escherichia coli	Gardnerella vaginalis
	Group β hemolytic streptococcus	Pseudomonas aeruginosa	Fusobacterium spp
	Staphylococcus pyogenes	Proteus spp	Bacteroides fragilis
	Staphylococcus epidermidis	Klebsiella spp	Peptostreptococcus spp
	Methicillin-resistant Staphylococcus aureus		Prevotella spp

Skin preparation: Presence of skin microflora increases the risk of contamination of the surgical site. This increases the risk of SSI. Alcohol or aqueous based solution of chlorhexidine can be used to reduce SSI. Alcohol or aqueous based solution of povidone iodine can be used when use of chlorhexidine is contraindicated.

Preoperative skin wash: Full body shower or bath with plain soap or antimicrobial soap is recommended. It should be done on the day before or on the day of surgery.

Vaginal cleansing: It is not mandatory, though vagina harbors several micro-organisms. It may be done in a selected case before hysterectomy or any vaginal surgery. Vaginal cleansing with chlorhexidine (4%) or povidone iodine may be done (ACOG).

Hair removal: It is needed routinely. Shaving is not recommended. Hair clipping to be done when needed. Razors should not be used.

Skin closure: Usual methods are to be followed. Skin suturing is preferred compared to use of staples.

Subcutaneous tissue closure: It reduces the risk of hematoma or seroma formation and also wound separation. This is recommended when subcutaneous fat is < 2 cm deep.

Gloves: Gloves to be worn to reduce SSI. Double gloving protects the surgeon as it reduces the risk of needle-stick injury.

Hand washing: Use of chlorhexidine or povidone iodine for hand washing reduces the load of skin flora. This reduces the risk of SSI. Surgical team members should wash their hands with antiseptic solution and single use nail brush before the first operation. Hand scrubbing should be done for a minimum of 3 minutes.

Surgical drapes: There is no difference in the incidence of SSI whether reusable or disposable drapes are used.

Steps of cesarean section: Standard principles of surgery and hemostasis are sufficient to reduce the SSI. Uterine closure either in one or two layers, nonclosure of visceral and parietal peritoneum have not shown to influence the rate of SSI.

- **Operative:** Patient homeostasis during surgery to maintain
  ♦ To maintain body temperature (NICE-2008)
  ♦ Maintain optimum oxygenation
  ♦ Optimum oxygenation during major surgery and in the recovery period
  ♦ Hemoglobin oxygen saturation to be maintained ≥ 95%
  ♦ Preoperative glycemic control (110-159) mg/dL (6.1-8.8 mmol/L) is ideal.

Use of drain: It reduces intra-abdominal collection. Its use is helpful to reduce SSI and postoperative morbidity in a selected cases. However drain can cause complications (trauma, sepsis) also.

Negative pressure wound therapy: It is used in a sealed wound dressing attached to pump. It creates a negative pressure environment (80-125 mm Hg). It stimulates development of granulation tissue, improves blood flow, reduces wound edema, improves wound circulation and prevents wound contamination. It may be used in high-risk women in primarily closed surgical incision.

Postoperative factors: Postoperative wound care with removing and changing the dressings to be done after 48 hours. Wound cleaning should be done with sterile saline. Patient may have shower safely 48 hours after surgery. Using antibiotics for a prolonged period in the postoperative period does not reduce SSI. Moreover it may result in development of antibiotic resistance. Perioperative antibiotics, good glycemic control and early mobilization are more useful for the enhanced recovery after surgery (ERAS).

Commonly used prophylactic antobiotics in obstetrics and gynecological surgery		
Indication	**Antibiotics**	**Comments**
Cesarean section	IV cefazolin cefazolin 2 g or cefuroxime 1.5 g + metronidazole 500 mg	Patient allergic to penicillin: clindamycin 400 mg IV + gentamycin 5 mg/kg
Abdominal hysterectomy	IV cefazolin 2 g or cefuroxime 1.5 g + metronidazole 500 mg or co-amoxiclav 1.2 g	Patient allergic to penicillin: clindamycin 400 mg IV + gentamycin 5 mg/kg
Vaginal hysterectomy	IV cefazolin 2 g or cefuroxime 1.5 g + metronidazole 500 mg or co-amoxiclav 1.2 g	Patient allergic to penicillin: clindamycin 400 mg IV + gentamycin 5 mg/kg
Perineal procedures (CPT, vaginal lacerations)	IV cefuroxime 1.5 g + metronidazole 500 mg or co-amoxiclav 1.2 g, followed by oral co-amoxiclav 625 mg 8-hourly for 5 days	Patient allergic to penicillin: gentamycin 5 mg/kg + metronidazole 500 mg, followed by oral clindamycin 300–460 mg 6-hourly for 5 days
MRSA-positive patients	IV teicoplanin 400 mg IV + gentamycin 5 mg/kg	

(IV: intravenous; MRSA: methicillin-resistant *Staphylococcus aureus*)
Source: Committee Opinion: ACOG-2015.

Classification of Surgical Site Infection (CDC, ACS, NSQIP-2011)

A. *Superficial incisional*
   ♦ Involves superficial tissues only
   ♦ Develops within 30 days of operation
   ♦ Clinical features
      • Purulent discharge with positive bacteria in culture
      • Pain, tenderness, redness or localized swelling
   ♦ **Diagnosis:** Made by a surgeon or a physician.

B. *Deep incisional*
- Involve abdominal wall muscles and fascia
- Develops within 30 days of operation
- Clinical features
  - Purulent discharge from deep tissues, not from organ/space component
  - Temperature ≥38°C, localized pain, tenderness
  - Detection of abscess by reoperation or radiology.

C. *Organ/space involvement*
- Develops within 30 days of operation
- Detection of abscess or infection involving the organ or space by direct examination, during re-operation, radiologically or on histology
- Bacteria recovered from the fluid/tissue in that organ/space
- Purulent discharge through drain/stab wound from the organ/space.

Classification of a wound

- **Clean wound:** Wound is in sterile condition where no organism, no inflammation present. During surgery no respiratory, alimentary or genitourinary tracts are entered.
- **Clean contaminated wound:** A wound made in sterile condition, but in which the respiratory, alimentary or genitourinary tracts is entered under controlled condition and no contamination observed.
- **Contaminated wound:** Any wound, in which there is a major break in sterile technique, or gross spillage from the GI tract, or in which acute and non-purulent inflammation is encountered or an open wound that is more than 12 to 24 hours old.
- **Dirty or infected wound:** Wounds with devitalized tissues with organisms pre-existing in the field before surgery.

Interventions for Preventions of Surgical Site Infection (SSI)

Summary of Management

A. **Preoperative**
- To reduce HbA1c levels to <7% before operation
- Improvement of nutritional status and level of hemoglobin
- To control any preoperative infections (respiratory/urinary tract).

B. **Perioperative**
- Removal/clipping of hair
- Thorough antiseptic scrub of hands, forearms of the surgical team members
- Preparation of the skin around the operative site with antiseptic agents (povidone iodine/chlorhexidine)
- Use of prophylactic antibiotics.

C. **Intraoperative**
- To reduce dead space
- To follow standard principles of asepsis
- Use of surgical drains (selective)
- Use of antibiotics (prophylactic/therapeutic as needed)
- To maintain intraoperative normothermia.

D. **Postoperative**
- To maintain plasma glucose < 200 mg/dL on postoperative day-1 or day-2
- To monitor wound healing and early detection of SSI.

MANAGEMENT OF SURGICAL SITE INFECTIONS

Common modes of presentation for a patient with SSI are: fever (>38°C), wound discharge (purulent or seropurulent), signs of inflammation (erythema, tenderness, induration) at the site of incision. Examination of the wound should be done. Sutures should removed, drainage of pus, seroma to be done. Swabs are to be taken from the wound. Investigations are to be organized.

Investigations for a patient with SSI
- Complete blood count, blood cultures, CRP
- Urine: Routine, microscopic, culture and sensitivity
- Plasma glucose and HbA1C
- Imaging studies (USG): to exclude any intra-abdominal collection
- CT—when USG is inconclusive

- **Antibiotic regimens:** Broad spectrum (covering: aerobics and anaerobics) to start with. It may be changed based on the culture report.

Common sites of wound infections following surgery [(a) cesarean section, (b) hysterectomy] **are:** • Abdominal wound, • Vaginal cuff cellulitis, • Pelvic cellulitis and • Pelvic abscess.

Necrotizing fasciitis (*See* Clinics in Obstetrics, Section 2, Ch 15): It is a rare variety of SSI. Overall incidences is 1.8-2 in 1000 cases following cesarean delivery. It is a polymicrobial infection (aerobic and anaerobic).

The first line antibiotics may be combination of: amoxycillin and clavulanic acid or cephalosporin and metronidazole. This combination is preferred to cover *S. aureus* and the anaerobes. Clindamycin or vancomycin can be given as an alternative. Patients not responding by 24–48 hours with this therapy, may be considered for gentamicin in addition, (provided the renal function is normal).

In spite of this, there may be failure of response to commonly used antibiotics. The wound induration is more. There is presence of gas within the tissues. Wound crepitus may be felt on clinical examination. Imaging studies CT may reveal gas in the soft tissues. This condition is rapidly progressive. In such situations, the antibiotics that should be used are: Penicillin G, aminoglycoside and clindamycin to cover the wide bacterial range (gram-positive, gram-negative and the anaerobes). Surgical debridement of the wound to be done.

Suggested Reading

1. Ban KA, Minei JP, Laronga C, Harbrecht BG, Jensen EH, Fry DE, et al. American College of Surgeons and Surgical Infection Society: Surgical Site Infection Guidelines, 2016. Update J Am Coll Surg. 2017;224(1):59–74.
2. Haas DM, Morgan S, Contreras K, Enders S. Vaginal preparation with antiseptic solution before cesarean section for preventing postoperative infections. Cochrane Database Syst Rev. 2018;7(7):CD007892.
3. Kurz A, Sessler DI, Lenhardt R. Perioperative normothermia to reduce the incidence of surgical-wound infection and shorten hospitalization. Study of wound infectioN ANd temperature group. N Engl J Med. 1996;334:1209-15.
4. Mangram AJ, Horan TC, Pearson ML, Silver LC, Jarvis WR. Guideline for prevention of surgical site infection, 1999. Hospital Infection Control Practices Advisory Committee. Infect Control Hosp Epidemiol. 1999;20(4):250-78.
5. National Collaborating Centre for Women's and Children's Health (UK) Surgical Site Infection: Prevention and Treatment of Surgical Site Infection RCOG Press; 2008.
6. National Institute For Health and Care Excellence (NICE). Surgical site infections: prevention and treatment. NICE guideline [NG 125]. London: NICE 2019. p. 1–28.
7. Rosenthal VD, Richtmann R, Singh S, Apisarnthanarak A, Kübler A, Viet-Hung N, et al. Surgical site infections, International Nosocomial Infection Control Consortium (INICC) report, data summary of 30 countries, 2005–2010; Infect Control Hosp Epidemiol. 2013;34(6):597–604.
8. Tanner J, Norrie P, Melen K. Preoperative hair removal to reduce surgical site infection. Cochrane Database Syst Rev. 2011;(11):CD004122.
9. World Health Organization (WHO). Antibiotics of choice for surgical antibiotic prophylaxis. Geneva: WHO; 2018. p. 1–28.

Chapter 50: Endoscopy in Gynecology (Laparoscopic Surgery)

Q. Energy source used for hemostasis in endoscopy surgery are:
a. Radiofrequency electricity is the most versatile method
b. Laser coagulation and cutting are the ideal one
c. Ultrasonic scalpel (harmonic) is the best
d. Stapling or knot tying is the better alternative.

Ans. a. T   b. F   c. F   d. F

- **Radiofrequency electricity:** It can be used either by monopolar or bipolar instrument. With optimum power settings tissues can be heated, desiccated and coagulated (Fig. 50.1). Ideally, the vessels should be compressed within the blades of a bipolar forceps and then the electrode is to be activated. This helps the vessel walls to seal by desiccation and coagulation when continuous low-voltage current is used (coaptive coagulation). *In a bipolar forceps, when tissues between the blades are completely desiccated, there is no flow of electricity. This can reduce the problem of lateral thermal spread*. Automated generators are available that can stop pulse energy automatically. Laser and radiofrequency electrical sources of energy convert electromagnetic energy to mechanical energy, which is then turned into thermal energy.

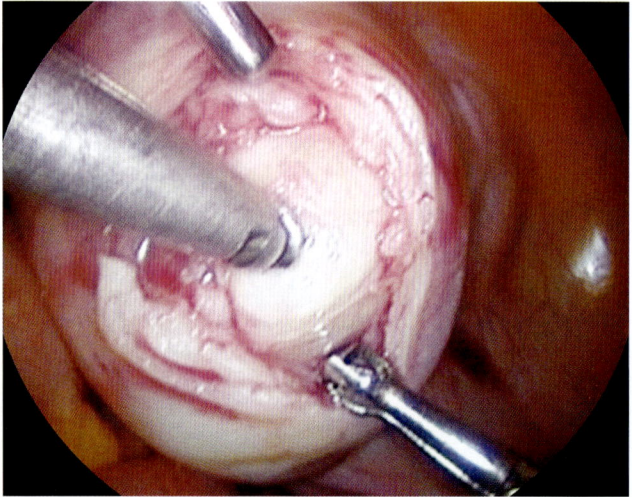

Fig. 50.1: Laparoscopic myomectomy. Enucleation of myoma is being done with a myoma screw.

High-current density energy, once delivered to tissues, the intracellular temperature rises >100°C and then intracellular water rapidly vaporizes. When this energy is *used in a linear fashion, tissue cutting effect is seen*. When radiofrequency energy with low-power density is used, effects such as desiccation and tissue coagulation are observed. **Monopolar** electrosurgical instruments with narrow ends generate high power density required to vaporize or cut tissues.

- **Laser energy:** It can be used to vaporize and cut tissues. KTP (potassium titanyl phosphate) and Nd:YAG lasers are used for cutting. CO_2 laser cannot be used effectively. KTP and Nd:YAG lasers, though much effective than CO_2 laser, have much higher risk of lateral thermal injury. Moreover, they are expensive.

- **Harmonic ultrasonic energy (harmonic scalpel):** It is a device used for coagulation and cutting of tissues. Electrical energy from the generator causes piezoelectric ceramics in the transducers (handpiece) to convert electrical energy into mechanical motion which is transferred to the blade extender. The ultrasonic wave is amplified as it travels down the blade tip, where it produces a maximum motion at 55,000 cycles/second. This results in simultaneous coagulation and cutting of tissues. No energy passes through the patient as opposed to that of electrosurgical instruments.

Tissue effects with harmonic ultrasonic
  - **Coaptation** involves transfer of mechanical energy to tissues. The internal mechanical friction breaks the hydrogen bonds and causes protein denaturation. A sticky coagulum is formed that seals the vessels at temperature <100°C.
  - **Cavitation** occurs when the blade vibrates (50–100 microns). The cell water is vaporized and subsequently the cells rupture. There is minimum lateral thermal injury.

  This device reduces the need of frequent instrument change, as it coagulates and cuts the tissues simultaneously.

- **Hemostatic clips** can be applied with a specially designed clip applicator. Clips are generally used for

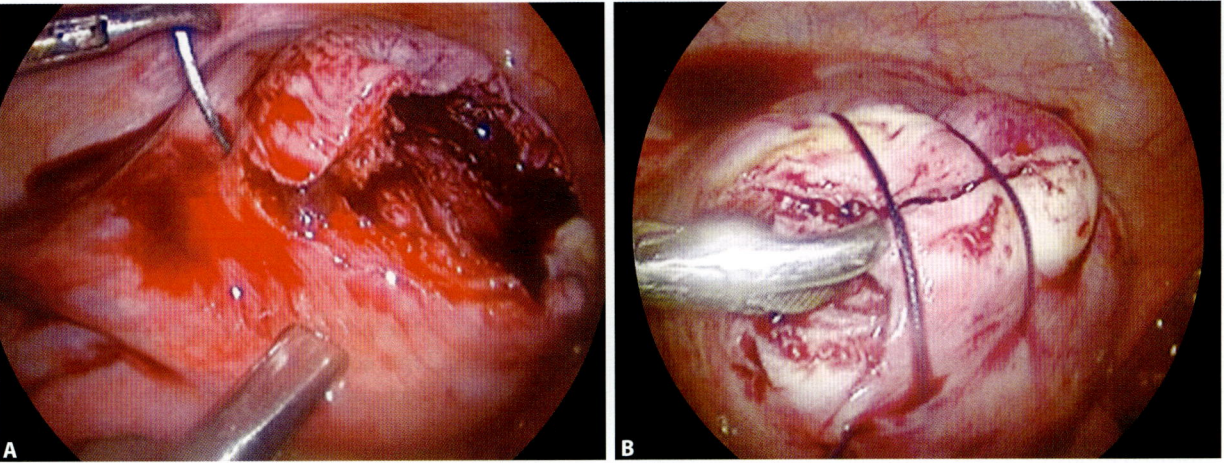

Figs. 50.2A and B: (A) Laparoscopic myomectomy; (B) Myoma bed is being sutured.
Courtesy: Dr P Kotdawala, Ahmedabad.

vessels of 4 mm diameter or more. It is of special benefit, when a large vessel close to an important structure (ureter) is to be ligated. Cost of stapling devices is high. Staplers cannot be used at all sites of bleeding, whereas electrodiathermy energy sources are of versatile use.

- ***Laparoscopic suturing:*** Intracorporeal suturing is done within the peritoneal cavity. This is similar to open surgery using the instruments. Extracorporeal knots are either (Figs. 50.2A and B) pre-tied (endoloops) or created outside and then pushed inside the peritoneal cavity by knot pusher.

A surgeon needs to develop the skills with a number of combination methods of hemostasis to be used as and when required. There is no evidence that one device is best and safe in comparison to others.

Suggested Reading

1. Herrmann A, De Wilde RL. Laparoscopic myomectomy—the gold standard. Gynecol Minim Invasive Ther. 2014;3(2):31–8.
2. La Chapelle CF, Bemelman WA, Bongers MY, et al. A multidisciplinary evidence-based guideline for minimally invasive surgery: part 2—laparoscopic port instruments, trocar site closure, and electrosurgical techniques. Gynecol Surg. 2013;10(1):11–23.
3. Lavazzo C, Mamais I, Gkegkes ID. Robotic assisted vs laparoscopic and/or open myomectomy: systematic review and meta-analysis of the clinical evidence. Arch Gynecol Obstet. 2016;294:5-17.
4. Lim CS, Mowers EL, Mahnert N, et al. Risk Factors and Outcomes for Conversion to Laparotomy of Laparoscopic Hysterectomy in Benign Gynecology. Obstet Gynecol. 2016;128:1295-305.
5. Payne TN, Dauterive FR, Pitter MC, et al. Robotically assisted hysterectomy in patients with large uteri: outcomes in five community practices. Obstet Gynecol. 2010;115:535-42.
6. Pellegrino A, Damiani GR, Trio C, et al. Robotic Shaving Technique in 25 Patients Affected by Deep Infiltrating Endometriosis of the Rectovaginal Space. J Minim Invasive Gynecol. 2015;22:1287-92.
7. Pluchino N, Litta P, Freschi L, et al. Comparison of the initial surgical experience with robotic and laparoscopic myomectomy. J Med Robot. 2014;10:208-12.

Chapter 51: Prevention of Urinary Tract Injuries in Gynecological Laparoscopic Surgery

Benefits of laparoscopic surgery in gynecology has been well established. The distinct advantages are:
- Shorter hospital stay
- Quicker recovery
- Improved exposure and visualization.

Majority of the gynecologic operation including gynecology oncology could be done with laparoscopy. As is known, complications may arise with laparoscopic surgery. Urinary tract injury is not uncommon in gynecological laparoscopic surgery. A gynecological surgeon must know the measures of prevention and management of such complications when they arise.

Q.1 What are the different laparoscopic surgeries done in gynecology?

Ans. Majority of the diagnostic and therapeutic procedures in the areas of general gynecology (fibroids, endometriosis), infertility (ovarian, tubal, uterine pathology), oncology (uterine, ovarian) and urogynecology are done by laparoscopy.

Q.2 What different sites of urinary tract injuries that may occur in gynecologic laparoscopy?

Ans.
i. Injury to bladder
ii. Injury to the ureter
iii. A combination of the both.

Q.3 What are the different pelvic pathologies that may cause urinary tract injures?

Ans.
1. **Pelvic endometriosis** (moderate-to-severe variety)
2. **Pelvic adhesions**—causing distorted pelvic anatomy.
   Patients with previous history of:
   a. Pelvic or lower abdominal surgery
   b. Pelvic inflammatory disease
   c. Radiation therapy
3. **Carcinoma of genital organs**
   a. Ovarian carcinoma
   b. Cervical carcinoma
   c. Colon carcinoma
4. **Obesity**
5. **Pelvic organ prolapse.**

Q.4 What is the prevalence of urinary tract injury in gynecologic surgery?

Ans. Overall incidence of bladder injury varies between 0.02% and 8.3%.

Q.5 What are the different types of urinary tract injuries that may occur during laparoscopic surgery?

Ans. During entry into the peritoneal cavity
1. **Direct trauma:**
   a. Injury to the bladder—during pneumoperitoneum with Veress needle
   b. Bladder injury with trocar and cannula through suprapubic port
2. **During surgery:**
   a. Ureteric injury during surgery, due to its proximity to the genital organs
   b. Injury due to electrodiathermy may occur to any of the organs.

Q.6 What are the common sites of ureteric injury in gynecologic laparoscopy?

Ans. Important anatomical locations where ureteric injury is more common are:
- At the level of infundibulopelvic ligament—where ureter runs parallel to ovarian vessels at the same place. Ureter forms the posterior boundary of ovarian fossa. Any inflammatory or malignant processes will involve the ureter.
- Deep in the pelvis, below the level of ischial spine, where ureter lies lateral to the peritoneum of uterosacral ligament.
- At the level of internal cervical os, 1.5 cm lateral to the cervix where uterine artery crosses the ureter from above.
- Over the anterior vaginal fornix, within the ureteric tunnel of cardinal ligament (tunnel of Wertheim) where it turns anteriorly and medially to enter the bladder.
- Where it traverses through the musculature of bladder (intravesical part).
- Any congenital malformation (duplex ureter) makes it more vulnerable to injury at any of these sites.

Q.7 What is the overall incidence of ureteric injury at gynecological laparoscopic surgery?

Ans. Over all incidence <1% to as high as 21% depending upon the pelvic pathology and the type of surgery (deep infiltrating endometriosis and laparoscopic hysterectomies).

Q.8 What are the common causes of urinary tract injury during laparoscopic surgery?

Ans: The common causes are due to electrothermal injury:
   a. Inadvertent tissue contact—with the ureter, bladder or the bowels
   b. Failure insulation of the instruments causing tissue contact and thermal injury
   c. Direct coupling: Spread of electrical current from one instrument to the other in contact. This causes spread of current to the other tissues and damage.
   d. Capacitive coupling.

Injuries are often not detected during the operations as such visceral injuries may occur beyond the surgeons view. Delayed tissue necrosis and break down occur. Manifestations are usually late.

Measures to prevent urinary tract injuries during laparoscopic surgery
- Thorough knowledge of pelvic anatomy in relation to uterus, cervix, ureter, bladder, urethra and the pelvic vessels are essential
- Thorough understanding of elctrosurgery
- Technique must be precise with correct tissue identification
- Insertion of secondary trocars must be under direct vision
- Bladder must be kept empty with a Foley's catheter during the entire period of surgery. Outlines of bladder may be delineated by filling the bladder with 200–300 mL of dye stained normal saline whenever in doubt
- Safety measures of electrosurgical use must be strictly followed

Safety measures of electrosurgical use
- The surgical field must be under direct vision and in the central field of the screen
- All instruments must be checked for insulation before use

Measures for prevention of injury due to laparoscopic electrosurgical energy sources (generators)
- Instruments must be properly insulated
- Optimum power setting for electrosurgical energy sources (generators)
- Use of bipolar electrosurgical equipments are preferred, whenever possible
- For monopolar equipments, use of low-voltage electrical waveform is preferred
- Intermittent and short activation of instruments are safer
- Activation of electrosurgical equipments should not be done when two instruments are in contact or in close proximity.
- Safety in the use of generators, instruments, insulation, inadvertent tissue contact and avoiding direct and capacitative coupling are essential
- The heel and tips of bipolar forceps are kept under direct vision when activated
- Seeing the catheter, the bag at the end of a procedure to detect any inadvertent injury to the bladder or ureter

Chapter 52: Management of Urinary Tract Injuries Following Laparoscopic Surgery

Identificaiton of Urinary Tract Injury with Laparoscopic Surgery

During Operation

- Intraoperative detection of any visceral injury (bladder, ureter) can reduce the morbidity to a large extent.
- The risk of litigation are also less. Simultaneous detection and repair may need the multidisciplinary team specialists (urologist, radiologist) involvement.

Bladder injury can be directly recognized by:

- Visualization or by seeing the urine leakage
- Noting hematuria and seeing the catheter and the balloon
- Intraoperative cystoscopy could be helpful where diagnosis is in doubt.

Instillation of about 200 mL of diluted normal saline solution of methylene blue or indigo carmine is done in to the bladder to identify the site and also the extent of injury. Cystoscopy examination is helpful to detect bladder injury when the site of injury in the retropubic space (space of Retzius) following a difficult suprapubic trocar insertion. Cystoscopic examination can also detect an injury at the trigone of the bladder. Bladder injury at the level of the trigone may increase the risk of the ureters. The laparoscope may also be introduced through the bladder rent to inspect the ureteral orifices over the trigonal area. Ureteric injury is not uncommon during pelvic surgery.

Measures to prevent ureteric injury during laparoscopic surgery

- Thorough knowledge of the anatomy of the ureter with its course
- To maintain the safe use of electrosurgical units
- Preoperative assessment of the course of the ureters in a case with: gross pelvic pathology [deep infiltrating endometriosis (DIE), pelvic adhesions] using IVU or MRI need to be done
- Inspecting the ureter during laparoscopic surgery with its peristalsis
- Electrosurgery to be avoided in close proximity of the ureter
- Ureterolysis can be performed preserving the blood supply within the adventitia
- Ureteric stenting (lighted stents, uriglow) can be helpful in cases with distorted pelvic anatomy (pelvic adhesions, deep infiltrating endometriosis)
- Illuminating ureteroscopy can be used to identify the location of the ureter
- Adequate dissection of the bladder from the uterus and cervix during laparoscopic hysterectomy will keep the bladder and ureter away from the uterine vessels

Types of ureteric injury

- Thermal (burn)
- Ligation
- Laceration
- Transection
- Resection
- Crushing
- Angulation (kinking)

Common sites of ureteric injuries

- At the brim of the pelvis where it forms the posterior boundary of the ovarian fossa
- At the base of the broad ligament, lateral to the cervix. Electrothermal injury is common at this level while coagulating the uterine artery
- Over the vaginal fornix, where the ureter turns medially to enter the bladder

Identificaiton of ureteric injury during laparoscopic pelvic surgery

- Laparoscopy is helpful to detect the transection of the ureter with leakage of urine
- Cystoscopic visualization of the ureteric orifices and to look for urine jets. Urine jets rule out, obstruction but not the other types of injury
- Presence of blood or air in the catheter or in the urine bag
- Indigo carmine given IV, color the urine turning to blue by 5–10 minutes. Subsequent cystoscopic and laparoscopic examination is helpful to detect the site of injury
- Insertion of a ureteric stent (cystoscopically) and inspecting the ureteric course laparoscopically is useful to detect any ureteric obstruction (hydronephrosis) or any injury. Ureteric stent can prevent kinking of the ureter
- Ureteroscopy is helpful to identify the site and extent of the injury
- Intravenous urography (IVU) is helpful to the diagnosis.

IDENTIFICATION OF URETERIC INJURY IN THE POSTOPERATIVE PERIOD

Clinical suspicion of injury is essential

Clinical presentation of the patient
- Delayed recovery in the postoperative period
- Pain and tenderness in the flank
- Hematuria
- Oliguria
- Vaginal discharge (watery)
- Formation of urinoma (formation of a cyst with urine in the retroperitoneal space)
- Features of sepsis
- Features of electrolyte imbalance

Cases with thermal injury to the ureter may result fistula formation, usually after 10–14 days. This is due to delayed ischemic necrosis of the ureter.

Ultrasonography, MRI or CT can evaluate presence of hydronephrosis, urinomas and abscess, CT intravenous urogram (CT-IVU) can locate site of injury. In cases where ureteral injury remains undetected, may resolve spontaneously. In about 25% of cases with unrecognized ureteral injuries result in eventual loss of the ipsilateral kidney.

Management of Urinary Tract Injuries Following Laparoscopic Gynecological Surgery

Management of ureteric injuries could be done by:
1. Laparotomy or
2. Laparoscopy.

A. **Cases for conservative management are:**
   i. Minimal crushing
   ii. Needle injury.
B. **Ureteral stenting**: Cases with ureteric obstruction, major crush injury, ligature injuries are managed with ureteral stenting for a period of 3–6 weeks.
C. **Cases with major ureteric injuries (transection, resection)**
   i. **Injury at the upper third of the ureter**: End-to-end anastomosis (ureteroureterostomy) is done.
   ii. **Injury at the middle third of the ureter** either a ureteroureterostomy or a transureteroureterostomy (end-to-side anastomosis of the injured ureter with the healthy ureter of the opposite side is done) (Fig. 52.1).
   iii. **Injury at the lower third of the ureter**: Ureteroneocystostomy (implantation of the ureter into the bladder) is done (Figs. 52.2 and 52.3A to C). To make the reimplantation tension free, a psoas hitch or a Boari flap can be made. In both these techniques, the bladder is mobilized to make the reimplantation tension free (Figs. 52.3A to C).

In **Boari method**, the dome of the bladder is cut into an oblique flap with a wide base. The flap is brought towards the ureter as a tunnel and the cystostomy is closed extending up to the ureter. In **psoas hitch method**, the bladder is fixed to the iliopsoas muscle tendon to make the implantation tension free.

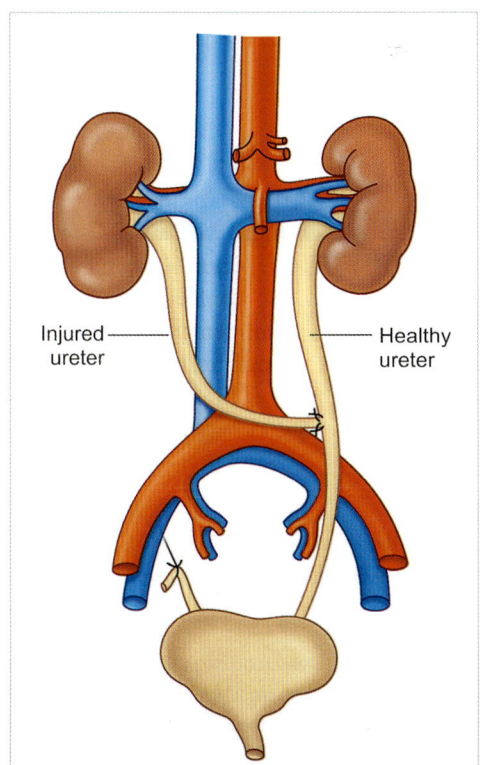

Fig. 52.1: Transureteroureterostomy is done in a case where the ureteric injury occurred in the middle-third of the ureter. Anastomosis has been done with the end of the injured ureter to the side of the healthy ureter (end-to-side anastomosis).

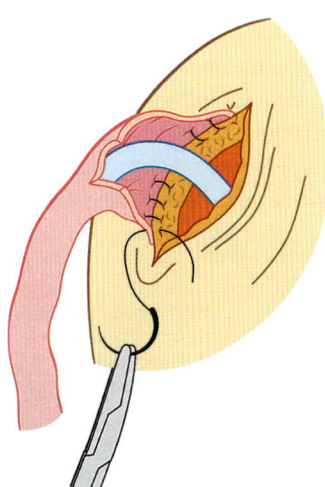

Fig. 52.2: Technique for ureteroneocystostomy. The distal ureter is spatulated for 1 cm. The bladder is opened (1–2 cm) on the posterolateral wall. A stent is introduced within the ureter and the anastomosis is completed over the stent. The bladder needs to be refilled to ensure watertight closure.

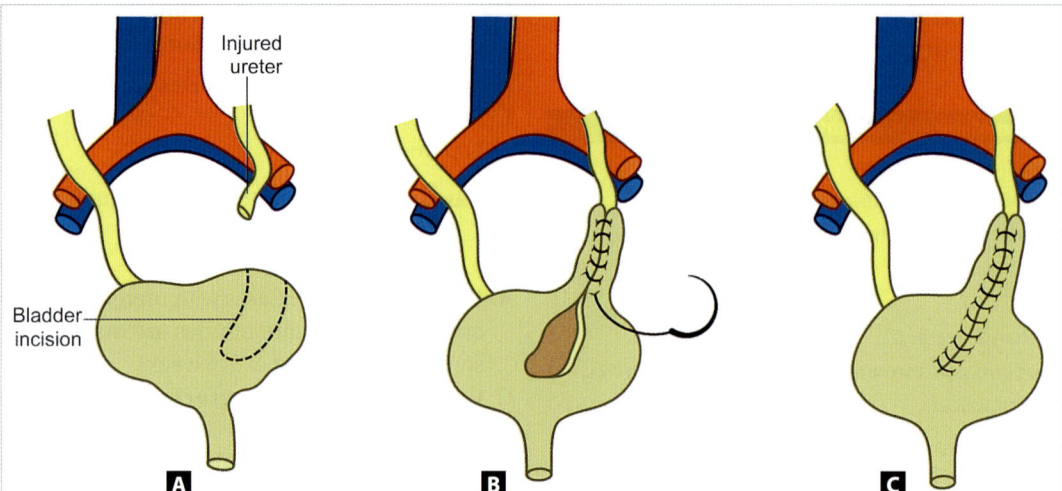

Figs. 52.3A to C: (A) Boari flap (Ureteroneocystostomy): Reimplantation of the ureter into the bladder is done. (A) Wide-based flap is made on the anterior bladder wall; (B) The flap is brought towards the injured ureter to make an anastomosis possible without any tension over the anastomotic site; (C) The bladder wall incision is closed. The tubular pattern of bladder wall closure allowed 10–12 cm of additional length of the ureter.

Principles of surgery for the management of ureteric injuries
- Careful and adequate dissection of ureter to be done and at the same time to avoid devascularization
- Ureteric mobilization may be needed for anastomosis
- Ureteric anastomosis should be:
    - Tension free
    - Watertight
    - Ureteric ends must be trimmed obliquely and spatulated
- Fine (delayed) absorbable sutures (vicryl : 4-0, 5-0) are used
- Interrupted sutures are used
- A suction catheter is placed retroperitoneally at the site of anastomosis
- Anastomosis is done over a double J stent
- Bladder catheter is used

Surgical methods of ureteric repair
- **Ureteric obstruction due to ligature**: Deligation and assessment of viability, stent placement
- **Partial transection**: Repair of the ureter over a ureteric stent
- **Thermal injury of the ureter:**
    Mild injury: Stenting for drainage of urine and to prevent stenosis
    Deep thermal injury: May need resection and reanastomosis
- **Transection**: Upper third—ureteroureterostomy over a ureteral stent
- **Resection**: Middle third—transureteroureterostomy (end-to-side anastomosis)
- **Lower third**: Ureteroneocystostomy

Suggested Reading
1. Alkatout I, Schollmeyer T, Hawaldar NA, Sharma N, Mettler L. Principles and safety measures of electrosurgery in laparoscopy. JSLS. 2012;16:130–9.
2. Bai SW, Huh EH, da Jung J, Park JH, Rha KH, Kim SK, Park KH. Urinary tract injuries during pelvic surgery: incidence rates and predisposing factors. Int Urogynecol J Pelvic Floor Dysfunct. 2006;17:360–4.
3. Gilmour DT, Baskett TF. Disability and litigation from urinary tract injuries at benign gynecologic surgery in Canada. Obstet Gynecol. 2005;105:109–14.
4. Ostrzenski A, Radolinski B, Ostrzenska KM. A review of laparoscopic ureteral injury in pelvic surgery. Obstet Gynecol Surv. 2003;58:794–9.
5. RCOG; 2008a [http://www.rcog.org.uk/files/rcog-corp/uploaded-files/GT49Preventing LaparoscopicInjury2008.pdf].
6. Royal College of Obstetricians and Gynaecologists. Preventing Entry-Related Gynaecological Laparoscopic Injuries. Greentop Guideline No. 49. London.
7. Shirk GJ, Johns A, Redwine DB. Complications of laparoscopic surgery: How to avoid them and how to repair them. J Minim Invasive Gynecol. 2006;13:352–9.

Chapter 53: Place of Prophylactic Salpingectomy or Salpingo-oophorectomy in Current Gynecologic Practice

TYPES OF OVARIAN CARCINOMAS

Nearly 80% of all ovarian cancers are epithelial in origin. Epithelial ovarian cancers (EOCs) are the important cause of death from gynecological malignancy. Of all the epithelial ovarian neoplasms the important subtypes are: (a) Serous: 68%, (b) Clear cell: 13%, (c) Endometroid: 9% and (d) Mucinous: 3%.

Serous adenocarcinomas are further divided into:
- Type 1 or low grade (LGSOC)
- Type 2 or high grade (HGSOC)

Most deaths are from HGSOC (20 times higher than LGSOC). The lifetime risk of developing EOC is 1 in 68 (1.4%) by 75 years of age. Of the several high-risk factors for EOC, the important ones are: (a) Advanced age and (b) Family history.

Q.1 What is the risk with family history of ovarian cancer?

Ans. Nearly 5–10% of all ovarian cancers are associated with inherited genetic abnormality. Mutation in BRCA1, BRCA2, genes (most common) and mutations in mismatch repair genes (MLH1, MSH2 and MSH6) are associated. High rate (100%) of p53 mutations are associated with HGSOC.

The inherited ovarian cancers are commonly observed in young women. They are often bilateral and are high grade serous in type.

Q.2 What is the current concept in the pathogenesis ovarian carcinoma?

Ans. Nonuterine pelvic high grade serous carcinomas are currently considered as secondary to distal fallopian tube carcinomas. Other supportive hypotheses for ovarian carcinogenesis are:
- ***Incessant ovulation theory (Fatallah-1971):*** Repeated ovulatory trauma to the ovarian surface epithelium is a promoting factor causing error in cell replication. Women having repeated ovulations (ovulation inductions) with gonadotropins (gonadotropin hypothesis) are at increased risk of EOC. On the other hand women with COCs (suppression of ovulation) are at lower risk.
- ***Hormonal hypothesis:*** Excess estrogen stimulation of ovarian surface epithelium increases the risk, whereas progesterone stimulation is protective to ovarian carcinogenesis.
- Distal tubal intraepithelial carcinoma (DTIC) as the origin (see below).

Q.3 How the high grade serous ovarian cancers are etiologically related to distal tubal intraepithelial carcinoma (TIC)?

Ans. Currently, there are several evidences to support that distal fallopian tube is the primary site of HGSOC. The possibility is that fallopian tube is involved early in the disease process of the HGSOCs.
- Adult epithelial stem cells are essential for cell repair through clonal growth of cells and self-renewal. These process make the cells susceptible to DNA damage and subsequent development of cancers.
- The amount of such stem like epithelial cells are almost double in the distal fallopian tube compared to the proximal end of the tube. With this, the distal fallopian tube initiates the neoplastic transformation. Locally elevated levels of inflammatory cytokines in the distal fallopian tube also promote the process of malignant transformation.
- However presence of coexisting intraepithelial carcinoma is a prerequisite for the diagnosis of primary tubal carcinoma.
- Incorporation of Müllerian epithelium into the ovary.

The mechanisms of incorporation of Müllerian epithelium into the ovary:
- Exfoliation of tubal mucosal cells over the ovarian surface results in formation of endosalpingiosis, cortical inclusions or endometriosis. This may occur with formation of adhesions/contact of the tube with the ovary.
- Müllerian cells undergoing metaplastic change over the ovarian surface epithelium.
- Molecular abnormality is the other pathway of ovarian carcinogenesis. At the molecular level, different mutations are observed for both the cases of LGSOC and HGSOC. Important one are: BRCA1, BRCA2, KRAS, BRAF, HER2 and p53.

TABLE 53.1: Difference between high grade serous ovarian cancers (HGSOC) and low grade serous ovarian cancers (LGSOC).

LGSOC	HGSOC
■ Associated gene mutations of KRAS or BRAF are observed in about 75% of cases ■ HER2 mutations are also observed ■ There is no mutation with p53 gene	■ Extremely high rate of p53 mutations (almost 100%) ■ BRCA mutations (BRCA1 and BRCA2) ■ Absence of KRAS, BRAF or HER2 mutations

- The incorporated cells on the ovarian surface, may give rise to neoplastic changes. The common tumors are serous tumors (either benign, borderline, low grade serous adenocarcinomas, endometrioid or clear cell tumors). Development of high grade serous ovarian cancers are rare with the mechanism of surface implantation.

There may be malignant transformation of the distal tubal mucosa through p53 mutations (p53 signatures). This may be the other pathway in the development of tubal intraepithelial carcinoma (TIC) lesions. These TIC cells may spread locally in the tubal wall, exfoliate on the surface of the ovary, in the peritoneal cavity (peritoneal serous adenocarcinoma) or there may be a combination of these. Based on these evidences the association of the fallopian tube and HGSOC are considered as indisputable.

Q.4 How high grade serous ovarian cancers (HGSOC) differ from that of low grade serous ovarian cancers (LGSOC)?

Ans. These two cancers (HGSOC and LGSOC) differ at molecular level also besides their response to therapy and in terms of five-year survival rate (Table 53.1).

Intense over expression of p53 is known as ***p53 signatures***. Serous tubal intraepithelial carcinoma (STIC) lesions are the precursors of HGSOC. There has been a link between STIC and HGSOC.

There is a significant impact in clinical outcomes and response to chemotherapy in this group of HGSOC. HGSOC are a separate histological subgroup based on molecular pathology. The overall 5-year survival rate of ovarian carcinoma is 43%.

Q.5 How the risk of ovarian carcinoma be reduced?

Ans. High risk women having BRCA mutation:
- Bilateral salpingo-oophorectomy provides the maximum reduction of risk for ovarian carcinoma (100%).
- It also reduces the risk of breast carcinoma (50%).
- Bilateral salpingectomy with delayed oophorectomy may be an alternative cost-effective strategy for women with BRCA mutation carriers.
- Ongoing epidemiological studies are likely to add strength to the current transitional research evidence to and change surgical practice.

Prophylactic (opportunistic) bilateral salpingectomy in low-risk women (without BRCA mutation) who have completed their families, should be carefully considered with conservation of ovaries at the time of gynecological surgery. This gives the benefit of risk reduction in one hand and at the same time it protects the woman from the disadvantages of surgical menopause.

Q.6 What is the current evidence in this field?

Ans. Evidence in human subjects are lacking. Trials in mice it is positive. But arguments is, 'if we wait until we have evidence before we offer the operation then, we will never generate evidence'.

Suggested Reading

1. Crump CP, Drapkin R, Miron A, et al. The distal fallopian tube: a new model for pelvic serous carcinogenesis. Curr Opin Obestet Gynecol. 2007;19:3-9.
2. Karst AM, Drapkin R. Ovarian cancer pathogenesis: a model in evolution. J Oncol. 2010:932371.
3. Liu J, Cristea MC, Frankel P, et al. Clinical characteristics and outcomes of BRCA-associated ovarian cancer: genotype and survival. Cancer Genet. 2012;205:34-41.
4. Narod SA. Salpingectomy to prevent Ovarian Cancer. A concurrent series. Curr Oncol. 2013;20:145-7.
5. National Cancer Institute. Surveillance, Epidemiology, and End Results Program (SEER) Stat Fact Sheets: Ovary Cancer. [online] Available from [http://seer.cancer.gov/statfacts/html/ovary.html]. [Accessed June, 2016].
6. Royal Australian and New Zealand. College of Obstetricians and Gynecologists. Managing the adnexae at the time of hysterectomy for benign gynecological disease. College Statement C-Gyn 25. Melbourne, Australia: RANZCOG; 2012.
7. Seidman JD, Sherman ME, Bell KA, et al. Salpingitis, salpingoliths, and serous tumors of the ovaries: Is there a connection? Int J Gynecol Pathol. 2002;21(2):101-7.
8. Society of Gynecologic Oncology (2013). SGO Clinical Practice Statement: Salpingectomy for Ovarian Cancer Prevention. Chicago: SCOG. [online] Available from [https://www.sgo.org/clinicalpractice/guidelines/sgo-clinical-practice-statement-salpingectomy-for-ovarian-cancerprevention] [Accessed June, 2016].

Chapter 54: Surgical Management of Polycystic Ovarian Disease

Polycystic ovarian syndrome (PCOS) is a common endocrine disorder affecting 8–10% of women of reproductive age, 2018 ESHRE/ASRM (Rotterdam) criteria, PCOS is defined as a syndrome of ovarian dysfunction along with the cardinal features of hyperandrogenemia and polycystic ovary morphology. It is the most common cause of anovulatory infertility (75%). PCOS is associated with menstrual abnormality (oligomenorrhea and amenorrhea, irregular bleeding). There is significant metabolic abnormality. Insulin resistance and compensatory hyperinsulinemia, dyslipidemia are common.

The most commonly performed ovarian surgery is **laparoscopic ovarian diathermy** (LOD). LOD is considered as a surgical method of indication for ovulation induction in cases where medical method [aromatase inhibitors/clomifene citrate (CC)] has failed. Clomifene-resistant cases where there is failure of ovulation even on incremental doses, (50–150 mg) of CC therapy, are also considered for LOD. The CC is commonly used as the first-line therapy for ovulation induction, in cases with PCOS. However, LOD could be used as the first-line therapy for ovulation induction in this group of women where there is other indications for laparoscopy. Advantages and disadvantages of LOD compared with follicle stimulating hormone (FSH) are shown in Table 54.1.

TABLE 54.1: Surgical versus medical therapy in cases with PCOS.

Advantages	Disadvantages
- Results are comparable to gonadotropin therapy - Avoids the complexity of monitoring as needed during gonadotropin therapy - Single treatment may result in repeated ovulatory cycles and has the benefit of successive pregnancies - Avoids the risks of OHSS - Risks of multiple pregnancies are less	- This is a surgical procedure and is done under general anesthetic - Risks of adhesion formation - Risks of premature ovarian failure (rare) - Complications of surgery - The procedure is expensive

Q.1 What are the objectives of LOD?

Ans. The extent of thermal energy *to be used* and number of punctures to be made in each ovary are important to get the best results. This is also important to minimize the damage to the ovary. Most centers prefer four punctures per ovary at 30 W for 5 seconds per puncture. This is found to be the optimum number required to get the satisfactory result.

Important steps of LOD
- Three-puncture laparoscopy is done (one main port and the other two side ports).
- Ovarian ligament is grasped with a pair of atraumatic forceps.
- The ovary is lifted up away from the bowel.
- A specially designed monopolar electrodiathermy needle is used (Figs. 54.1A and B).
- The probe is applied at right angle to the antimesenteric surface of the ovary.
- The probe should be away from ovarian hilum and the fallopian tube.
- Power is adjusted to avoid damage to the ovary. It is set at 30 W (coagulating).
- The full length of the needle is pushed into the capsule to the depth of 6–8 mm.
- Electricity is activated for 5 seconds.
- Four punctures are usually made in each ovary.
- The ovary and the peritoneal cavity is irrigated with saline before releasing the ovarian ligaments.
- A crystalloid solution is instilled in the peritoneal cavity at the end of the procedure.

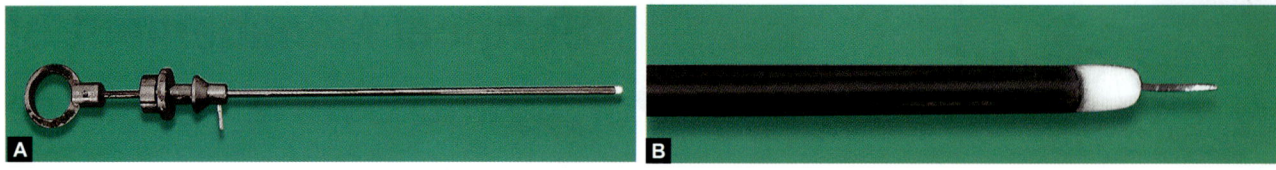

Figs. 54.1A and B: (A) LOD needle; (B) The pointed needle is seen when pushed out.

Q.2 How the LOD Works?

Ans. The mechanism of action of LOD is due to the damage of androgen-producing tissues in the ovary. There is decrease in circulating levels of androgens. There is also fall in the levels of androgenic follicular microenvironment. This helps in follicular growth and maturation. There is fall in estrogen levels also. This results in rise in serum FSH levels. This effect coupled with a decrease in local androgen concentrations, would convert the intrafollicular microenvironment from being androgen dominant to one that is estrogen dominant. This removes the intraovarian block to follicular maturation and allows follicular growth, maturation, and ultimately ovulation.

Q.3 What are the complications of laparoscopic ovarian surgery?

Ans. Intraoperative complications of LOD include bleeding from the ovary at the cautery points and thermal injury to the bowel and injury to the utero-ovarian ligament. Iatrogenic adhesion formation following the LOD may occur. Adhesion formation is usually prevented by reducing thermal injury to the ovarian surface and repeated irrigation of the ovaries. Crystalloid solution (normal saline) is used to irrigate the ovaries and the pelvis. Some amount (500 mL) of normal saline may be left in the peritoneal cavity at the end of the procedure. Iatrogenic development of premature ovarian insufficiency (failure) is another risk. This is possibly due to the excessive destruction of the normal ovarian tissues or due to inadvertent damage of the ovarian blood supply (rare). This risk can be largely reduced by minimizing the number of punctures made on the ovarian surface and by avoiding diathermy away from the ovarian hilum.

Q.4 Who are the women that respond poorly with LOD?

Ans.
a. Obese women (BMI> 35 kg/m²)
b. Hyperandrogenemia (testosterone > 4.5 nmol/L)
c. Free androgen index high (FAI >15)
d. Women with long history infertility (> 3 years)

Keypoints

- LOD is used for ovulation induction in women with PCOS when she is found CC resistant or CC failure.
- LOD is as effective as gonadotropins for successful ovulation induction and pregnancy. It has minimum risks of OHSS.
- Four punctures per ovary at 30 W for 5 seconds per puncture using a monopolar diathermy needle is optimum.
- About two-thirds of women ovulated after LOD and 50% conceive within 12 months.
- About one-third of the patients may get the benefit of LOD even after the next pregnancy.
- Postoperative adhesion formation can be minimized by avoiding thermal injury to the ovarian surface and by ample irrigation of the pelvis.
- Women with BMI > 35 kg/m² testosterone > 4.5 nmol/L, free androgen index (FAI) >15 and/or infertility for > 3 years are often resistant to LOD.

Suggested Reading

1. Armar NA, McGarrigle HH, Honour J, Holownia P, Jacobs HS, Lachelin GC. Laparoscopic ovarian diathermy in the management of anovulatory infertility in women with polycystic ovaries: endocrine changes and clinical outcome. Fertil Steril. 1990;53:45-9.
2. Asunción M, Calvo RM, San Millán JL, Sancho J, Avila S, Escobar-Morreale HF. A prospective study of the prevalence of the polycystic ovary syndrome in unselected Caucasian women from Spain. J Clin Endocrinol Metab. 2000;85:2434-8.
3. Felemban A, Tan SL, Tulandi T. Laparoscopic treatment of polycystic ovaries with insulated needle cautery—a reappraisal. Fertil Steril. 2000;73:266-9.
4. Gjonnaess H. Polycystic ovarian syndrome treated by ovarian electrocautery through the laparoscope. Fertil Steril. 1984;41: 20-5.
5. Hull MG. Epidemiology of infertility and polycystic ovarian disease: endocrinological and demographic studies: Gynecol Endocrinol. 1987;1:235-45.
6. Naether OG, Fischer R, Weise HC, Geiger-Kötzler L, Delfs T, Rudolf K. Laparoscopic electrocoagulation of the ovarian surface in infertile patients with polycystic ovarian disease. Fertil Steril. 1993;60: 88-94.
7. Rotterdam ESHRE/ASRM-sponsored PCOS Consensus Workshop Group. Revised 2003 consensus on diagnostic criteria and long-term health risks related to polycystic ovary syndrome. Fertil Steril. 2004;81(1):19-25.

Chapter 55: Bariatric Surgery in Gynecology and Obstetrics

Q.1 What is the relevance of this problem and the importance of pregnancy management for such patients?

Ans. Obesity is a growing problem in the developed world and also in many other countries including India. Obesity poses problems in achieving pregnancy, its successful continuation also causes problems in labor and puerperium. Operative interventions, weight reduction or bariatric surgery is becoming the common procedure to overcome this situation. Pregnancy following surgery may face nutritional and many surgical complications. These complications may affect the pregnancy outcome adversely. It is essential that obstetricians should be aware of these procedures, the need of counseling and management of women who undergo the bariatric surgery and conceive subsequently.

Q.2 What is the magnitude of the problem of obesity?

Ans. Most centers consider BMI = weight in kg/(height in meters) is equal 30 or more is obesity. With this cut off value the prevalence of obesity in US has been reported to range between 16% and 50%. Obesity is an epidemic in US as one study revealed 66% adults were either overweight or obese. Women, with a pregnancy BMI > 30 or a pregnancy weight more than 200 pounds, have been used to stratify risk during pregnancy. In India, exact data is difficult to quote, but the BMI values of > 25 and > 30 are considered overweight and obese, respectively. Overall prevalence of obesity in India is 16% (ICMR 2013–2014).

Q.3 Discuss the different complications of obesity in pregnancy.

Ans. See Clinics in Obstetrics, Section 2, Chapter 8.

Q.4 Discuss the different fetal and neonatal effects of obesity in pregnancy.

Ans. See Clinics in Obstetrics, Section 2, Chapter 8.

Q.5 Mention the different modes of management for obesity in pregnancy.

Ans.
- *Nonsurgical methods* are initially done. These includes—dietetic restriction, exercise, behavioral changes and pharmacotherapy. Patients with BMI < 40, are usually considered for nonsurgical method of management.
- *Surgical method (bariatric surgery):* Considered for women with BMI ≥ 40, woman with associated comorbidities (hypertension, ischemic heart disease) are considered for bariatric surgery even if BMI is < 40.

Bariatric surgery has been started since 1960s.

Q.6 How much is the success of bariatric surgery?

Ans. Bariatric surgery is a highly effective therapy especially for women with morbid obesity. Bariatric surgery significantly improves the obesity and the associated comorbidities. It improves the quality of life also.

Q.7 What is the principle of bariatric surgery in the management of obesity?

Ans. The objective is to reduce the body weight. It can be done in two ways:
1. Restriction and
2. A combined method of restrictive and malabsorptive operations.

Q.8 What is the type of operation commonly done these days?

Ans. The combined method is commonly done. It is the Roux-en-Y gastric bypass procedure. An adjustable gastric banding (restrictive) and Roux-en-Y gastric bypass (malabsorptive) is done.

The proximal stomach is separated from the remaining part of the stomach with staples. In banding procedure, a fluid-filled band is placed around the stomach close to the fundus. This reduces the volume of the functional stomach. These methods could be performed by laparoscopy or laparotomy. Many other techniques like biliopancreatic diversion (malabsorptive) or jejunoileal bypass (malabsorptive) were used.

Q.9 What is the place of bariatric surgery at present?

Ans. Presently increasing numbers of bariatric surgical procedures are performed in each year. The majority of the procedures are done in women (80%) of which about 50% are done for women of reproductive age (with the mean age of 40 years). Interestingly bariatric surgery is also being done in adolescents with morbid obesity.

Q.10 What is the effect of surgery on future fertility and obesity?

Ans. Bariatric surgery is most effective for morbid obesity and to improve the quality of life. There is significant improvement of reproductive behavior of women with obesity. Improvement of PCOS, hyperinsulinemia, hyperandrogenemia, obesity, irregular menses are there. Improvement of fertility is also observed. However, bariatric surgery should not be recommended as a treatment of infertility. Due to the effects of compromised absorption (malabsorptive surgery), the patient may develop nutritional deficiencies (vitamin and minerals).

Unintended pregnancies are high in these women as the absorption of combined oral contraceptive is low.

Q.11 What are the effects of surgery on health in their subsequent pregnancies?

Ans. Weight reduction either by medical or surgical method has got significant impact on women's health to improve the maternal comorbidities especially diabetes and hypertension and the quality of life. One systematic review of pregnancy after bariatric surgery described decreased rates of gestational diabetes and pre-eclampsia. However, late complications of bariatric surgery like intestinal obstruction, gastrointestinal hemorrhage, have been observed during pregnancy.

Q.12 What are the effects of bariatric surgery on perinatal outcome?

Ans. Bariatric surgery is not associated with increased perinatal death. Congenital abnormalities are not increased. Macrosomia (birth weight > 4 kg) was less. Babies of lower mean birth weights or small gestational age were observed, especially after Roux-en-Y gastric bypass.

Q.13 What should be contraceptive counseling in the patients following bariatric surgery?

Ans. Pregnancy rates following bariatric surgery are improved significantly. There is an increased risk of combined oral contraceptive failure after bariatric surgery. These women should therefore be counseled for nonoral administration of hormonal contraception. Woman is advised not to become pregnant within 12–24 months of bariatric surgery till the full weight loss is achieved. Woman needs closed monitoring as regard maternal weight gain, nutritional status and fetal growth.

Q.14 What is the concern for nutritional status during pregnancy in a woman who has undergone bariatric surgery?

Ans.
- The woman may suffer from nutritional deficiencies especially after malabsorptive surgery (Roux-en-Y gastric bypass).
- The common deficiencies are protein, iron, vitamin B_{12}, folate, vitamin D and calcium.
- The woman needs evaluation for these micronutrients at the start of pregnancy. Investigations including complete hemogram, serum ferritin, calcium and vitamin D at each trimester of pregnancy are to be done.
- Oral supplementation has to be continued. If there is no improvement based on laboratory data, parenteral route supplementation should be done. Consultation with a nutritionist should be done.
- Folic acid supplementation (0.4 mg/day) may be increased to prevent birth defects. Whereas vitamin A should be limited to 5,000 IU/day during pregnancy to reduce the risk of birth defects.
- Postpartum monitoring should also be continued especially for the women who are breastfeeding.
- Women having restrictive surgical procedures (adjustable gastric banding procedure) may be allowed more oral intake by adjusting the band (by removing the fluid from the band). This 'active band management' procedure is found to improve woman's nutritional status.

Q.15 What are the special care during the antenatal period for women who had undergone bariatric surgery?

Ans.
- Complications of bariatric surgery should be diagnosed early. These may be anastomotic leak, bowel obstructions band erosion, internal hernias, band migration and abdominal pain.
- Dumping syndrome can occur after gastric bypass procedures. It is due to fluid shifts from the intravascular compartment into the bowel lumen following ingestion of high glycemic carbohydrates.

Symptoms: Abdominal cramps, bloating, nausea, vomiting, diarrhea, hypoglycemia (due to hyperinsulinemia), tachycardia and palpitations. Women with dumping syndrome should avoid 50/75 g oral glucose screening test in pregnancy.
- The absorptive surface of the intestine is decreased. Extended release preparations are avoided instead oral solution and rapid release preparations are used. Drugs like NSAIDs are to be avoided to minimize gastric ulcerations.

Q.16 What special management issues are to be maintained during labor and delivery for women who underwent bariatric surgery?

Ans.
- Women that they remained obese even after bariatric surgery, should be managed similar to that of an obese women (*See* Clinics in Obstetrics, Ch 8).

- Cesarean delivery rates are higher after bariatric surgery (up to 62%). However, bariatric surgery itself should not be considered an indication for cesarean delivery. Otherwise, bariatric surgery itself should not alter the course of management during labor and delivery from a normal woman.

Suggested Reading

1. Colquitt J, Clegg A, Loveman E, et al. Surgery for morbid obesity. Cochrane Database Syst Rev. 2005;(4):CD003641.
2. Ehrenberg HM, Dierker L, Milluzzi C, et al. Prevalence of maternal obesity in an urban center. Am J Obstet Gynecol. 2002;187(5):1189-93.
3. Maggard MA, Yermilov I, Li Z, et al. Pregnancy and fertility following bariatric surgery: a systematic review. JAMA. 2008;300(19):2286-96.
4. National Center for Health Statistics. Health, United States, 2007 With Chartbook on Trends in the Health of Americans. Hyattsville; 2007.
5. Ogden CL, Carroll MD, Curtin LR, et al. Prevalence of overweight and obesity in the United States, 1999-2004. JAMA. 2006;295(13):1549-55.
6. Patel JA, Patel NA, Thomas RL, et al. Pregnancy outcomes after laparoscopic Roux-en-Y gastric bypass. Surg Obes Relat Dis. 2008;4(1):39-45.
7. Pradeepa R, Anjana RM, Joshi SR, et al. Prevalence of generalized & abdominal obesity in urban & rural India—the ICMR-INDIAB study (Phase-I) [ICMR-INDIAB-3]. Indian J Med Res. 2015;142(2):139-50.

56 Chapter — Robotic Surgery in Gynecology

Q. Robotic surgery:
  a. It is a facilitated laparoscopy having a computerized interface between patient and surgeon
  b. From technologic point of view, robotic and laparoscopic surgery are the same
  c. Robotic movements are intuitive
  d. Learning curve for robotic surgery is long
  e. Prior laparoscopic surgery skill is essential for robotic surgery

Ans. a. T   b. F
     c. T   d. F
     e. F

Robotic technology facilitates the laparoscopic surgery with the use of a computer interface. Robotic technology enhances surgeon's ability with superior accuracy, dexterity, performance (suturing), shorter working times and reduces the number of complications compared to conventional laparoscopic surgery.

TECHNOLOGY AND INSTRUMENTS USED IN ROBOTIC SURGERY

The surgeon controls the robotic arms with his two hands. Foot switches (five) to control are clutch, camera, focus, energy sources (monopolar and bipolar-cutting and coagulation).

Robotic technology: The surgeon sits at the console which is away from the patient. The assistant sits by the side of the patient. The stereoscopic view of robotic laparoscopy is different from laparoscopic image. Robotic system consists of a robotic column with robotic arms (Figs. 56.1A to C) and a surgeon's console.

The robotic column has three or four robotic arms. The robotic arms work in a direction towards the robotic column. The robotic arms hold the robotic instruments with the robotic trocars (Figs. 56.2A and B).

In gynecologic surgery, the robotic column placed between the patient's legs or lateral to the legs to get access to the vagina, rectum or urethra.

Docking: In robotic laparoscopic surgery docking is defined as the attachment of the robotic arms to the robotic trocars inserted in the patient. Mean docking time of about 3 minutes is observed and it is improved with progressive number of surgery.

Robotic laparoscopic surgery is especially useful in obese patients, surgery for gynecologic oncology—endometrial cancer, cervical cancer, retroperitoneal lymphadenectomy for advanced ovarian cancer and robotic pelvic exenteration operation.

Special advantages are: Operation time is similar compared to laparoscopic surgery, reduced blood loss, shorter hospital

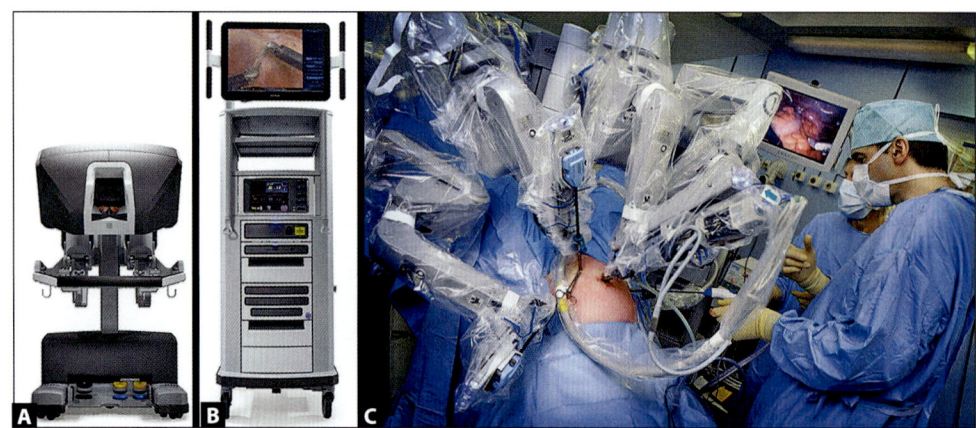

Figs. 56.1A to C: (A) Robotic console with foot pedals and the hand controls. Hand controls are used to manipulate the instruments and to move, rotate and focus the camera. The foot pedals are used to activate the energy sources and to move the camera; (B) Telestration monitor; (C) Robotic column: It is placed between the patient's legs while doing the pelvic surgery.

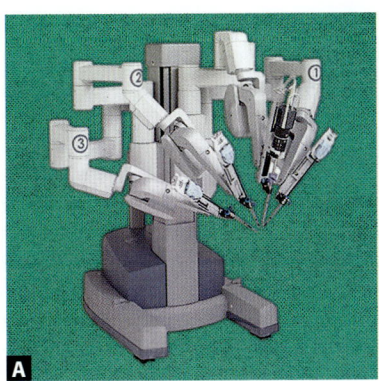
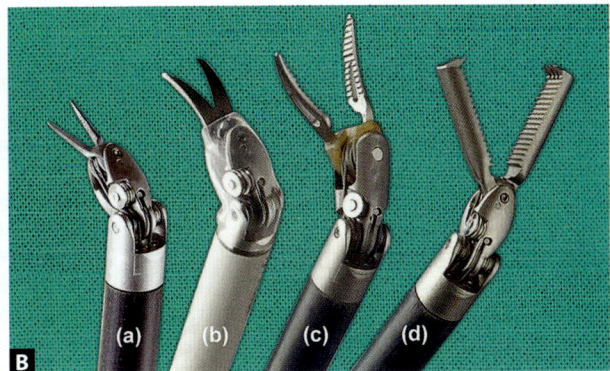

Figs. 56.2A and B: (A) Robotic column with robotic arms; (B) Commonly used robotic instruments: (a) Maryland bipolar, (b) Hot shears, (c) Prograsp forceps (fenestrated), (d) Cobra grasper.

stay, higher number of lymph nodes removed and similar rate of postoperative complications. Tumor recurrence is not different compared to laparoscopic surgery.

TECHNOLOGICAL AND OTHER ADVANTAGES OF ROBOTIC SURGERY

Advantages on the Part of the Surgeon

- **Surgeon** sits on the console, which is situated away from the operation site. He controls the robotic arms with hands and foot switches for camera and energy sources. Surgeon's arms and hands are in a comfortable position.
- **Docking** is the process of attaching the robotic arms to the robotic trocars inserted in the patient. One assistant sits with the patient in the theater. Assistant does the docking. The assistant is trained in robotics, so as to help the procedure (using vessel-sealing device, suction, irrigation) whenever needed.
- **Surgeon's morbidity** due to prolonged surgery (as observed in laparoscopy) is less.

Technological Advantages

- Robotic image is stereoscopic (3D) which is different from laparoscopic view.
- Robotic movements are intuitive. The instrument tips are articulated such as to have seven degrees of movements. It mimics the movements of human wrist and fingers. So, any complex maneuver can be done within a limited space.
- It helps suturing and intracorporeal knot tying with ease unlike that of laparoscopy.
- High precision and absence of tremor are of particular benefits in cases of ureteric anastomosis, fistula repair or retroperitoneal lymphadenectomy.
  The **third generation robotic system**, da Vinci Si model (2009), have a resident teaching console, where a trainee can learn robotic technology directly from the surgeon.
- Increased accuracy and enhanced dexterity are the distinct benefits compared to laparoscopic surgery.
- Robotic surgery has the benefits as the movements of the instrument tip are intuitive. In laparoscopic surgery, the movements are counter intuitive which is opposite to the movements of the surgeon's hands.
- Significant reduction in surgeon's morbidity and stress compared to laparoscopic surgery. In robotic surgery, the surgeon sits on a console whereas in laparoscopic surgery the surgeon stands in a strained position with hands and shoulders for a long time.

COMPLICATIONS OF ROBOTIC SURGERY

- Due to lack of tactile feedback, injury may occur to any organ unless done under visual control.
- Unwanted resistance due to collision of the robotic arms may occur.
- Prolonged pressure of the robotic arms on the patient's thighs or arms may cause injury.
- Sudden loss of pneumoperitoneum may result in pulling the instruments off the anterior abdominal wall. This is due to the fact that robotic trocars are fastened to the robotic arms and with that of robotic column.

DISADVANTAGES OF ROBOTIC SURGERY

- Robotic columns and its arms are heavy and risks of injury are there.
- Absence of tactile feedback.
- Repositioning of robotic column and arms when needed increases surgical time.
- Operating room must be spacious (6,000 sq feet or more) to accommodate equipments and the surgical team.
- The assistants must be versed with robotic surgery to comply with the required maneuvers, as the surgeon is away and sitting at the console.
- Cost (both initial or maintenance) is prohibitive for robotic programs.

LIMITATIONS OF LAPAROSCOPIC SURGERY

- Long-learning curve
- Longer operative time
- Counterintuitive hand movements
- Limited degrees of instrument motion
- Ergonomic difficulty and there is tremor amplification.

OVERALL ADVANTAGES OF ROBOTIC SURGERY

- 3D visualization
- More accurate instrument movements
- Instrument movements mimics to complex hand movements
- Enhanced dexterity without tremor
- Faster suturing
- Shorter learning curve.

Suggested Reading

1. Pitter MC, Anderson P, Blissett A, et al. Robotic-assisted gynaecological surgery-establishing training criteria; minimizing operative time and blood loss. Int J Med Robot. 2008;4(2):114-20.
2. van der Schatte Olivier RH, Van't Hullenaar CD, Ruurda JP, et al. Ergonomics, user comfort, and performance in standard and robotic-assisted laparoscopic surgery. Surg Endosc. 2009;23(6):1365-71.

(For more references *See* Ch 50)

Interventional Radiology in Obstetrics and Gynecology

Interventional radiology is currently being carried out in the management of many areas in obstetrics and gynecology. Embolotherapy can obviate the need of many major operations like myomectomy or hysterectomy.

PLACE OF INTERVENTIONAL RADIOLOGY IN OBSTETRICS

- *Uterine artery embolization (UAE)* in the management of postpartum hemorrhage (PPH) (primary and secondary) is an effective intervention. It is an alternative to hysterectomy. In many hospitals, it is now routinely used in the management of PPH where resources and expertize permit. *Cases of PPH due to atonicity,* following cesarean section are effectively managed with UAE.
- Cases with placenta previa and accreta where placenta is morbidly adherent to the uterine wall, often bleeds profusely following delivery either vaginal or cesarean section. Such problems are commonly faced in cases with prior cesarean delivery. Care plans could be organized in such cases for doing UAE procedure electively just prior to the operation.
- UAE is considered as the most effective management for hemorrhage caused by uterine vascular malformations (uterine artery malformation, arteriovenous malformation, arteriovenous fistula formation, gynecologic malignancies including GTDs or aneurysm formation). These women suffer from profuse secondary PPH. Diagnosis of such vascular malformations is often difficult. Doppler study may be helpful in few situations. Uterine vascular angiography is the gold standard in the diagnosis. UAE is the most effective management to control the abnormal bleeding in these cases. Uterine arteriovenous malformation (AVM) can be congenital or acquired. **Congenital AVM** have multiple feeding vessels and multiple draining veins with an intervening nidus. On the contrary, acquired AVMF, usually have one feeding artery and one draining vein without a nidus. The congenital form can cause intractable PPH. Common conditions in obstetrics and gynecology that are associated with acquired AVM are:
  A. Endometrial or cervical carcinoma, gestational trophoblastic neoplasia (GTN)
  B. Pseudoaneurysm of the uterine artery. It is mostly following trauma to the uterine artery
  C. Cesarean section, often due to lateral extension of the incision. Pseudoaneurysm lacks the three layers of an arterial wall. Pseudoaneurysm is very fragile. It can rupture even with an increase of blood pressure. It can cause heavy uterine bleeding or PPH.

Diagnostic tests for AVM: A. Angiography is considered the gold standard investigation in the diagnosis of vascular (arteriovenous) malformations; B. Ultrasonography with the use of color Doppler has shown to be an important diagnostic tool. Color Doppler usually demonstrate the blood flow within the lesion and a "to-and-fro" phenomenon. This sign of "to-and-fro" differentiates the pseudoaneurysm from other common pelvic lesions like hematomas or fibroids.

Benefits of UAE: Besides the therapeutic benefit of control of hemorrhage, preservation of the uterus and the fertility are the other important benefits. The overall success rate of UAE is 90–95%. Pregnancies have been reported following UAE for treatment of PPH.

UAE in gynecology: UAE has been done in cases with fibroid uterus (Fig. 57.1). It reduces the size, vascularity and problems of bleeding and pressure effects of the tumor. However, complications are also reported. Other uses of selective UAE in gynecology are:
a. To control hemorrhage after abdominal and vaginal hysterectomy
b. Hemorrhage from cervical cancer
c. Hemorrhage from ectopic pregnancy (Fig. 57.2)
d. Retroperitoneal hemorrhage.

Procedure: Both the uterine arteries are selectively catheterized through the femoral artery under fluoroscopic guidance. It is done via percutaneous catheterization through the femoral artery. Angiography identifies the anatomy and the possible source of hemorrhage. A temporary agent, gelatin sponge, is typically used to reduce the perfusion pressure and to stop the hemorrhage. It also allows eventual recanalization. Polyvinyl alcohol particles are used to embolize the vessels. The exact size of the particulate emboli depends on the type of agent. Sizes ranging between 300 to 900 microns are commonly used as it avoids the risk of passing through the utero-ovarian collaterals. This method is simple. It is done by a skilled interventional radiologist under local anesthesia.

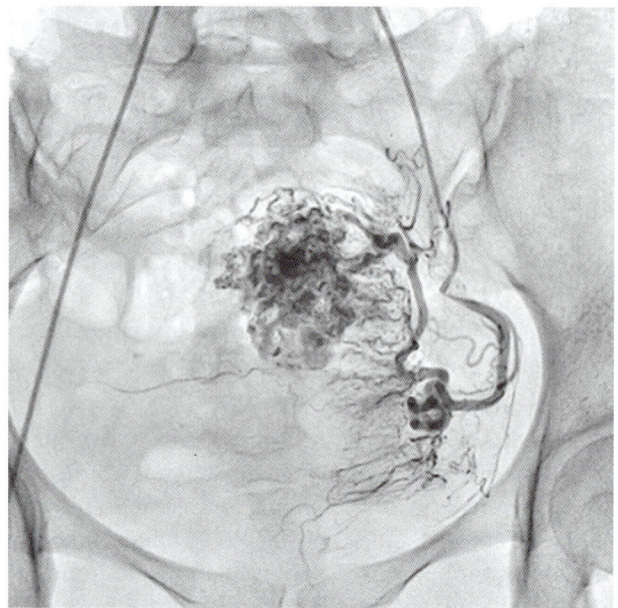

Fig. 57.1: Uterine artery embolization in a case of huge uterine fibroid.

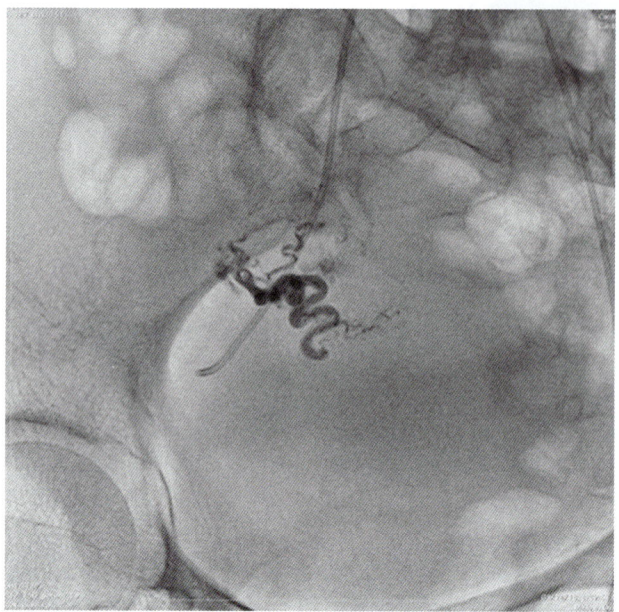

Fig. 57.2: Uterine artery embolization in case with cornual ectopic pregnancy.

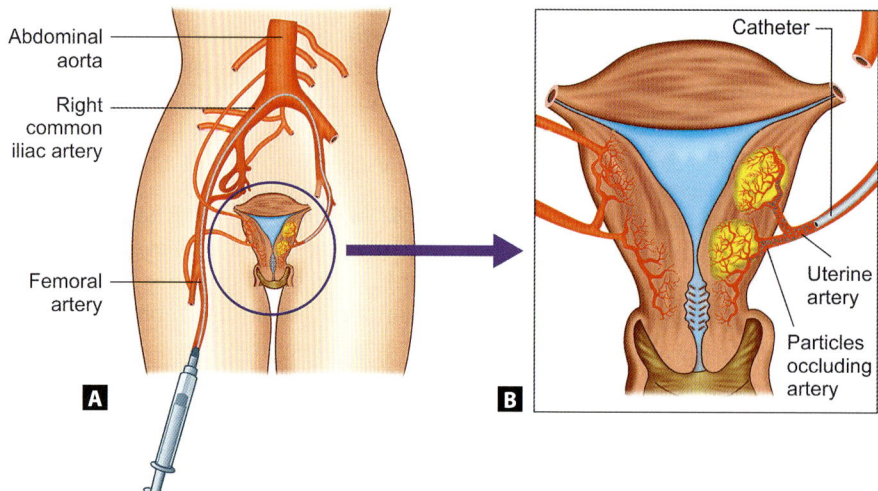

Figs. 57.3A and B: Uterine artery embolization. (A) Pelvic angiography is done through femoral artery catheterization; (B) Uterine artery embolization is done through the catheter.

Contraindications of UAE
- Pregnancy
- Active pelvic infection
- Allergy to contrast media
- Desire for future pregnancy
- Undiagnosed pelvic mass
- Pedunculated myoma

Overall success rate of UAE: About 96–98% (Figs. 57.3A and B).

Benefits are: Improvement of menorrhagia, reduction in volume and size of fibroids (60%), conservation of uterus. Successful pregnancies have been reported following UAE.

Complications of UAE
- **Common complications:** Low-grade fever, pain, pelvic infection, injury to femoral and iliac arteries and ischemia of buttock.
- **Other complications:** Following treatment of uterine fibroids: Abdominal pain, fever, vaginal discharge, nausea, vomiting, amenorrhea, bladder necrosis, sepsis (<1%) and ovarian failure (<5%).
- **Future pregnancy complications:** Miscarriage, preterm delivery, fetal growth restriction (FGR), PPH and increased risk of cesarean delivery.
- However, regarding future fertility and pregnancy following UAE, more studies are awaited.

Suggested Reading

1. Abu-Yousef MM, Wiese JA, Shamma AR. The "to-and-fro" sign: duplex Doppler evidence of femoral artery pseudoaneurysm, AJR Am J Roentgenol. 1988;150:632.
2. Brown BJ, Heaston DK, Poulson AM, Gabert HA, Mineau DE, Miller FJ Jr. Uncontrollable postpartum bleeding: a new approach to hemostasis through angiographic arterial embolization. Obstet Gynecol. 1979;54:361-5.
3. Burchell RC, Creed F, Rasoulpour M, Whitcomb M. Vascular anatomy of the human uterus and pregnancy wastage. BJOG. 1978;85:698-706.
4. Butori N, Coulange L, Filipuzzi L, Krausé D, Loffroy R. Pseudoaneurysm of the uterine artery after cesarean delivery: management with superselective arterial embolization. Obstet Gynecol. 2009;113:540-53.
5. Helvie MA, Rubin JM, Silver TM, Kresowik TF. The distinction between femoral artery pseudoaneurysms and other causes of groin masses: value of duplex Doppler sonography. AJR Am J Roentgenol. 1988;150:1177-80.
6. Pelage JP, Le Dref O, Jacob D, Soyer P, Herbreteau D, Rymer R. Selective arterial embolization of the uterine arteries in the management of intractable post-partum hemorrhage. Acta Obstet Gynecol Scand. 1999;78:698-703.
7. Sieber PR, Bladder necrosis secondary to pelvic artery embolization: case report and literature review, J Urol. 1994;151:422.
8. Soncini E, Pelicelli A, Larini P, Marcato C, Monaco D, Grignaffini A. Uterine artery embolization in the treatment and prevention of postpartum hemorrhage. Int J Gynaecol Obstet. 2007;96:181-5.
9. Vedantham S, Goodwin SC, McLucas B, Mohr G. Uterine artery embolization: an underused method of controlling pelvic hemorrhage. Am J Obstet Gynecol. 1997;176:938-48.
10. Wells I. Internal iliac artery embolization in the management of pelvic bleeding. Clin Radiol. 1996;51:825-7.

Section 7: Maternal Sepsis

Section Outline

- Ch. 58. Maternal Sepsis: Prevention, Recognition and Management
- Ch. 59. Guidelines for use of Antimicrobials/Antibiotics in Gynecology

Chapter 58: Maternal Sepsis: Prevention, Recognition and Management

BACKGROUND

- Sepsis remains the third leading cause of maternal death in India.
- Common etiological factors are infections due to: bacterial, viral or fungal
- Important issues for diagnosis and management are:
  - Early detection
  - Evaluation of the patient and to organize investigations
  - Start of antibiotics
- **The aim is to:**
  - Prevent sepsis with the use of prophylactic antibiotics
  - Recognise sepsis and treat through the Sepsis 6 pathway (see below).
- Organ dysfunction secondary to sepsis is now identified using **Red Flag** Criteria (see below).
- **Sequential organ failure assessment (SOFA) score** is used to assess the severity and prognosis of sepsis mainly by the critical care settings. Score < 2 is suggestive of poor outcome
- **qSOFA score** is useful in assessing the suspected sepsis in the acute setting.
- This is done by assessing: systolic BP < 100 mm Hg, altered mentation and RR >22/min. Score < 2 is abnormal.

Q.1 How to define sepsis?

Ans. Sepsis is a syndrome caused by dysregulated inflammatory response to infection, which can lead to multiple organ dysfunction and ultimately death. (*Third International Consensus Definitions for Sepsis and Septic Shock, February 2016*).

Q.2 What is septic shock?

Ans. **Septic shock:** Sepsis with persistent hypotension and requiring ionotropic support or lactate ≥2 mmol/L despite adequate fluid resuscitation.

Q.3 What is maternal sepsis?

Ans. **Maternal sepsis:** A life-threatening condition defined as organ dysfunction resulting from infection during pregnancy, childbirth, post-abortion or postpartum period (World Health Organization, 2017).

Q.4 What are the different risk factors for maternal sepsis?

Ans. A. Conditions not related to pregnancy
B. Conditions related to pregnancy

Non-pregnant	Pregnancy related risk factors
■ Obesity	■ Primiparous
■ Impaired glucose tolerance/diabetes	■ Multiple pregnancy
■ Anemia	■ Amniocentesis and other invasive intrauterine procedures
■ History of pyelonephritis/ UTI	■ Prolonged rupture of membranes
■ History of pelvic infection/STI	■ Preterm pre-labor rupture of membranes (PPROM)
■ Immunocompromised status (e.g., HIV)	■ All forms of operative vaginal delivery
■ Pre-existing medical problem (e.g., asthma, hematological, renal disorders, heart failure)	■ Complications of cesarean section: wound hematoma, infection
	■ Retained products of conception after miscarriage, termination of pregnancy
	■ Manual removal of placenta

Sepsis Recognition

Q.5 Who are the women that should be screened for sepsis?

Ans. Any women who is clinically ill should be screened. Sepsis 6 pathway should be initiated and completed to recognise sepsis if she belongs to **Red Flag** criteria or **Amber Flag** criteria (see below).

Sepsis Pathway

- Send all the investigations including 2 sets of paired blood cultures and give antibiotics within one hour of diagnosis. Two sets of paired blood cultures increase the probability of finding the microorganism from 50% to 85%.
- For every hour of delay in giving antibiotics, there is cumulative increaze of 7.5% of mortality (over background mortality of 60%).

Further Management of Sepsis

- To continue Modified Early Obstetric Warning Score (MEOWS) assessment every 30 minutes
- To perform serial lactate to assess response to treatment
- To identify the source of sepsis

- To start thromboprophylaxis: If it is contraindicated, apply intermittent compression device (Flowtron).
- If anemic with Hb < 7 g/dL transfuse blood: aim for target Hb = 7–9 g/dL.

Q.6 What are the signs of septic shock?

Ans.
- Systolic blood pressure persistently below 90 mm Hg.
- Reduced level of consciousness despite resuscitation
- Respiratory rate over 25 breaths per minute or a need for respiratory support.
- Lactate not reduced by more than 20% of initial value within 1 hour of fluid resuscitation.

Q.7 How to manage the complications?

Ans.
- If the condition deteriorates or does not improve, consider additional or alternative IV antibiotics.
- Consider additional imaging study to aid diagnosis and target treatment.
- If pregnant, consider delivery to assist resuscitation measures.
- Closed-space infections need surgical drainage, including evacuation of retained products of conception.
- Most commonly identified microorganisms among direct causes are *E. coli* and Group A *Streptococcus* (GAS).

Multi-disciplinary Team Management of Septic Shock/Severe Sepsis

Sepsis screening tools
Risk factors for sepsis in pregnancy - Recent trauma/surgery/invasive procedure - Impaired immunity (e.g. diabetes, steroids, chemotherapy) - Indwelling lines/broken skin
Common sites of infection: - Infected cesarean wound - Chorioamnionitis/endometritis - Respiratory - Breast abscess - Urine - Abdominal pain, distension
ANY marker of RED FLAG PRESENT? - Objective evidence of altered mental state - Systolic BP ≤ 90 mm Hg (or drop of >40 from normal) - Heart rate ≥130 per minute - Respiratory rate ≥ 25 per minute - Needs O$_2$ to keep SpO$_2$ ≥ 92% (88% in COPD) - Skin: mottled/ashen/cyanotic - Not passed urine in 18 hours (0.5 mL/kg/hr if catheterized)	Red Flag Sepsis present: to start bundle (see below)

Contd...

Contd...

ANY AMBER FLAG PRESENT?	
- Behavioral/mental status change - Acute deterioration in functional ability - Respiratory rate 21–24 - Heart rate 100–129 - Systemic BP 91–100 mm Hg - Has had invasive procedure in last 6 weeks (e.g. CS, forceps delivery, ERPC, cerclage, CVs, miscarriage, termination of pregnancy) - Temperature < 36°C - Has diabetes or gestational diabetes - Prolonged rupture of membranes - Offensive vaginal discharge - Non-reassuring CTG/fetal tachycardia > 160	- Get assessment by a doctor - Is urgent referral to hospital required? - Start ongoing management plan (including observation frequency and planned second review)

No Amber flag = routine care/consider other diagnosis

Complete all actions within one hour: *THE SEPSIS SIX*.
1. **Ensure clinical review by the senior**
2. **Oxygen therapy** Start if O$_2$ saturations less than 92%, aim for O$_2$ saturations of 94–98%
3. **Obtain IV access and take blood** Blood cultures, blood glucose, lactate, full blood count, serum-urea, creatinine, electrolytes, CRP and clotting, lumbar puncture if indicated
4. **Give IV antibiotics** Maximum dose broad spectrum therapy; consider (*See* Clinical in Obstetrics, Section 7, Ch 71)
5 **Give IV fluids** Give fluid bolus of 500 mL NICE recommends using lactate to guide further fluid therapy
6. **Monitor** Use MEOWS, measure urinary output, this may require a urinary catheter, repeat lactate at least once per hour if initial lactate elevated or if clinical condition changes

Red Flag after one hour—involve the consultant

Essential Investigations

Q.8 What are the investigations to organize?

Ans.
- Full blood count (FBC)
- Venous blood gas for lactate (part of sepsis 6 pathway)
- Follow amber and red flag guidance on sepsis 6 pathway for blood tests to be done
- Blood: Group and Save (G+S)
- Blood cultures – 2 sets (take 3 sets only if infective endocarditis suspected)
- Mid-stream urine (MSU) or catheter specimen urine (CSU) for culture and sensitivity
- Low vaginal swab (LVS)

Q.9 What are the additional investigations to be done?
Ans. Selectively could be done if clinically indicated:
- **Endometritis/chorioamnionitis:** High vaginal swab (HVS); low vaginal swab (LVS) and rectal swab for GBS and GAS culture
- **Pelvic inflammatory disease:** Endocervical swabs for chlamydia (use PCR detection kit) and gonorrhea (swab in charcoal medium)
- **Chest infection:** Sputum cultures, urine for culture test
- **Wound infection:** wound swab
- **Headache/photophobia:** Lumbar puncture for CSF

Q.10 What is the place of imaging?
Ans. Cases with severe sepsis imaging are needed to determine focus of infection
- Chest X-ray (CXR)
- Ultrasound (USG) abdomen and pelvis
- Computed tomography (CT) chest (+/- CTPA) or abdomen
- Magnetic resonance imaging (MRI)

Table 58.1: Clinical presentations in general for a woman with sepsis.

Central nervous system - Altered consciousness/confusion	**Cardiovascular** - Tachycardia - Hypertension - Prolonged capillary refill - Warm or cool peripheries
Respiratory - Tachypnea - Hypoxia	**Renal** - Oliguria - Anuria
Gastrointestinal - Abnormal LFT's - Reduced albumin	**Metabolic** - Lactic acidosis - Hypo/hyperglycemia - Hypocalcemia

Hematology
- WBC abnormal count
- DIC
  ♦ Reduced platelets
  ♦ Increased PT/APTT
  ♦ Increased D-dimer
  ♦ Reduced fibrinogen
	Skin
	- Hyperthermia
	- Hypothermia

TABLE 58.2: Organ site of sepsis and the clinical findings.

Central nervous system - Headache - Neck stiffness - Photophobia	**Cardiovascular** - Murmur
Respiratory - Consolidation - Pleural effusion - Sore throat, cervical lymphadenopathy	**Renal** - Dysuria - Loin pain - Hematuria
Gastrointestinal - Abdominal pain/tenderness	**Joints** - Swelling/redness/tenderness
Breast changes - Tenderness, engorgement, lump, axillary lymphadenoapthy	**Skin** - Cellulitis - Rash, splinter hmorrhages - Wounds
Hematology - Neutropenia	**Postnatal** - Uterine tenderness - Uterine subinvolution - Offensive lochia discharge - Perineal/cesarean wound discharge or breakdown
Obstetric (antenatal) - Uterine tenderness - Fetal tachycardia - Offensive liquor	

Table 58.3: Clinical diagnosis.

Central nervous system - Meningitis - Encephalitis - Sinusitis - Cerebral abscess	**Cardiovascular** - Endocarditis
	Breast - Mastitis - Abscess
Respiratory - Pneumonia - Empyema - Bronchiectasis	**Renal** - UTI - Pyelonephritis
Gastrointestinal - Peritonitis (upper or lower perforation) - Appendicitis - Cholecystitis - Diverticulitis	**Joints** - Septic arthritis
	Skin - Cellulitis - Endocarditis - Wound infection
Hematology - Neutropenic sepsis	

Obstetrics
- Antenatal
  ♦ Chorioamnionitis
- Postnatal
  ♦ Endometritis
  ♦ Retained products of conception
  ♦ Pelvic collection
  ♦ Perineal or abdominal wound infection	

Suggested Reading

1. Maternal sepsis update: current management and controversies – The Obstetrician & Gynaecologist, Volume 22, issue 1 https://obgyn.onlinelibrary.wiley.com/doi/10.1111/tog.12623
2. MBRRACE UK: Saving Lives, Improving Mothers Care – 2014, 2017, 2018, 2019, 2020. https://www.npeu.ox.ac.uk/mbrrace-uk
3. NICE NG121. Intrapartum care for women with existing medical conditions or obstetric complications and their babies (updated April 2019) https://www.nice.org.uk/guidance/ng121

4. NICE Quality Standards QS 161. https://www.nice.org.uk/guidance/qs161
5. Royal Berkshire NHS Foundation Trust
6. RCOG guidelines; Green-top guideline No. 64a & 64b. https://www.rcog.org.uk/en/guidelines-research-services/guidelines/gtg64a/ https://www.rcog.org.uk/en/guidelines-research-services/guidelines/gtg64b/
7. Singer M, Deutschman CS, Seymour CW, et al. The Third International Consensus Definitions for Sepsis and Septic Shock (Sepsis-3). JAMA. 2016;315(8):801-10.
8. UK sepsis trust – clinical tools https://sepsistrust.org/professional-resources/clinical-tools/

Chapter 59: Guidelines for use of Antimicrobials/Antibiotics in Gynecology

Gynecological infections, clinical presentations, investigations, and the treatment.

Type of Infections	Clinical Presentations	Investigations	Treatment Recommendations — First Choice	Alternatives	Comments
Trichomonas vaginalis (TV)	- Vaginitis associated with frothy, greenish-yellow discharge, vulval soreness/itching, dysuria - TV is almost exclusively STI. - TV is associated with high prevalence of co-infection with other STIs.	- HVS for smear microscopy - HVS/Cx/CCU for *Chlamydia trachomatis*, n. gonorrhoeae, *herpes simplex*, trichomonas vaginalis, polymerase chain reaction test	PO metronidazole 400 mg 12 hourly for 5 days (Metronidazole is safe to use in pregnancy)	There is no suitable alternative to PO metronidazole for TV	- Screening of sexual contacts for all STIs and treatment for TV irrespective of results is indicated - Routine screening or treatment of asymptomatic women is not indicated
			- **Breastfeeding** should be withheld during treatment and for 12–24 hours after the last dose to reduce infant exposure to metronidazole		
Bacterial vaginosis (BV)	- Thin, gray/white, homogenous discharge - Fishy/offensive odor - Not associated with soreness itching or inflammation	- Vaginal pH >4.5 **Microscopy:** - Wet mount microscopy for Clue cells - A smear of discharge sent to lab for gram-stain	PO metronidazole 400 mg 12 hourly for 5 days	**Breastfeeding** - Intravaginal metronidazole gel (0.75%) once daily at night for 5 days OR - Intravaginal clindamycin cream (2%) once daily at night for 7 days	- Antibiotic treatment for BV is indicated for symptomatic women only - Routine screening for, or treatment of, asymptomatic women for BV to reduce perinatal complications is not indicated
***Chlamydia trachomatis* (CT) Gonorrhoea: *Neisseria gonorrhoeae* (NG)**	- Vaginal discharge - Dysuria without significant bacteriuria or persistent dysuria despite successful treatment of bacteriuria	'High risk for STI' - CT/NG screening in the first trimester: ST-LVS, urine for CT/NG PCR; - ToC 3–4 weeks post-treatment; - Re-testing in 3 months	IM ceftriaxone 500 mg STAT + PO azithromycin 1 g single dose	IM spectinomycin 2 g single dose + PO azithromycin 1 g single dose	- Please refer to Suraksha clinic (STI) for the partner management
Malaria	- Fever, headache, malaise - GI disturbances: Nausea, abdominal pain, vomiting, diarrhea - H/o travel to malaria—endemic area in previous 6 days–6 months, regardless of antimalarial prophylaxis	- Thick and thin blood films - Rapid diagnostic test - 3 negative diagnostic samples over 24 hours are required to exclude malaria - Blood film may be negative in complicated falciparum malaria due to high parasite load in placenta	**Uncomplicated malaria in the first trimester:** Quinine + Clindamycin **Uncomplicated malaria in the 2nd and 3rd trimester:** Artemether-lumefantrine (Riamet®) PO **Severe malaria in any trimester:** Artesunate IV		

1. Accreditation Standards for Hospitals (5th edition) April 2020. National Accreditation Board for Hospitals and Healthcare Providers (NABH). New Delhi. https://www.nabh.co/images/Standards/NABH%205%20STD%20April%202020.pdf (accessed on 22/09/2021).
2. Royal Berkshire NHS Foundation Trust; 2020.

Section 8: Practice of SBA and EMQs

Section Outline

Ch. 60. Model Questions and Answers for Practice of SBA
Ch. 61. Model Questions and Answers for Practice of EMQs

Chapter 60: Model Questions and Answers for Practice of SBA

PART I MRCOG: GYNECOLOGY
SINGLE BASED ANSWER (SBA)

This page provides some examples of SBA. For each question, select the single most appropriate answer from the 5 options listed.

Q.1 A 30-year-old woman with history of previous three recurrent miscarriages was investigated. Combined laparoscopy and hysteroscopy revealed bicornuate uterus.
She was successful to have her fourth pregnancy and that continued to 35 weeks. Which obstetric phenomenon has an increased association with bicornuate uterus?
a. Placental abruption b. Pre-eclampsia
c. Placenta previa d. Breech presentation
e. Fetal congenital malformations

Ans. d. Breech presentation.
Presence of bicornuate uterus is associated with increased risk of recurrent fetal loss, preterm labor and malpresentation (breech).

Q.2 A 39-year-old woman presents to clinic with secondary amenorrhea. A pregnancy test is negative. Her BMI is 25 kg/m². She is otherwise fit and well. Blood tests are ordered with the following results:

Follicle-stimulating hormone (FSH): 73 IU/L
Luteinizing hormone (LH): 56 IU/L
Estradiol (E_2): <70 nmol/L
Anti-Mullerian hormone level (AMH): <1.2 U/L

What is the most likely diagnosis?
a. Asherman's syndrome
b. Imperforate hymen
c. Kallmann syndrome
d. Premature ovarian failure
e. Turner syndrome

Ans. d.

Q.3 A 68-year-old woman is referred to the gynecology clinic. A GP had arranged an ultrasound scan because the woman had some lower abdominal pain. This showed a 3.5 cm multilocular cyst in the right ovary but no other concerning features.
A serum CA125 is requested, and this is found to be 50 u/mL.
The risk of malignancy index (RMI) for this woman is:
a. 0 b. 2
c. 50 d. 150
e. 175

Ans. d.

Q.4 You are called to the gynecology ward by a very concerned FY1 doctor. A 48-year-old woman who had a hysterectomy the day before has had a postoperative full blood count with the following result:
1. Hb: 7.2 2. Hematocrit: 23%
3. WBC: 9.6 4. Platelets: 278
The preoperative Hb was 12.3, so the FY1 doctor is very concerned. The patient is well with stable observations. The catheter bag is full.

What is the most likely diagnosis?
a. Excessive IV fluids b. Hemolysis
c. Laboratory error d. Normal results
e. Postoperative bleeding

Ans. a.

Q.5 Women with obstetric cholestasis often experience intense pruritus.
Which drug, that is commonly prescribed in obstetric cholestasis, effects the greatest improvement in pruritis?
a. Chlorpheniramine
b. Cholestyramine
c. Dexamethasone
d. S-adenosylmethionine
e. Ursodeoxycholic acid

Ans. e.

Q.6 Patients with sickle-cell anemia have HbS rather than HbA.
The formation of HbS is due to a mutation in which globin chain:
a. α b. β
c. δ d. γ
e. ε

Ans. b

Q.7 A 30-year-old woman is referred to the gynecology clinic with menorrhagia, dysmenorrhea, dyspareunia and pelvic pain.
An ultrasound scan is arranged with the following report and image:
- Normal uterus and right ovary
- Within the left ovary there is a structure with a ***ground glass appearance*** measuring 25–30 mm
- Small amount of free fluid in the pouch of Douglas (POD).

What is this structure most likely to be?
a. Follicular cyst
b. Corpus luteum cyst
c. Dermoid cyst
d. Ovarian carcinoma
e. Endometrioma

Ans. e.

Q.8 What is the usual genetic origin and arrangement in a partial molar pregnancy?

Ploidy	Maternal genes	Paternal genes
a. Diploid	1 set	1 set
b. Diploid	2 sets	0 set
c. Diploid	0 set	2 sets
d. Triploid	1 set	2 sets
e. Triploid	2 sets	1 set

Ans. d.

Q.9 To which class of antiretroviral medication does the drug atazanavir belong?
a. CCR5 antagonist/entry inhibitor
b. Integrase inhibitor
c. Non-nucleoside reverse transcriptase inhibitor
d. Nucleoside reverse transcriptase inhibitor
e. Protease inhibitor

Ans. e.

Q.10 The Jarisch-Herxheimer reaction may manifest as fever, rigors and hypotension.
Typically, this reaction follows antibiotic treatment of which infection?
a. Chlamydia
b. Gonorrhea
c. Molluscum contagiosum
d. Syphilis
e. *Trichomonas vaginalis*

Ans. d.

Q.11 An anxious patient had an intravenous bolus of midazolam prior to colposcopic treatment.
Following treatment she is excessively drowsy, with a low respiratory rate and hypotension.
Which drug would you administer?
a. Adrenaline
b. Buprenorphine
c. Flumazenil
d. Naloxone
e. Pseudoephedrine

Ans. c.

Q.12 Acyclovir is an analog of which nucleoside?
a. Adenosine
b. Cytidine
c. Guanosine
d. 5-methyluridine
e. Uridine

Ans. c.

Q.13 Which muscle is demonstrated in red in the diagram below?
a. Gluteus maximus
b. Gluteus minimus
c. Obturator internus
d. Vastus lateralis
e. Pyriformis

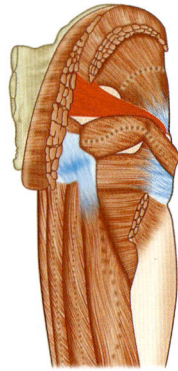

Ans. e.

Q.14 Which anatomical structure can be used to distinguish between the body of the uterus and the cervix?
a. Broad ligament
b. Ovarian ligament
c. Round ligament
d. Sacrospinous ligament
e. Uterosacral ligament

Ans. e.

Q.15 At which vertebral level is the bifurcation of the aorta?
a. L1
b. L2
c. L3
d. L4
e. L5

Ans. d.

Q.16 Which structure makes a dimple in the skin of the buttock at S2?
a. Posterior inferior iliac spine
b. Posterior superior iliac spine
c. Sacrococcygeal ligament
d. Sacrospinous ligament
e. Supraspinal ligament

Ans. b.

Q.17 What is the value of the submentobregmatic diameter in a normal term infant?
 a. 7.5 cm
 b. 8.5 cm
 c. 9.5 cm
 d. 10.5 cm
 e. 11 cm
Ans. c.

Q.18 The middle rectal artery is a branch of which artery?
 a. Anterior division of the internal iliac artery
 b. Posterior division mesenteric artery
 c. Inferior mesenteric artery
 d. Abdominal aorta
 e. Pudendal artery
Ans. a

Q.19 Which muscle of the anterior abdominal wall has a free edge that forms the inguinal ligament?
 a. External oblique muscle
 b. Internal oblique muscle
 c. Transversus abdominis muscle
 d. Rectus abdominis muscle
 e. Pyramidalis
Ans. a.

Q.20 The facial nerve splits into several major branches in the parotid gland, into how many branches does it split?
 a. 2
 b. 3
 c. 4
 d. 5
 e. 6
Ans. d.

Q.21 What is the most common cause of hyperthyroidism in reproductive age?
 a. Graves disease
 b. Thyroid follicular carcinoma
 c. Thyroiditis
 d. Toxic adenoma
 e. Toxic multinodular goiter
Ans. a.

Q.22 Which peptide of 31 amino acids is removed from proinsulin in the Golgi apparatus?
 a. A peptide
 b. B peptide
 c. C peptide
 d. D peptide
 e. E peptide
Ans. c.

Q.23 What is the main site of secretion of angiotensin-converting enzyme in the body?
 a. Adrenal
 b. Kidney
 c. Liver
 d. Lung
 e. Spleen
Ans. d.

Q.24 What is the embryological origin of the cells in the thyroid gland that produce calcitonin?
 a. Eustachian tube
 b. Foramen cecum
 c. Rathke's pouch
 d. Thyroglossal duct
 e. Ultimobranchial body
Ans. d.

Q.25 Which neurons in the hypothalamus are inhibited by leptin to give a feeling of satiety?
 a. α-melanocyte-stimulating hormone containing neurons
 b. GnRH containing neurons
 c. Neuropeptide Y containing neurons
 d. Somatostatin containing neurons
 e. VEGF containing neurons
Ans. c.

Q.26 Which enzyme converts pregnenolone to progesterone in the steroid synthesis pathway?
 a. 11 hydroxylase
 b. 17 hydroxylase
 c. 21 hydroxylase
 d. 3 hydroxysteroid dehydrogenase
 e. 5 reductase
Ans. d.

Q.27 From where in the body is cholecystokinin secreted?
 a. Duodenal mucosa
 b. Gallbladder
 c. Liver
 d. Pancreas
 e. Spleen
Ans. a.

Q.28 Which protein binds 20% of estradiol in the plasma?
 a. Albumin
 b. Fibrinogen
 c. Lipoprotein
 d. Sex-hormone binding globulin
 e. Transferrin
Ans. a.

Q.29 Which enzyme is deficient in 95% of cases of congenital adrenal hyperplasia?
 a. 11 hydroxylase
 b. 17 hydroxylase
 c. 21 hydroxylase
 d. 3 hydroxysteroid dehydrogenase
 e. 5 reductase
Ans. c.

Q.30 What is the half-life ($t_{1/2}$) of ethinyl estradiol?
 a. 3 hours
 b. 8 hours
 c. 15 hours
 d. 20 hours
 e. 36 hours
Ans. e.

Q.31 200 women with polycystic ovary syndrome but otherwise healthy are followed-up over a 10-year period. 100 women are taking metformin and 100 are taking placebo.

After 10 years, the women are assessed for the development of type 2 diabetes.
In the metformin group, 20 women have type 2 diabetes.
In the placebo group, 40 women have type 2 diabetes. What is the relative risk of developing diabetes for women who take metformin?
- a. 0.1
- b. 0.2
- c. 0.4
- d. 0.5
- e. 1.0

Ans. d.

Q.32 16 patients have their diastolic blood pressure measured in an antenatal clinic. The mean diastolic BP is 70 mm Hg, with a standard deviation of 12 mm Hg.
What is the standard error of the mean in this population?
- a. 1.33
- b. 3
- c. 4
- d. 4.375
- e. 5.83

Ans. b.

Q.33 What type of data are the ABO blood group?
- a. Discrete
- b. Interval
- c. Nominal
- d. Ordinal
- e. Ratio

Ans. c.

Q.34 What kind of error occurs when the null hypothesis is incorrectly rejected?
- a. β error
- b. γ error
- c. δ error
- d. Type I error
- e. Type II error

Ans. d.

Q.35 What statistical test is used to compare the medians of two groups of nonparametric data?
- a. Analysis of variance
- b. Kruskal-Wallis test
- c. Mann Whitney U test
- d. Sign test
- e. Student's test

Ans. c.

Q.36 In statistical tests, what is an alternative name for the β level?
- a. False-negative rate
- b. False-positive rate
- c. Negative predictive value
- d. Power
- e. True-negative rate

Ans. b.

Q.37 In a forest plot of a meta-analysis, the odds ratio of each contributing study is represented by a square. What is the size of the square proportional to?
- a. Age of the study
- b. Confidence interval of the study
- c. Number in the study
- d. Odds ratio of the study
- e. Weighting used in the meta-analysis

Ans. e.

Q.38 Following an episode of hypoglycemia, glucagon is released. Which metabolic pathway is activated initially?
- a. Gluconeogenesis in hepatocytes
- b. Gluconeogenesis in cells of pancreas
- c. Glycogenolysis in hepatocytes
- d. Glycogenolysis in cells of pancreas
- e. Lipolysis

Ans. c.

Q.39 Which compound is tested for in the Guthrie spot to screen for cystic fibrosis in the newborn?
- a. Chloride
- b. Free thyroxine
- c. Immunoreactive trypsinogen
- d. Medium-chain acyl-CoA dehydrogenase
- e. Phenylalanine

Ans. d.

Q.40 What is the correct order of potency of estrone, estradiol and estriol from strongest to weakest?
- a. Estradiol, estrone, estriol
- b. Estradiol, estriol, estrone
- c. Estriol, estrone, estradiol
- d. Estriol, estradiol, estrone
- e. Estrone, estradiol, estriol

Ans. b.

Q.41 What is the most prevalent cation in the intracellular fluid?
- a. Ca_2^+
- b. Ca^-
- c. HCO_3
- d. K^+
- e. Na^+

Ans. d.

Q.42 Which vitamin facilitates the absorption of iron from the gut?
- a. Vitamin A
- b. Vitamin B_1
- c. Vitamin B_{12}
- d. Vitamin C
- e. Vitamin K

Ans. d.

Q.43 Where in the body is angiotensin I converted to angiotensin II under the influence of angiotensin-converting enzyme?
- a. Adrenal cortex
- b. Blood vessel wall
- c. Kidney
- d. Liver
- e. Lung

Ans. e.

Q.44 A woman presents with a short history of vaginal spotting and cramping abdominal pain after 7 weeks of amenorrhea. A few days earlier she had a positive result on a home pregnancy test. The cervix is closed on examination. An ultrasound scan shows an intrauterine gestational sac. A fetal pole with cardiac activity is seen. What is the most likely diagnosis?
   a. Complete miscarriage
   b. Incomplete miscarriage
   c. Inevitable miscarriage
   d. Septic miscarriage
   e. Threatened miscarriage

Ans. e.

Q.45 In a trial where the null hypothesis is false (i.e., there is a real difference present) but a small trial does not find a statistically significant difference, what error is most likely to have occurred?
   a. Confidence interval error
   b. External validity error
   c. P value error
   d. Type I error
   e. Type II error

Ans. e.

Q.46 A 23-year-old woman attends the genitourinary medicine (GUM) clinic with an offensive discharge. Triple swabs are taken and the endocervical swab yields the following result.
   Large numbers of Gram-negative diplococci identified.
   Which organism is most likely to be causing the infection?
   a. *N. gonorrhoeae*
   b. *Chlamydia trachomatis*
   c. *Trichomonas vaginalis*
   d. *Candida albicans*
   e. *Treponema pallidum*

Ans. a.

Q.47 Concerning magnetic resonance imaging (MRI):
   a. MRI uses ionizing radiation
   b. In T_1-weighted images, water containing tissues appear white
   c. The international system unit used to measure magnetic field strength is tesla (T)
   d. In T_2-weighted images, bone appears bright
   e. Pregnancy is a contraindication

Ans. c. MRI uses magnetic field and not ionizing radiation. T_2-weighted images, bone and fat appear dark.

Q.48 The posterior pituitary gland:
   a. Synthesizes oxytocin
   b. Releases vasopressin into the hypophyseal circulation
   c. Secretes prolactin
   d. Is known as adenohypophysis
   e. Both oxytocin and vasopressin are octapeptides

Ans. b.

Q.49 The nerve that traverse through the superficial inguinal ring:
   a. Nerve to the pectineus
   b. Genitofemoral nerve
   c. Ilioinguinal nerve
   d. Obturator nerve
   e. Femoral Nerve

Ans. c.

Q.50 The following are the correlations of embryonic germ cell layers with the tissues differentiated:
   a. Ectoderm: Bones
   b. Ectoderm: Kidney
   c. Endoderm: Endocrine glands
   d. Mesoderm: Peripheral nervous system
   e. Mesoderm: Pituitary gland

Ans. c.

Q.51 A woman with premature menopause has a dual-energy X-ray absorptiometry (DEXA) scan to assess her bone mineral density.
   What t score is considered to be diagnostic of osteoporosis?
   a. +2.5
   b. +1.5
   c. 0
   d. –1.5
   e. –2.5

Ans. e.

Q.52 A 24-year-old woman attends a genitourinary medicine clinic with vaginal discharge. Swabs are taken and she is found to be infected with Chlamydia.
   Which antibiotic is an effective treatment for Chlamydia in a single dose?
   a. Azithromycin
   b. Doxycycline
   c. Erythromycin
   d. Tetracycline
   e. Vancomycin

Ans. a.

Q.53 Which artery may be ligated in cases of massive postpartum hemorrhage where conservative measures have failed to stop the bleeding?
   a. Common iliac artery
   b. External iliac artery
   c. Inferior mesenteric artery
   d. Internal iliac artery
   e. Ovarian artery

Ans. d.

Q.54 A 42-year-old woman has an ultrasound scan which shows a simple 5 cm cyst in her left ovary.
   Which blood test is now required?
   a. α-fetoprotein
   b. CA-125
   c. β-hCG
   d. Lactate dehydrogenase
   e. No blood test required

Ans. e.

Q.55 What percentage of complete hydatidiform moles arise as a consequence of duplication of a single sperm following fertilization of an 'empty' ovum?
   a. 5%
   b. 10%
   c. 30%
   d. 50%
   e. 75%

Ans. e.

Q.56 A woman attends the early pregnancy unit. It is 6 weeks since her last menstrual period and she had a positive pregnancy test 2 weeks ago.
She presents with a heavy per vaginam (PV) bleed. An ultrasound scan is arranged with the following report:
Normal size uterus with endometrial thickness 5 mm. No evidence of a gestational sac. Both ovaries appear normal. No free fluid.
What is the most likely diagnosis?
   a. Complete miscarriage
   b. Ectopic pregnancy
   c. Incomplete miscarriage
   d. Heterotopic pregnancy
   e. Missed miscarriage

Ans. a.

Q.57 Which physical principle does MRI use to form an image?
   a. Stimulated emission of radiation
   b. Acceleration of electrons
   c. Vibration of a piezo-electric crystal
   d. The alignment of protons in water
   e. Conversion of low frequency current to high frequency current

Ans. d.

Q.58 A 70-year-old preoperative patient who is taking lisinopril for hypertension, has an ECG performed. What electrolyte disturbance is most likely to be present?
   a. Hyponatremia
   b. Hypernatremia
   c. Hypokalemia
   d. Hyperkalemia
   e. Hypomagnesemia

Ans. a.

Q.59 Following a surgical evacuation of the uterus, you receive the following report:
The sample contains hydropic villi with hyperplasia of villous trophoblast. No evidence of fetal parts.
What is the correct course of action?
   a. Arrange to re-evacuate the uterus
   b. Commence the COCP immediately
   c. Refer to a regional trophoblastic disease center
   d. Advise that is fine to try and conceive immediately
   e. Take no action

Ans. c.

Q.60 What is the mechanism of action of mifepristone?
   a. Selective estrogen receptor modulator
   b. Progesterone agonist
   c. Progesterone antagonist
   d. β2-agonist
   e. Cyclo-oxygenase inhibitor

Ans. c.

Q.61 What class of drug is tranexamic acid?
   a. Cyclo-oxygenase inhibitor
   b. Anti-fibrinolytic
   c. Progestagen
   d. Anti-androgen
   e. Estrogen

Ans. b.

Q.62 Immunoglobulin G consists of how many peptide chains:
   a. 2
   b. 3
   c. 4
   d. 5
   e. 6

Ans. c.

Q.63 What type of muscarinic receptors are found on the detrusor muscle?
   a. M1
   b. M2
   c. M3
   d. M4
   e. M5

Ans. c.

Q.64 Which complement protein is the most abundant, and whose cleavage results in activation of the lytic sequence?
   a. C1
   b. C2
   c. C3
   d. C4
   e. C5

Ans. c.

Q.65 Which cell type is the effector cell of the adaptive immune system?
   a. Basophil
   b. Eosinophil
   c. Lymphocyte
   d. Macrophage
   e. Monocyte

Ans. c.

Q.66 Which cell type is responsible for the majority of antibody production?
   a. B cells
   b. Cytotoxic T cells
   c. Helper T cells
   d. Macrophages
   e. Plasma cells

Ans. e.

Q.67 Which subtypes of the human papillomavirus are responsible for the majority cases of genital warts?
   a. HPV 16
   b. HPV 18
   c. HPV 16, 18
   d. HPV 6, 11
   e. HPV 43, 53

Ans. d.

Q.68 What is the epithelial lining of the labia majora?
  a. Columnar
  b. Cuboidal
  c. Stratified squamous, keratinized
  d. Stratified squamous, non-keratinized
  e. Transitional
Ans. d.

Q.69 What is the root value of the obturator nerve?
  a. L1, 2, 3
  b. L2, 3, 4
  c. L3, 4, 5
  d. L4, 5, S1
  e. L5, S1, 2
Ans. b.

Q.70 At which receptor is ondansetron, an antagonist?
  a. $5-HT_{1a}$
  b. $5-HT_{1b}$
  c. $5-HT_{1c}$
  d. $5-HT_2$
  e. $5-HT_3$
Ans. e.

Q.71 Approximately how many times higher is the intratesticular concentration of testosterone compared to plasma?
  a. 10
  b. 30
  c. 100
  d. 300
  e. 1,000
Ans. e.

Q.72 Which neurotransmitter is antagonized by atropine?
  a. Acetylcholine
  b. Adrenaline
  c. Dopamine
  d. Noradrenaline
  e. Serotonin
Ans. a.

Q.73 Which embryonic structure fail to fuse completely resulting in the development of bicornuate uterus?
  a. Metanephric duct
  b. Mesonephric duct
  c. Paramesonephric duct
  d. Promesonephric duct
  e. Vitelline duct
Ans. c.

Q.74 At which gestation does plasma volume reach its maximal level?
  a. 12/40
  b. 16/40
  c. 24/40
  d. 38/40
  e. 32/40
Ans. e.

Q.75 What is the oxygen consumption of the fetus at term?
  a. 10 mL/min
  b. 20 mL/min
  c. 40 mL/min
  d. 80 mL/min
  e. 100 mL/min
Ans. b.

Q.76 You are asked to see a 21-year-old woman for preconceptual care. She was diagnosed with generalized tonic-clonic epilepsy 4 years ago. This is poorly controlled. She is currently on sodium valproate and levetiracetam.
What is the next step in her management?
  a. Arrange an MRI
  b. Arrange an EEG
  c. Commence aspirin 75 mg
  d. Commence folic acid 5 mg
  e. Review medication
Ans. e. To consider the risks of antiepileptic drugs (AEDs) and use the lowest effective dose for each AED, avoiding polytherapy and commencing folic acid.

Q.77 In order to help plan the capacity required for providing future maternity services, you are asked to design a study to establish the incidence of vaginal birth following previous cesarean section. The study will require establishing the mode of delivery in women who have either had only vaginal delivery or have had a cesarean section in at least one previous pregnancy. You review the epidemiological study methods that may be appropriate for this type of study.
Which type of research study should you choose?
  a. Case control
  b. Cohort
  c. Cross sectional
  d. Ecological
  e. Survey
Ans. b. The answer is cohort study. Cohort studies are longitudinal and follow subjects with or without exposure to a certain characteristic over time. The groups are then compared, e.g., for the development of a particular disease. Cohort studies can be used to measure incidence rates and relative risks.

Q.78 A woman has an instrumental delivery of a baby weighing 3,950 g in her first pregnancy. A Grade 3C tear of the anal sphincter is identified. An appropriate overlapping repair using 3/0 PDS is performed. Prior to discharge, she asks about the long-term risk of fecal or flatal incontinence.
What percentage risk would you advise?
  a. 10%
  b. 20%
  c. 30%
  d. 40%
  e. 50%
Ans. d.

PART II MRCOG: GYNECOLOGY
SINGLE BASED ANSWER (SBA)

Practice SBA: Some examples of the SBA format are given below. Remember that for each question, you need to select the single most appropriate answer from the five options listed.

Q.1 You have been asked to obtain consent from a 32-year-old woman with cyclical pelvic pain for a diagnostic laparoscopy under general anesthesia. What would you advise her regarding the overall risk of a serious complication?
  a. 1 in 50
  b. 1 in 100
  c. 1 in 250
  d. 1 in 500
  e. 1 in 1,000

Ans. d.

Q.2 A 28-year-old woman undergoes extensive laparoscopic surgery in the lithotomy position. She presents after 2 days with unresolved right-sided foot drop and paraesthesia over the calf and dorsum of the right foot.
Damage to which nerve is the most likely cause?
  a. Common peroneal
  b. Femoral
  c. Ilioinguinal
  d. Lateral cutaneous of the thigh
  e. Obturator

Ans. a.

Q.3 A 19-year-old woman was seen in the gynecology clinic with a history of excessive growth of facial hair, she needs to wax every 2–3 weeks. Her menstrual periods last 7–8 days every 24–35 days. There is no change in her voice. Her BMI is 28 kg/m². Examination shows: Ferriman-Gallwey grade 2–3 hirsutism over chest and abdomen. A pelvic ultrasound showed no abnormality. Her day 2 hormone tests showed luteinizing hormone level 7.4 IU/L, follicle-stimulating hormone level 5.2 IU/L, serum testosterone level 2.3 nmol/L, SHBG 24 nmol/L.
What is the most likely diagnosis?
  a. Adrenocorticotropic hormone (ACTH) tumor
  b. Androgen-producing ovarian tumor
  c. Cushing's syndrome
  d. Idiopathic hirsutism
  e. Polycystic ovary syndrome

Ans. d. Diagnostic criteria for PCOS in presence of at least two of the three following criteria: Polycystic ovaries [either 12 or more peripheral follicles or increased ovarian volume (greater than 10 cm³)], oligo or anovulation, clinical and/or biochemical signs of hyperandrogenism. Testosterone level will be raised in Cushing's syndrome, ACTH tumor and virilizing ovarian tumor.

Q.4 A 34-year-old woman complains of heavy periods. She is trying to get pregnant so you prescribe mefenamic acid for her, knowing it is very effective in reducing the blood flow.
What type of drug is this?
  a. Cyclo-oxygenase inhibitor
  b. Derivative of 17α-ethinyl testosterone
  c. Gonadotropin-releasing hormone agonist
  d. Plasminogen activator inhibitor
  e. Synthetic steroid hormone

Ans. a.

Q.5 A 45-year-old woman with history of vulval itching and soreness for past 2 years attends the gynecology clinic. She is a smoker. She gives a history of using high-potency steroid ointment previously with no symptom relief. A biopsy in the clinic reports vulval intraepithelial neoplasia (VIN) 3. You counsel her for excision of the lesion.
What percentage of VIN ultimately have unrecognized invasion detected on excision?
  a. 5%
  b. 10%
  c. 15%
  d. 20%
  e. 25%

Ans. d. Ref: RCOG Green Top Guideline No. 58, 2011

Q.6 A 55-year-old woman is due to come in for total abdominal hysterectomy and bilateral salpingo-oophorectomy for a large mucinous ovarian cyst. She takes sequential hormone replacement therapy (HRT) for menopausal symptoms.
You discuss with her the risk of venous thromboembolism. How long prior to surgery should she stop HRT?
  a. 2 weeks
  b. 3 weeks
  c. 4 weeks
  d. 5 weeks
  e. 6 weeks

Ans. c.

Q.7 A 22-year-old woman presents to the early pregnancy unit with mild left iliac fossa pain. Examination is normal. She has a positive urine pregnancy test. Her serum human chorionic gonadotropin (hCG) is 700 IU/L.
A transvaginal ultrasound scan reports:
'Bulky anteverted uterus with a 2 mm cystic area centrally located within the endometrial cavity. Both ovaries have normal ultrasonic appearances. There are no adnexal masses or free fluid in the pelvis.'
What is the most appropriate management?
  a. Diagnostic laparoscopy +/– proceed
  b. Methotrexate therapy
  c. Serum hCG (human chorionic gonadotropin) measurement in 48 hours
  d. Serum progesterone
  e. Ultrasound scan in 7 days

Ans. c. This is a pregnancy of unknown location (PUL). Ultrasound findings suggest a pseudosac. A true gestational sac would be eccentrically located and have a double decidual sac sign (two concentric rings surrounding an anechoic sac). The visualization of the yolk sac is the critical landmark of the gestational sac. Performing serial serum hCG measurements is the next most appropriate step to guide further management.

Q.8 A 70-year-old woman had noticed that her voice has deepened and she has increasing hair on her face over the last 3 years. Serum testosterone is elevated at 7.2 nmol/L and DHEAS (dehydroepiandrosterone) and urinary 17 ketosteroids are normal.
   Which of the following is the most likely diagnosis?
   a. Adrenal carcinoma
   b. Congenital adrenal hyperplasia
   c. Ovarian hyperthecosis
   d. Polycystic ovary syndrome
   e. Sertoli-Leydig cell tumor

Ans. c.

Q.9 A 45-year-old woman underwent total abdominal hysterectomy for heavy menstrual bleeding. She has received treatment for cervical intraepithelial neoplasia (CIN) 3 and is on annual smears. Hysterectomy specimen has reported no CIN. What would be the management plan?
   a. Continue annual smears
   b. Human papillomavirus testing
   c. No follow-up
   d. Vault smear in 6 months
   e. Vault smear in 12 months

Ans. d.

Q.10 A 30-year-old woman presents to the infertility clinic with primary infertility and dysmenorrhea and is found on ultrasound to have a 6-cm endometrioma in the left ovary.
   What is the most appropriate initial management?
   a. Gonadotropin-releasing hormone agonist for 6 months
   b. *In vitro* fertilization
   c. Intrauterine insemination
   d. Laparoscopic drainage of the endometrioma
   e. Laparoscopic excision of the endometrioma

Ans. e.

Chapter 61: Model Questions and Answers for Practice of EMQs

EXTENDED MATCHING QUESTIONS (EMQs) IN GYNECOLOGY

EMQs have considerable advantages over the Multiple Choice Questions (MCQs). EMQs need application of knowledge in a clinical scenario. MCQs only test the memory with simple factual recall without any clinical context.

The models of EMQs given in the book are to help the medical students for their preparation. Few models of EMQs are given from RCOG for exact standard.

The answersheet is numbered 1–20 and against each number there are twenty lozenges labeled from A to T. Each question in the question booklet will consist of an option list (with same type of letter to reflect the answersheet). A lead-in statement (which tells the candidate clearly what to do) is there and then a list of one to five questions (each numbered, again to match the answersheet). Candidate is expected to judge each particular question and to answer by boldly blackening out the letter that corresponds the single best answer in the option list. In the examination, the option list may provide 10–14 answer options. The option lists will nearly always be in alphabetical or numerical order for ease of reference.

The candidate is expected to select the single answer that fits best. There may be several possible answers but only the most likely one from the option list must be chosen.

The model of a complete answersheet is shown with the EMQs section dealt below:

Marking: Incorrect answers are not penalized. Each correct EMQs answer will be scored one mark. Candidate is encouraged to fill one lozenge for each of the 20 answers. Marking of two or more boxes for one question, no mark is awarded even if one of the answers is correct. Any mistake must be erased clearly and completely.

Examples of the EMQs Format

EMQs Sample 1. Theme: Neuroendocrinology in relation to reproduction

Options:
A. Follicle stimulating hormone (FSH)
B. Gonadotropin releasing hormone (GnRH)
C. Calcitonin
D. Insulin
E. Luteinizing hormone (LH)
F. Oxytocin
G. Cortisol
H. Parathyroid hormone
I. Prolactin
J. Thyroxine
K. Growth hormone

Instructions: For each action described below, choose the single most likely causative hormone from the above option list. Each option can be used once, more than once or not at all.

Q.1 Causes hyperglycemia through lipolysis and opposing the effects of insulin.
Q.2 Function is essential for growth and development of central nervous system (CNS) and skeletal system.
Q.3 Induces aromatization in granulosa cells to convert androgens to estrogen.
Q.4 Continued stimulation may cause gonadotropic cells downregulation.
Q.5 Lowers plasma calcium concentration by reducing bone resorption.
Q.6 Inhibits glycogenolysis, increases glycolysis and promotes glycogenesis.
Q.7 Stimulates deposition of cartilage at the ends of bones.
Q.8 Initiates milk let-down reflex.
Q.9 Sustained and peak level augments ovulation.
Q.10 Enhances urinary excretion of calcium.

The answersheet area will look like this and correct responses are to be put as shown below:

	[A]	[B]	[C]	[D]	[E]	[F]	[G]	[H]	[I]	[J]	[K]	[L]	[M]	[N]	[O]	[P]	[Q]	[R]	[S]	[T]
1	[A]	[B]	[C]	[D]	[E]	[F]	[■]	[H]	[I]	[J]	[K]	[L]	[M]	[N]	[O]	[P]	[Q]	[R]	[S]	[T]
2	[A]	[B]	[C]	[D]	[E]	[F]	[G]	[H]	[I]	[■]	[K]	[L]	[M]	[N]	[O]	[P]	[Q]	[R]	[S]	[T]
3	[■]	[B]	[C]	[D]	[E]	[F]	[G]	[H]	[I]	[J]	[K]	[L]	[M]	[N]	[O]	[P]	[Q]	[R]	[S]	[T]
4	[A]	[■]	[C]	[D]	[E]	[F]	[G]	[H]	[I]	[J]	[K]	[L]	[M]	[N]	[O]	[P]	[Q]	[R]	[S]	[T]
5	[A]	[B]	[■]	[D]	[E]	[F]	[G]	[H]	[I]	[J]	[K]	[L]	[M]	[N]	[O]	[P]	[Q]	[R]	[S]	[T]
6	[A]	[B]	[C]	[■]	[E]	[F]	[G]	[H]	[I]	[J]	[K]	[L]	[M]	[N]	[O]	[P]	[Q]	[R]	[S]	[T]
7	[A]	[B]	[C]	[D]	[E]	[F]	[G]	[H]	[I]	[J]	[■]	[L]	[M]	[N]	[O]	[P]	[Q]	[R]	[S]	[T]
8	[A]	[B]	[C]	[D]	[E]	[■]	[G]	[H]	[I]	[J]	[K]	[L]	[M]	[N]	[O]	[P]	[Q]	[R]	[S]	[T]
9	[A]	[B]	[C]	[D]	[■]	[F]	[G]	[H]	[I]	[J]	[K]	[L]	[M]	[N]	[O]	[P]	[Q]	[R]	[S]	[T]
10	[A]	[B]	[C]	[D]	[E]	[F]	[G]	[■]	[I]	[J]	[K]	[L]	[M]	[N]	[O]	[P]	[Q]	[R]	[S]	[T]

EMQs Sample 2. Theme: pelvic blood vessels and collateral circulation

Options:
- A. Common iliac artery
- B. External iliac artery
- C. Anterior division of internal iliac artery
- D. Main trunk of internal iliac artery
- E. Middle rectal artery
- F. Uterine artery
- G. Ovarian artery
- H. Inferior epigastric artery
- I. Inferior gluteal artery
- J. Superior rectal artery
- K. Superior vesicle artery
- L. Inferior rectal artery
- M. Internal pudendal artery

Mrs AR, 27-year-old multiparous lady suffers from atonic postpartum hemorrhage, following forceps delivery. Decision was made to go for bilateral ligation of iliac arteries as the bleeding continued in spite of all medical measures. Regarding establishment of collateral circulation, the following points were discussed.

Instructions: For each question presented below choose the single most appropriate option from the list above. Each option may be used once, more than once or not at all.

Q.11 Which iliac vessels are to be ligated?

Q.12 Which other vessel anastomoses with superior rectal artery?

Q.13 Which vessel does inferior epigastric arise from?

Q.14 Which other vessel anastomoses with the uterine artery?

Q.15 Which vessel runs above and anterior to the ureter?

Q.16 Which vessel does internal pudendal artery arise from?

Q.17 Which vessel does inferior rectal artery arise from?

Ans. 11 = C, 12 = E, 13 = B, 14 = G, 15 = F, 16 = C, 17 = M.

EMQs Sample 3. Theme: Physiology of menstruation

Options:
- A. Follicle stimulating hormone (FSH)
- B. Luteinizing hormone (LH)
- C. Estradiol (E2)
- D. Progesterone (PGN)
- E. Sex hormone binding globulin (SHBG)
- F. Estriol (E3)
- G. Gonadotropin releasing hormone (GnRH)
- H. Androstenedione
- I. Inhibin
- J. Dehydroepiandrosterone

Instructions: For each of the following case presentation below, select the hormone most likely to be responsible in the options above. Each option may be used once, more than once or not at all.

Q.18 A 7-year-old girl presents with isosexual precocious puberty. She started menstruation also. Details of investigations revealed accelerated bone maturation. Endocrine assay revealed the case as the constitutional variety.

Q.19 A 22-year-old woman is being investigated for her inability to conceive. She is instructed to maintain the basal body temperature (BBT). The chart showed a rise of core body temperature by 1°F. (See Dutta's Textbook of Gynecology, 8th Edition, p. 195).

Q.20 A 29-year-old woman is being treated for primary infertility. She had regular menstrual cycle. She had been instructed to perform urine test using a kit at home on daily basis for 5 consecutive days in each cycle, depending on her cycle length. (See Dutta's Textbook of Gynecology, 8th Edition, p. 195).

Q.21 A 40-year-old woman with irregular cycles seeks investigations for her inability to conceive. Her doctor feels to perform a blood test to see her ability to conceive as regard the functional status of the ovary. (See FSH in Dutta's Textbook of Gynecology, 8th Edition, p. 200, 442).

Q.22 A 28-year-old woman attends the infertility clinic after 3 years of her marriage. Speculum examination was done for cervical smear. At the same time cervical mucus was taken for fern test, which showed characteristic fern-tree appearance. (See Dutta's Textbook of Gynecology, 8th Edition, p. 93).

Ans. 18 = G, 19 = D, 20 = B, 21 = A, 22 = C.

EMQs Sample 4. Options for Questions 23–24

- A. Atrophic vulvovaginitis
- B. Benign mucous membrane pemphigoid
- C. Paget's disease
- D. Contact dermatitis
- E. Eczema
- F. Herpes simplex infection
- G. HIV infection
- H. Human papillomavirus infection
- I. Lichen planus
- J. Lichen sclerosus
- K. Lichen simplex chronicus
- L. Psoriasis
- M. Vulval intraepithelial neoplasia
- N. Vulvodynia

Instructions: For each clinical scenario below, choose the single most likely diagnosis from the list above. Each diagnosis may be used once, more than once, or not at all.

Q.23 A 23-year-old woman presents with a two-year history of vulval, perineal and perianal irritation. The vulva is red, excoriated and there are areas of white, thickened skin. Application of 3% acetic acid shows areas of mosaic and coarse punctuation.

Q.24 A 68-year-old woman presents with vulval irritation, soreness and dysuria. On examination, the vulvar skin looks white. Vulvar biopsy revealed hyperkeratosis and thinning of the epithelium. There is hyalinization and chronic inflammatory cell infiltrate in the subepithelial zone.

Ans. 23 = M, 24 = J.

EMQs Sample 5. Options for Questions 25–27

- A. Damage to bladder/ureter
- B. Damage to bowel
- C. Failure rate 1 in 200
- D. Failure to gain entry into abdominal cavity
- E. Failure to identify disease
- F. Failure to visualize uterine cavity
- G. Hemorrhage requiring blood transfusion
- H. Hemorrhage requiring return to theater
- I. Laparotomy
- J. Pain
- K. Premature menopause
- L. Removal of ovaries
- M. Urinary retention
- N. Uterine perforation
- O. Vaginal bleeding

Instructions: For each of the case histories described below, choose the single most relevant complication that you must discuss with the patient when taking consent prior to surgery from the above list of options. Each option may be used once, more than once or not at all.

Q.25 A 52-year-old woman with frequent heavy periods is listed for diagnostic hysteroscopy. She has had two children both delivered by cesarean section. She is hypertensive and her body mass index (BMI) is 26 kg/m^2.

Q.26 A 56-year-old woman is scheduled for laparotomy and possible bilateral salpingo-oophorectomy for an ovarian mass. She had a total abdominal hysterectomy at the age of forty for fibroids and is in discomfort with an ovarian mass which measures 15 cm in diameter on ultrasound examination.

Q.27 A 48-year-old nulliparous woman is scheduled for vaginal hysterectomy because of menorrhagia. Her uterus is enlarged equivalent to 14 weeks' gestation.

Ans. 25 = N, 26 = A, 27 = G.

EMQs Sample 6. Options for Questions 28–32

- A. Wide local excision and biopsy
- B. Radical hysterectomy
- C. Wide local ablation
- D. Total abdominal hysterectomy with bilateral salpingo-oophorectomy
- E. Radical vulvectomy with bilateral inguino-femoral lymphadenectomy
- F. Debulking (cytoreductive) surgery
- G. Chemotherapy
- H. Trachelectomy
- I. Radiotherapy
- J. Concurrent chemoradiation

Instructions: For each of the clinical case presentation given below, select the most appropriate treatment from the list of options. Each option may be used once, more than once or not at all.

Q.28 Mrs AR, 32-year-old parous woman presents with moderate dyskaryotic smear. Subsequent colposcopy revealed well-defined area of acetowhite epithelium at the transformation zone. Colposcopy-directed biopsy confirmed CIN III. (See Dutta's Textbook of Gynecology, 8th Edition, p. 271)

Q.29 Mrs A, 67-year-old lady presents with vulval sore and discharge. Clinical examination revealed a 3 × 4 cm ulcerated lesion on inspection. Inguinal lymph nodes were enlarged. Biopsy from the lesion confirmed squamous cell carcinoma of the vulva. (*See* Dutta's Textbook of Gynecology, 8th Edition, p. 280)

Q.30 A 48-year-old lady presents with an abdominal mass of 20 weeks size. Serum CA-125 was 1020 IU/mL. She underwent laparotomy where stage IIIa. Ovarian cancer was diagnosed. (*See* Dutta's Textbook of Gynecology, 8th Edition, p. 317)

Q.31 A 39-year-old multiparous woman presents with postcoital bleeding. On speculum examination, cervix appeared abnormal. Punch biopsy confirmed squamous cell carcinoma of the cervix. FIGO staging made the case stage IIIb. (*See* Dutta's Textbook of Gynecology, 8th Edition, p. 287)

Q.32 A 57-year-old nulliparous woman, known to be diabetic and hypertensive, presents with postmenopausal bleeding. Hysteroscopy and endometrial biopsy revealed well-differentiated adenocarcinoma of the endometrium. (*See* Dutta's Textbook of Gynecology, 8th Edition, p. 299)

Ans. **28** = A, **29** = E, **30** = F, **31** = J, **32** = D.

Section 9: History in Obstetrics and Gynecology

Section Outline

Ch. 62. History in Obstetrics and Gynecology

Chapter 62: History in Obstetrics and Gynecology

HISTORY IN OBSTETRICS AND GYNECOLOGY

List of eminent personalities with their contributions in Obstetrics and Gynecology has been presented in this section. Sometimes questions are asked by the examiner in relation to such personalities with their contributions. Failure to answer such question is not going to fail the candidate, but certainly this improves the impression of the candidate if he or she could answer it.

Fallopio, Gabriele (1523–1563): He was the Professor of Surgery, Anatomy and Botany at the University of Padua, Italy. He described the fallopian tubes (Oviducts) in 1561.

Chamberlen, Peter (1601–1683) obstetric forceps: The modern obstetric forceps is the modification of original forceps designed by Chamberlen. Much had been written about the Chamberlen family (*See* Dutta's Textbook of Obstetrics, 9th Edition, p. 531). William Chamberlen was a Huguenot Surgeon in Paris. He fled to England in 1569 due to religious persecution. He had two sons, Peter (elder) and Peter (younger). The son of Peter (younger) was also named Peter (1601–1683). He was known as Dr Peter as he received medical degrees from Padua, Oxford and Cambridge. Forceps were kept secret within the family for about a century. Four pairs of Chamberlen forceps are now on display at the RCOG, London.

de Graaf, Regnier (1641–1673): He was born in Holland and worked as an Anatomist and Physician in France. He described graafian follicle (mature ovarian follicle) in 1672 (*See* Dutta's Textbook of Gynecology, 8th Edition, p. 69).

Bartholin, Caspar (1655–1738): He was the Professor of Anatomy, Medicine and Physics at the University of Copenhagen. He described Bartholin's gland (greater vestibular glands) in 1677 (*See* Dutta's Textbook of Gynecology, 8th Edition, p. 2).

Douglas, James (1675–1742): Anatomist and 'male midwife' working in London. He was the physician to Queen Caroline, the wife of George II. He is remembered by his descriptions:
- ***Pouch of Douglas:*** Rectovaginal pouch (*See* Dutta's Textbook of Gynecology, 8th Edition, p. 16).
- ***Semicircular fold of Douglas:*** Lower arcuate margin of the posterior rectus sheath, situated below the level of umbilicus.

Wolff, Kaspar (1733–1794): Professor of Anatomy and Physiology at St Petersburg. He described Wolffian duct (mesonephric duct) in 1759 (*See* Dutta's Textbook of Gynecology, 8th Edition, p. 27).

Naegele, Franz Carl (1778–1851): Franz Carl Naegele is remembered for three things: Pelvic deformity, Naegele's obliquity (anterior asyclitism). Franz Carl Naegele was born in Dusseldorf, Germany. He was the Director at the University of Heidelberg, succeeding his father-in-law in the position.

Cloquet, Jules Germain (1790–1883): Professor of Anatomy and Surgery in Paris. He was the president of the French Academy of Medicine. He described the lymph gland of Cloquet (1817), which is the uppermost deep femoral node situated in the femoral canal (*See* Dutta's Textbook of Gynecology, 8th Edition, p. 22, 24, 510).

Christian Doppler, Johann (1803–1853): Austrian Physicist and Mathematician. Doppler effect of ultrasound was described by him in 1842.

Sims, James Marion (1813–1883): An American Gynecologist and is recognized by his pioneering work on vesicovaginal fistula repair. Some of his many other contributions are: ***Sims' Speculum, Sims' position and Sims' wire*** (*See* Dutta's Textbook of Gynecology, 8th Edition, p. 84, 528). Sims bought a malleable pewter spoon and fashioned it into a retractor for the posterior vaginal wall. This was the forerunner of ***Sims' Speculum*** (*See* Dutta's Textbook of Gynecology, 8th Edition, p. 528, Fig. 38.2). Sims made many contributions to surgery and Gynecology. In 1876, he was elected the President of American Medical Association and in 1880 became the President of the American Gynecological Society.

Sims published an account of his surgical technique in 1852 using ***silverwire as suture material*** for repair of vesicovaginal fistula (VVF). Sims' relentless pursuit of surgical cure of VVF was recognized almost a century later by ***John Chassor Moir***, a subsequent master of surgery of VVF. He died of coronary thrombosis on 13 November 1883. A bronze statue of James Marion Sims stands in Central Park, New York.

Spencer Wells, Thomas (1818–1897): He was a surgeon at the Samaritan Free Hospital for Women and Children, London (UK). He devised the clamp to place across the ovarian pedicles. He established himself as the most prolific ovariotomist of his era. In 1884, he was elected the President of Royal College of Surgeons (See Dutta's Textbook of Gynecology, 8th Edition, p. 540).

Braxton-Hicks, John (1825-1997): Obstetrician and Gynecologist at Guy's Hospital, London. He described intermittent painless uterine contractions during pregnancy. "Braxton-Hicks Contractions" in 1871. He also described bipolar (combined external and internal) version in 1860.

Hegar, Alfred (1830-1914): Professor of Obstetrics and Gynecology in Freiburg. He designed the metallic-graded cervical dilators, Hegar's dilator.

Allis Oscar Huntington (1836-1921): He was a surgeon at Presbyterian Hospital, Philadelphia, USA.

Emil Theodor Kocher (1841-1917): He was the Professor of Surgery, Berne, Switzerland. He was awarded Nobel Prize for Physiology or Medicine in 1909 for his work on the physiology, pathology and surgery of thyroid gland.

Pinard, Adolphe (1844-1934): Pinard was a great clinical teacher in Obstetrics during his time. He was the first to promote antenatal care and to establish the value of logical and systematic approach for abdominal palpation in pregnancy. His contributions in Obstetrics for the management of pregnancy and labor are many. Obstetric maneuvers—the external cephalic version, bringing down the extended leg in frank breech presentation, go by his name (Pinard's maneuvers). He is also remembered for the Pinard fetal stethoscope (See Dutta's Textbook of Obstetrics, 9th Edition, p. 622).

Friedrich, Schauta (1849-1919) radical vaginal hysterectomy: Schauta popularized the vaginal radical hysterectomy to reduce the operative mortality of abdominal procedure (See Dutta's Textbook of Gynecology, 8th Edition, p. 291). Schauta's technique was later modified by Alfred Amreich (1885-1972) to remove more pelvic connective tissues. This procedure is often known as **Schauta-Amreich operation**. He was head of the department in University of Vienna in 1891. Later on Schauta had disagreement with his assistant, Wertheim, who left him in 1897.

Deaver John Blair (1855-1931): He was Professor of Surgery at University of Pennsylvania Medical School, Philadelphia, USA.

Wertheim, Ernst (1864-1920): Gynecologist from Vienna. He described ***Wertheim's operation*** (***Radical hysterectomy***) in 1900 (See Dutta's Textbook of Gynecology, 8th Edition, p. 291, 507). He worked as assistant to ***Friedrich Schauta***. Later on, he became the Professor of Gynecology. Wertheim was an excellent sportsman particularly in skiing and skating. He died of influenza at 56 years of age.

Pomeroy, Ralph Hayward (1867-1925): Ralph Pomery developed the simple procedure of tubal ligation which goes by his name 'Pomeroy tubal ligation'. It was not Ralph himself but two of his colleagues Dr Eliot Bishop and WF Nelms, presented his technique at the New York State Medical Society on June 1929, 4 years after his death. This method is accepted as a simple, safe and effective method all over world.

Das Sir KN (1867-1936): Consultant Obstetrician and Gynecologist and Principal of Carmichael (now RG Kar) Medical College, Kolkata. He designed a special variety of long curved obstetric forceps suited for the Indian women, whose pelvis and baby sizes are comparatively small to the Western countries. This is popularly known as the Das's variety of obstetric forceps.

Pantaleoni, D Commander C (1869): Pantaleoni made the first report on the use of endoscope (hysteroscope) to diagnose and treat an intrauterine lesion in 1869. Initial works on hysteroscope was done by Philipp Bozzini in 1805.

Initial hysteroscopy use was made by paraffin lamp illumination as devised by Francis Cruse of Dublin in 1865. It took more than a century for diagnostic and operative hysteroscopy to become popular.

Andrews, Henry (1871-1942): Consultant Obstetrician and Gynecologist working at London Hospital. His name is associated with Brandt-Andrews maneuvers; which describes the procedure of delivery of the placenta by controlled cord traction and suprapubic pressure.

Krukenberg, Friedrich (1871-1946): Pathologist and Professor of Ophthalmology, Halle. He described Krukenberg tumor in 1896 (See Dutta's Textbook of Gynecology, 8th Edition, p. 325).

Bonney, William Francis Victor (1872-1953): Gynecologist at the Middlesex Hospital, the Chelsea Hospital for women and the Postgraduate Medical School, London. His contributions to Gynecology are manifold. He is mostly remembered for his conservative surgery for fibroids (myomectomy). Unfortunately, before he pioneered myomectomy, his wife had subtotal hysterectomy for fibroid uterus. His significant contributions are:

- ***Bonney's hood myomectomy:*** Myomectomy using anterior hood type incision to prevent adhesions (See Dutta's Textbook of Gynecology, 8th Edition, p. 507 and Bedside Clinics and Viva-Voce, p. 568).
- ***Bonney's myomectomy clamps:*** Special clamps used to compress the uterine arteries at the base of the broad ligament during myomectomy operation (See Dutta's Textbook of Gynecology, 8th Edition, p. 537, Fig. 38.22).
- ***Bonney's myomectomy screw (See Dutta's Textbook of Gynecology, 8th Edition, p. 536, Fig. 38.21):*** Special type of screw used to fix a big myoma after incising the capsule.

Traction is maintained when the myoma is enucleated out of its bed (myomectomy).
- **Bonney's test:** Elevation of bladder neck during vaginal examination. It was used as a diagnostic test for stress urinary incontinence and its success for repair surgery. Currently this test is not practiced.
- **Bonney's gynecological surgery:** Textbook of Operative Gynecology, first edition was in 1911.

Couvelaire, Alexandre (1873-1948) Paris Obstetrician: He described Couvelaire uterus (uteroplacental apoplexy) in 1911 (*See* Dutta's Textbook of Obstetrics, 9th Edition, p. 238).

Green-Armytage, Vivian Bartley (1882-1961): MB, worked as the captain in Indian Medical Service. He was the resident surgeon at Eden Hospital, Calcutta (1912). Later, he became the Professor of Obstetrics in the same department. He also worked in West London Hospital. He devised the forceps, 'Green-Armytage forceps' for holding the uterine incision margins and the angles during cesarean section (*See* Dutta's Textbook of Obstetrics, 9th Edition, p. 621, Fig. 42.29).

Papanicolaou, George Nicholas (1883-1962): He worked in New York hospital on exfoliative cytology for the diagnosis of cancer of the female genital tract. In collaboration with **Dr Herbert Trout**, he published their landmark work in 1941. Later, in 1947, **James Ire** simplified cell collection procedure with a wooden spatula. This is currently being used. In 1961, Papanicolaou became the director of the Miami Cancer Institute.

Asherman, Joseph (1889-1968): Gynecologist from Tel Aviv. Intrauterine adhesion (synechiae) associated with amenorrhea is recognized by his name Asherman's syndrome (*See* Dutta's Textbook of Gynecology, 8th Edition, p. 384). He was not the first to report the syndrome that bears his name. In fact, Asherman did not describe endometrial destruction and adhesions as the cause of amenorrhea. He described the amenorrhea to sclerosis of the internal os.

Foley, Frederick Eugene Basil (1891-1966)—Frederick Foley was a urologist in St Paul's Hospital, Minnesota. He devised a 'hemostatic bag' catheter, to provide hemostatic tamponade to the excised prostatic bed and for continuous drainage of bladder. It was originally a soft rubber catheter with a balloon sleeve of rubber around the shaft below the eye of the catheter. Currently, the catheter is made of latex which is less irritating to urethral mucosa. Frederick Foley died of lung cancer in 1966.

Meigs, Joseph (1892-1963): Professor of Gynecology at Harvard University. He described Meigs' syndrome in 1937 (*See* Dutta's Textbook of Gynecology, 8th Edition, p. 245).

Turner, Henry (1892-1970): Professor of Medicine, Oklahoma University, USA. He described Turner's syndrome, (Ovarian dysgenesis 45, XO) (*See* Dutta's Textbook of Gynecology, 8th Edition, p. 369). He became the doyen of clinical endocrinology in United States. He diagnosed his own lung cancer as inoperable. He worked until his death on 4th August, 1970.

Mitra, Subodh (1896-1961): Gynecological Cancer Surgeon and Vice-Chancellor, University of Calcutta, India. He is remembered for his new technique of operation, 'radical vaginal hysterectomy with bilateral extraperitoneal lymphadenectomy'. This operation is popularly known as 'Mitra's operation for cancer of the cervix (*See* Dutta's Textbook of Gynecology, 8th Edition, p. 291).

Shirodkar, VN (1899-1971): He was born in Goa, India. Gynecologist from Grant Medical College, Mumbai, India. He introduced 'Shirodkar's Stitch' cervical encirclage operation in 1955, for cases with cervical incompetence and recurrent midtrimester abortion (*See* Dutta's Textbook of Obstetrics, 9th Edition, p. 162). He was the President of the Federation of Obstetric and Gynecological Societies of India. He received the Honorary Fellowship of the Royal College of Obstetricians and Gynecologists (RCOG), London. He was a good golf and tennis player. He was awarded Padma Bhushan in 1960.

Vigneaud, Vincent Du (1901-1978): Revolution in the use of oxytocic drugs was made with the identification and synthesis of oxytocin in 1953. Working in the Department of Biochemistry of Cornell University Medical College, Vigneaud and his colleagues identified and synthesized the hormone oxytocin and also vasopressin. Du Vigneaud received Nobel Prize for chemistry in 1955 for his landmark research in identification and synthesis of posterior pituitary hormones.

Leventhal, Michael (1901-1971): American Obstetrician and Gynecologist. He along with **Stein, Irving** from Chicago, described **Stein-Leventhal syndrome (polycystic ovarian disease)** in 1935 (*See* Dutta's Textbook of Gynecology, 8th Edition, p. 384).

Palmer, Raoul (1905-1985): Raoul Palmer used his technique of laparoscopy in gynecology in 1943. Besides laparoscopy, he was also a noted surgeon for his skills in tubal and vaginal surgery, 'Palmer's Point' in laparoscopic surgery goes by his name (*See* Dutta's Textbook of Gynecology, 8th Edition, p. 517). He assisted Vivian Green Armytage, while in Paris, in vaginal hysterectomy operation.

Menon, K Krishna (1908-1988): Gynecologist from Madras (presently Chennai), served the Indian Medical Service in the Second World War. He was the Professor of Obstetrics and Gynecology at Madras Medical College and Stanley Medical College. He became the Director Professor of the Institute of Obstetrics and Gynecology at Madras Medical College and Government Hospital for Women and Children. He was a Visiting Professor in Britain and United States. Menon became the President of Federation of Obstetrics and Gynecological Societies of India in 1961 and honorary Fellow of the Royal College of Obstetricians and Gynecologists. He was awarded "Padma Shri" in 1973 by the President of India. Menon presented his results using, Lytic Cocktail in the management of eclampsia at the University College Hospital, London in 1960. He spoke with his own experience from the hospital that he worked. Menon's monumental work on "lytic cocktail" using phenothiazine and pethidine in eclampsia was published in Jr Obstet Gynecol, Br Common W.

Apgar, Virginia (1909-1974): Anesthetist working in America. She introduced 'Apgar Score' for assessment of cardiopulmonary and neurological status of the newborn at birth. This was described in 1953. Virginia Apgar's newborn score is used almost universally. She was apparently a fast walker, fast talker and a fast driver. She started flying lessons when she was 59 years old. Apgar was a popular musician and played cello and violin. Virginia Apgar died in her sleep on 7th August 1974.

Ayre, James Ernest (1910-1974): He is recognized by his contribution of a special spatula for collecting cervical smear 'Ayre's spatula' (*See* Dutta's Textbook of Gynecology, 8th Edition, p. 527). He was the director of Papanicolaou Cancer Research Institute, Miami, Florida.

Donald Ian (1910-1987): Professor of Obstetrics and Gynecology at Queen Mother's Hospital, Glasgow. He introduced the use of ultrasound, 'Sonar' in medicine. He was the author of the book, 'Practical Obstetric Problems'. Ian served in Royal Air Force as a Medical Officer from 1942-46. From the experience of the two World Wars, he thought of the echo sounding system that was used for antisubmarine detection. He worked with **Tom Brown**, a brilliant young engineer to produce the first contact compound sector scanner described in the Lancet in 1958.

Donald was an enthusiastic, ambitious and a revered man. His book, **Practical Obstetric Problems**, reflects his vast experience and the entertaining type of writing. He underwent cardiac surgery for rheumatic heart disease on three occasions. Besides all his medical carrier, Donald was an accomplished sailor, pianist and artist. He suffered repeated heart failures and died on 19 June 1987. Throughout the world, these days, ultrasound is in use in every hospital in almost every department—a great discovery by a great man.

Purandare, BN (1911-1990): Gynecologist from Mumbai, India, is recognized by his abdominal cervicopexy operation for cases with nulliparous prolapse (prolapse without a cystocele) (*See* Dutta's Textbook of Gynecology, 8th Edition, p. 184).

Steptoe, Patrick Christopher (1913-1988), Edwards, Robert Geoffrey (1925-2013): Patrick Steptoe was a consultant Obstetrician and Gynecologist in the district hospital Oldham, Lancashire, England. World's first test tube baby, Louise Joy Brown was born in 25 July, 1978. This was the culmination of 10 years collaborative research between **Patrick Steptoe** and **Robert Edwards** the two men residing 250 km apart. **Bob Edwards** was the geneticist and embryologist working at Cambridge. They faced criticism about the ethics. They worked against the hardship of fund and repeated failures to achieve implantation. Patrick Steptoe was a talented musician. After the retirement from the National Health Service (NHS), he worked at Bourn Hall to train others. He died on 21 March, 1988 from prostate cancer. Bob Edwards was born in Yorkshire, England. He received PhD in animal genetics in Edinburgh. He conducted further research on induction of ovulation and IVF in animals. This knowledge, in fact, led Edwards to meet Steptoe as his clinical partner. In 1968, Edwards approached Steptoe at Royal Society of Medicine, London, where Steptoe presented his work on gynecological laparoscopy. Bob Edwards was appointed the Scientific Director of the Bourn Hall Clinic in 1980.

The revolution in reproductive medicine made by Steptoe and Edwards came following the years of tenacious endeavor with limited resources and in the face of opposition (*See* Dutta's Textbook of Gynecology, 8th Edition, p. 206).

INDEX

Page numbers followed by *f* refer to figure, *fc* refer to flowchart, and *t* refer to table, respectively.

A

Abdominal incision 201
    types of 202*f*
Abnormal uterine bleeding 29, 64, 94, 96, 154, 209
    basic pathology of 98
    causes of 96
    classification of 94
    differential diagnosis of 95
    iatrogenic causes of 98
    management of 98, 99
    prevalence of 96
    severity of 96
Abortion
    aspiration 161*t*
    follow-up care of 160
    guidelines, WHO medical management of 158
    incomplete 162
    induced 159, 162
    management of 158, 162
    medical 157, 158, 160, 179
    methods of 157
    septic 162
    surgical 157-160
Acanthosis nigricans 75*f*, 78
Acne 78
Acquired immunodeficiency syndrome 50, 66
Actinomycin D 193
Activated protein C resistance 59
Add-back therapy 84
Adenocarcinoma 26, 26*f*
    endometrial 29
    primary peritoneal 38
    serous 225
Adenomyomectomy 88
Adenomyosis 7, 88, 90, 95, 96, 98, 140
    clinical features of 87
    diagnosis of 87
    management of 88, 89
    risks factors for 87
    surgical management of 88
    treatment of 7
    ultrasonographic diagnostic criteria of 87
    uteri 87
Adnexal mass 100, 101*f*, 102
    differential diagnosis for 100
    management of 100, 102
Adoption 117
Adrenal disease 12, 115
Adrenal gland 35
    androgen producing tumors of 78
Adrenogenital syndrome 13*f*, 44
    characteristic features of 13
    congenital 37
Alkali hematin 62

Alopecia 78, 190
Alpha-fetoprotein 102
Amenorrhea 3, 9, 98, 104, 113, 190
    induction of 104
    primary 12, 32, 36
    secondary 14, 32, 34
American Society for Reproductive Medicine 130*t*
Amniotic sac 207*f*
Anal canal 54
Anastrozole 88
Androgen 39, 74, 85
    binding proteins 123
    exogenous 78
    insensitivity syndrome 13
    metabolism 48
    role of 138
    sources of 36
Androgenic-anabolic steroid 78
Anencephaly 51
Anesthesia, local 160
Aneuploidy screening 138
Angiogenesis 191
Anovulation 98, 117, 189
Anovulatory dysfunctional uterine bleeding 98
Anovulatory infertility, problems of 16
Antiangiogenesis agents 191
Antibiotics 215
    broad-spectrum 147
    prophylactic 214
    regimens 216
Anticonvulsants 147
Antiemetic drugs 192
Antiestrogens 71
Anti-Müllerian hormone 89, 109, 116, 135, 137
    levels of 135
    physiological functions of 135
Antimuscarinic drugs 68
Antioxidant food supplement 124
Antiphospholipid antibody 58
    syndrome 57, 58, 60, 149
Antiretroviral therapy 148
    toxicities of 67
Antithrombin 59
Antral follicle count 115, 135
Aortic lymphadenectomy 26
APA syndrome, diagnosis of 60
Apgar score 268
Apoptosis 196
Aromatase inhibitors 71, 84, 88
Arterial cardiovascular disease 148
Arteriovenous malformation 97, 98
    diagnosis of 97
Artificial urinary sphincter 69
Asherman's syndrome 44
Aspirin, low-dose 138

Assisted reproductive technology 16, 18, 75, 107, 119, 124, 126, 130*t*, 133, 134
    cycle 89, 126, 127
    principle steps of 17
    different methods of 16
    health risks of 133
    procedure of 133
    steps of 127*t*
    treatment, adverse effects of 130*t*
Asthenospermia 123, 124
Asthma 92
Atresia 109, 111, 128
Autosomal chromosomal syndrome 52
Autosomal dominant inherited cancer 197
Azoospermia 124, 125
    classification 124
    testicular 124
    treatment 124

B

Bariatric surgery 229, 230
    place of 76
    principle of 229
Bartholin's gland 40, 265
Basal serum
    estradiol level 116
    inhibin B 135
Beta-human chorionic gonadotropin 181
Bevacizumab 191
Biopsy 29, 95, 185
    endometrial 62
    multiple peritoneal 185
    testicular 35
Bipolar electrosurgery 80
Bipolar radiofrequency endometrial ablation 210
Birth defects 67
Bladder injury 222
Blastocyst transfer 129
Bleeding 160
    disorders 65
    excessive 162
Blood 209
    loss, measurements of 62
    pressure 92
    transfusion 133
Boari flap 224*f*
Boari method 223
Body
    mass index 137
    surface area 192
    weight 137
Bone
    marrow depression 190
    mineral density 148
Bonney's gynecological surgery 267

Bonney's myomectomy 266
    clamps 266
    screw 266
Bonney's test 267
Botulinum toxin, injection of 69
Brachytherapy 194-196
Brain metastasis 178*f*
Brandt-Andrews maneuvers 266
Braxton-Hicks contractions 266
Breast
    atrophy of 78
    cancer 148
    disease, benign 92
    examination, clinical 11
    female 54
    self-examination 11
Breastfeeding 146, 148, 245
Bromocriptine therapy 36, 37
Burch colposuspension 46
Buserelin 126

C

Call-Exner body 51, 52
Camper's fascia 201
Cancer
    antigen 102
    cervix 97
    management of 23
    familial 29, 30
    gynecologic 197
    testicular 155
Carbohydrate intolerance 189
Carboplatin 191, 193
Carcinoma
    cervix
    management of 23
    pathogenesis of 22
    serum tumor markers of 25
    types of 21
    embryonal 102
Cardiac failure, congestive 211
Cardiovascular disease 76, 156
Catastrophic antiphospholipid syndrome 57
Cavitation 218
Cell death 196
Cellular pleomorphism 174
Centchroman (Saheli) 147
Cerebral
    canal 160, 207*f*
    funneling of 207*f*
    cancer 24, 183, 187, 195
    brachytherapy for 195
    elimination of 24
    radiotherapy for 195
    screening program 23, 41
    cap 162
    cerclage operation 206-208
    cytology screening 45
    ectopy 96, 98
    edema 211
    fibroid 10, 10*f*, 70
    incompetence 59, 206
    insufficiency 206
    intraepithelial neoplasia 32
    pathology 96
    preparation 160
Cervix 207*f*
    carcinoma of 21, 21*f*, 22-24, 24*f*, 25
    microinvasive cancer of 43
    squamous cell carcinoma of 21, 24
    ultrasonography of 207*f*
Cesarean delivery 133, 134
Cetrorelix 126
Chemoradiation, concurrent 23, 26
Chemotherapeutic drugs 193
Chemotherapy 149, 186, 190, 192
    prophylactic 49
    response, evolution of 192
Cherney incision 202
Chest infection 243
Chlamydia trachomatis 17, 65, 245
Chocolate cyst 8*f*, 82, 100, 100*f*
Chorioamnionitis 243
Choriocarcinoma 35, 47, 49, 102, 177*f*, 178*f*, 181
Chorionic villus sampling 52, 53
Clean wound 216
Clear cell carcinoma 171
Clitoris, enlargement of 78
Cloaca 38
Clomiphene 118
    citrate 138, 227
Coaptation 218
Cobra grasper 233*f*
Coffee bean nuclei 52
Colinidine 93
Colorectal cancer 29
Colporrhaphy, anterior 69
Colposcopy 51
Coma 211
Combined oral contraceptives 64, 70, 81, 84, 98, 126, 128, 135, 146, 163
    pill 6, 45
Complete mole, karyotype pattern of 10*f*
Computed tomography scan 29, 65
Condom 162, 163
Conformal radiation technique 195
Contaminated wound 216
Contraception 104, 143, 145, 152, 211
    advances in 145
    emergency 104, 162
    hormonal 147
    long-term reversible methods of 153
    methods of 149, 163
    permanent method of male 148
    post-abortion 162
Contraceptive
    long-acting reversible 148-150
    methods 162
    failure rates of 51
    pills, oral 137, 138
Contrast-enhanced computed tomography 97
Controlled ovarian stimulation 81, 121, 126, 138
Copper-bearing intrauterine device 163
Cornual ectopic pregnancy 236*f*
Coronary artery disease 117
Corporeal fibroids 70
Corpus luteum 31
    formation of 115
Corticosteroids 117
Couvelaire uterus 267

Craniopharyngioma 44
Cryopreservation, methods of 130
Cryosurgery 39
Cryptomenorrhea 12, 14, 15
Cushing's disease 78
Cushing's syndrome 78
Cut380 A 98, 145, 145*f*
Cyclooxygenase 99
Cyclophosphamide 186, 190
Cyst
    aspiration 80
    endometriotic 81
    multiple small 73*f*
    paraovarian 33, 101*f*
    simple 101
Cystectomy 80
Cystic fibrosis 124
    transmembrane regulator gene 124
Cystitis
    hemorrhagic 190
    interstitial 46, 83

D

Danazol 6, 88, 99
    side effects of 6
Deep dyspareunia 5
    causes of 37
Deep perineal pouch 39
Deep thermal injury 224
Dehydroepiandrosterone 117
Depot medroxyprogesterone acetate 70, 84, 163
Detrusor overactivity 46
Diabetes mellitus 92, 117, 189
    gestational 76, 118, 133
    juvenile 12
    non-insulin-dependent 74
Diaphragm 162, 163
Diarrhea 160
Diathermy 153, 155
Dienogest 84
Dirty wound 216
Distal tubal intraepithelial carcinoma 225
Docetaxel 193
Dominant follicle
    basically selection of 110
    emergence of 109
    selection of 115
Donor
    insemination 125
    oocyte 117, 131
Down's syndrome 52, 134
Doxorubicin 193
    hydrochloride liposome 191
Drugs 193
    adverse effects of 205
    dose calculation 192
    therapy 69
Dyschezia 83, 104
Dysfunctional uterine bleeding 105, 209
Dysgenetic gonads 14
Dysgerminoma 102
Dyslipidemia 74, 117, 189
Dysmenorrhea 83, 87, 104
    intractable 7*f*
    primary 49

Index

Dyspareunia 83, 87, 104
　causes of 8
　severe deep 8

E

Ectopy 37
Electrical vacuum aspiration 161
Elevated maternal serum alpha fetoprotein level 51
Embryo 130f
　cryopreservation of 130
　culture 129
　morphology 129
　quality, morphological assessment of 129
　transfer 117, 127, 130
　number of 130t
　procedure for 17, 130
Endocrine 109
　abnormalities 5
　factors 59, 61
Endodermal sinus tumor 102
Endometrial ablation 88, 99, 209
　indications for 210
　method 210
　procedures 211
Endometrial cancer 20, 29, 105, 167, 183, 189
　diagnosis of 20
　evaluation of 21
　management of 170, 172
　surgical staging of 197
　treatment of 167, 172, 173
Endometrial carcinoma 11, 19, 20, 26, 27, 27f, 31, 43, 96, 167f, 168, 170, 189
　diagnosis of 20
　high-risk factors for 26
　histological type of 26
　management of 168, 170
　surgical management of 170
Endometrial destruction
　commonly used first-generation methods of 210
　second-generation methods of 210
　techniques 210
Endometriomas 80-82
　laparoscopic cystectomy for 8
　large 82
　resection 85
Endometriosis 5, 7, 48, 80, 81, 83, 85, 104, 105, 120
　complications of 5
　deep infiltrating 83
　diagnosis of 83
　hysterectomy for 85
　mild 8, 80
　minimal 80
　moderate to severe 81
　severe 80
　sign of 83
　sites of 5
　surgical procedures for 85
　symptom of 83
　treatment of 53
Endometritis 243
Endometrium 9f, 26, 97
　antiproliferative effect on 104
　carcinoma of 26, 167
　complications of transcervical resection of 211
　ectopic 83
　evaluation of 97fc
　laser ablation of 210
　transcervical resection of 45, 63, 210
Epithelial ovarian
　cancer 28
　epidemiology for 28
　tumor 53
Epithelium, types of 45
Erythropoietin, synthetic 192
Estradiol 110
Estrogen 91
　dominant follicular microenvironment 111
　secretion 38
　therapy 91
　benefits of 91t
　route of 91
Ethamsylate 99
Ethinyl estradiol 146
Etoposide 191, 193
External beam radiation therapy 194

F

Facial hair
　excess growth of 3f
　male type of 75f
Fallopian tube 40, 50, 153f, 265
　cancer 97
　carcinoma of 36
Falope ring 153
Familial ovarian cancer 19, 101
Fascial interposition 155
Fatigue 191
Femoral artery catheterization 236f
Ferriman-Gallwey score 78
　modified 78f
Fertility
　awareness methods, use of 149
　conserving surgery 185
　preservation 175, 183
　sparing surgery 25, 175
　status 26
Fetal
　chromosomal abnormalities 58
　heart rate abnormalities, causes of 54
　malformations 52
　testis 37
　trisomy, risks of 134
Fever 160
Fibroid 90, 94f, 96, 140
　asymptomatic 70
　location of 70
　symptomatic 70
　uterus 7, 62f, 70
　management issues 70
Filshie clip 153, 153f
　loaded applicator 153f
Fimbrioplasty, laparoscopic 18f
First generation ablation techniques 63
Fitz-Hugh-Curtis syndrome 34
Fluid over load 211
Folic acid, administration of 124
Folinic acid 190
Follicle-stimulating hormone 44, 98, 109, 110, 112, 123, 126, 227
Follicular androgens, role of 138
Follicular atresia 109
Follicular growth 109, 110f, 111, 128
　monitoring of 17
　phases of 109, 110f
　process of 110
Folliculogenesis 109, 138
Frozen embryo transfer, endometrial preparation for 131

G

Gabapentin 93
Galactorrhea 115
Gamete intrafallopian transfer 127
Ganirelix 126
Gemcitabine 190
Genital organs
　carcinoma of 220
　development of 41, 49
　female 39, 47
Genital tract, developmental defect of 12
Genital tuberculosis 31, 33, 37, 39, 41, 118
Genitalia
　ambiguous 49
　external 38
Germ cell 109
　migration 109
　tumor 50, 53
　malignant 53
Gestational age
　duration of 157
　lower 133
Gestational trophoblastic disease 47, 149, 177, 180, 181
　follow up of 180
　management of 181, 182
　treatment of 179
Gestational trophoblastic neoplasia 97, 177, 181
Gestrinone 85, 99
Glands, endometrial 87
Glomerular filtration rate 191
Glucocorticoid receptor 104
Glutaraldehyde cross-linked collagen 69
Glycine overload 211
Gonadotropin 109, 118, 126t
　releasing hormone 44
　agonist 84, 117, 127, 137, 184
　analog 6, 16, 44, 64, 70, 81
　antagonist 84, 126-128, 138
　therapy 123
　stimulation 128, 137
　therapy, indications of 16
Gonads, development of 49
Gonorrhea 245
Goserelin 126
Graafian follicle 265
Granulocyte colony-stimulating factors 192
Granulosa cell 31
Greater vestibular glands 265
Growth
　factors 192
　hormone 109

Gynecological cancers 190
    radiotherapy in 194
Gynecological surgery, laparoscopic 223
Gynecology, endoscopy in 218

H

Hair
    growth 78
    rapid 78
    removal 215
Harmonic ultrasonic energy 218
Headache 243
Heart 91
    disease, ischemic 148
Heavy menstrual bleeding 62, 62f, 64, 209
    operative treatments for 63
    pharmacotherapy for 63
    surgical management of 209
Hegar's dilator 266
Hematocolpos 14, 14f
Hematuria 104
Hemolysis 211
Hemorrhage 211
Hemorrhagic disorder 64
Hemostatic clips 218
Heparin, unfractionated 60
Highly active antiretroviral therapy 67
Hilus cell tumor 78
Hirsutism 78
    ovarian causes of 35
Hobnail cells 52
Hormone replacement therapy 11, 46, 98
Hostile cervical mucus 124
Hot flushes 91
Human chorionic gonadotropin 177, 181, 184
Human growth hormone, role of 138
Human immunodeficiency virus 66
    infection, congenital 66
Human leukocyte antigen 57
Human menopausal gonadotropin 126
Human papillomavirus infection, pathogenesis of 22f
Human progesterone receptor 104
Human seminal fluid 42
Hydatidiform mole 9, 9f, 177
Hydrocephaly 10
Hydrosalpinx 17, 17f, 18, 119
Hydrothermal balloon ablation 210
Hydroxylase deficiency 13f
Hydroxysteroid dehydrogenase deficiency 78
Hyperammonemia 211
Hyperandrogenemia 4, 74, 78, 117, 189
    biochemical evaluation of 78
    clinical features of 78
    differential diagnosis of 78
    gestational 79
Hyperhomocysteinemia 59
Hyperinsulinemia 4, 37, 74
Hyperlipidemia 92
Hyperplasia 87, 95
Hyperplasia
    adrenal 35
    congenital adrenal 13f, 45, 78
    endometrial 11, 87
Hyperprolactinemia 115
Hypertension 92, 117
    gestational 133
Hyperthyroidism 98, 115
Hypertrophy 87
Hypogonadism 44
    hypergonadotropic 12, 115, 116
    hypogonadotropic 12, 115, 116
Hyponatremia 211
Hypothalamic-pituitary
    dysfunction 115, 117
    failure 115
Hypothesis, hormonal 225
Hypothyroidism 98, 115
Hysterectomy 11, 19, 26, 64, 72, 85, 88, 140, 212, 213
    abdominal 212
    benefits of 19
    bilateral oophorectomy during 19
    indication of 64, 189
    laparoscopic 212
    operation of 34
    radical 24, 24f, 168, 266, 267
    risks of 19
    robot-assisted 170, 213
    route of 64, 212
    total 34, 172
    abdominal 29, 100, 168, 189
    laparoscopic 170
    types of 22
Hysterosalpingography 60f
Hysteroscopy 20, 26, 29, 60f, 63, 65, 95
    advantages of 98
    limitations of 98

I

Idiopathic thrombocytopenic purpura 96
Ifosfamide 190
Immature oocytes, collection of 118
Immunotherapy 60
Implants 147, 150
In vitro fertilization 82, 117, 119, 124, 127
    cycle 17
    embryo transfer, indications of 16
    failure of 125
    insemination 129
    place of 81
    surrogacy 140
In vitro maturation 183
Indocyanine green 197
Infections 60, 96-98
    control of 158
    gynecological 245
    prevention of 158
    role of 121
    sites of 242
    types of 245
    viral 42
Infertility 3, 16, 17, 32, 80, 83, 87, 107, 113, 124
    causes of 5
    evaluation 113
    female 115
    male 123, 124
    management of 16, 113
    peritoneal factors for 120
    primary 16
    tubal factors for 118, 119
    unexplained 113, 121, 124, 125
Inflammatory bowel disease 83
Infracolic omentectomy 185
Inguinal canal 48
Injury, prevention of 221
Insemination 124
Insulin
    growth factor 109
    resistance 74
    sensitizers, place of 4
Intensity-modulated radiotherapy 194, 196
Internal iliac artery 40
    anterior division of 40
    bilateral ligation of 53
International Federation of Gynecology and Obstetrics 178, 209
    classifications 71, 71t
    early stage disease 167
    grading system 167
International Society for Minimally Invasive and Noninvasive Medicine 89
Intracavitary fibroids 71
Intracytoplasmic sperm injection 124, 127
    fertilization rate of 125
    procedure 125f
Intrauterine
    contraceptive devices 51, 98, 145, 150, 153, 162, 163
    fetal death 105
    insemination 16, 81, 120, 124, 127
Intravaginal radiation 168
Invasive carcinoma 22f
    cervix 39
    management of 22
Invasive moles 181
Isosexual precocious puberty, causes of 38

J

Jadelle® implant 148f
Joel-Cohen incision 203

K

Kallmann's syndrome 44, 123
Karyotype 45
Keratin pearls 52
Klinefelter's syndrome 113, 124
Kroener technique 153
Krukenberg tumor 32, 266

L

Labia majora 48
Labia minora 48
Labor, induction of 134
Lactate dehydrogenase 102
Laparoscopic ovarian
    diathermy 227
    drilling 4, 33, 51
    surgery 35, 51
    complications of 228
Laparoscopic surgery 6, 40, 80, 176, 218, 220-222
    limitations of 234
Laparoscopic uterosacral nerve ablation 85
Laparoscopic-assisted
    radical vaginal trachelectomy 26
    supracervical hysterectomy 213
    vaginal hysterectomy 170, 212

Index

Laparoscopy 60*f*, 65, 85, 120
    absolute contraindications of 39
    gynecologic 220
    indications of 85
Laparotomy 72, 174*f*, 175*f*, 176
    standard procedure of 175
Laser surgery 80
Leiomyoma 70, 87, 94*f*, 95, 98, 105, 221*f*
    management of 89
    subclassification of 94
Leptin 116
Lesions, endometriotic 85
Leucovorin 190
Leukemia 96
Leukopenia 190
Leuprorelin 126
Levator ani 40
Levonorgestrel-releasing intrauterine device 62, 64, 70, 84, 88, 91, 99, 145*f*, 152
Leydig cell 123
    tumor 78
Lippes loop 9*f*
Liver disease 98, 148
Low molecular weight heparin 60
Low-dose rate brachytherapy 194
Luteal phase defect 45, 122
    treatment for 122
Luteinizing hormone 44, 98, 109, 110, 112, 123
Lymph node
    approximate rate of 26
    dissection 29
    evaluation 172
    involvement 172
    para-aortic 29
    place of 29
Lymph vascular space involvement 189
Lymphadenectomy 168, 197
    bilateral extraperitoneal 267
    para-aortic 168, 172, 197
    place of 172

M

Madlener technique 153
Magnetic resonance imaging 27*f*, 29, 63, 65, 71, 83, 95, 97
Malaria 245
    severe 245
    uncomplicated 245
Malignancy 95
    gynecologic 183, 185, 194
    index, risk of 28
Marshall-Marchetti-Krantz procedure 69
Masculinization 78
Mass, presence of 100
Maternal sepsis 239, 241
Maternal serum alpha fetoprotein, low levels of 51
Matrix metalloproteinase 83
Mayer-Rokitansky-Küster-Hauser syndrome 12, 140
Maylard incision 202, 203
McCune-Albright syndrome 49
McDonald's operation 207
Medroxyprogesterone acetate 84, 99, 148
Meigs' syndrome 53, 267

Menopause 11, 19, 34, 46, 91
Menorrhagia 7*f*, 87, 96*f*
Menotropin 126
Menstrual cycle 31, 109, 111
    irregularities 78
    normal 48, 49
Menstruation 115
    abnormal 104
    cessation of 14
    normal 12
Mesonephric duct 265
Mesosalpinx 38
Metabolic syndrome 75, 117
Metallic-graded cervical dilators 266
Metformin 76, 117
    dose schedule of 76
    metabolic functions of 75
    therapy 75
Methotrexate 186, 190, 193, 205
Metrorrhagia 87
Microinvasive carcinoma cervix, management of 22
Microsurgical epididymal sperm aspiration 125
Midurethral retropubic tape 69
Mifepristone 45, 70, 85, 88, 104, 105, 160
Migraine 92
Minimally invasive surgery 85, 167, 170
Mirena 98
Miscarriage 17, 58, 60*f*, 76, 87, 133
    recurrent 57, 58, 60, 61, 76, 117, 140
Misoprostol administration
    buccal routes of 160*f*
    different routes of 160
    sublingual routes of 160*f*
Missed pills 146
    risks of 146
Mitotic catastrophe 196
Molar pregnancy 49, 149
    partial 149
    treatment of 179
Mucus debris 118
Mullerian duct system 50, 135
Multileaf collimator 194
Multiload 375 145, 145*f*
Mumps 113
Muscle transection incision 202*f*
Myolysis 72
Myoma 219*f*
    enucleation of 218*f*
    interstitial 120
    submucosal 120
Myomectomy 63, 64, 211, 266
    hysteroscopic 63, 212
    laparoscopic 72, 218*f*, 219*f*
    limitations of 90
Myometrium 26*f*, 27*f*
    evaluation of 97*fc*
    hypertrophic 98

N

Nafarelin 126
National Comprehensive Cancer Network 197
Natural killer cells 59
Nausea 160, 190, 191

Necrotizing fasciitis 216
Negative pressure wound therapy 215
Neisseria gonorrhoeae 245
Neoadjuvant chemotherapy 23, 29
    place of 29, 195
Neonatal intensive care unit 133
Neoplasia, nongestational 182
Neural tube defects 59
Night sweat 91
Non-descent vaginal hysterectomy 212
Non-invasive perinatal testing 134
Nonpolyposis colorectal cancer, hereditary 197
Nonsteroidal anti-inflammatory drugs 64, 81, 84
Norethisterone 84, 99
    acetate 84
    enantate 163
No-scalpel vasectomy 155, 155*f*
Nuclear atypia 174
NuvaRing 150

O

Obesity 4, 74, 92, 96, 133, 189, 220, 229, 230
    android 73
    central 74
    complications of 229
    gynecoid 73
    management of 229
    neonatal effects of 229
Obstetrics and gynecology, history in 263, 265
Olaparib 191
Oligoasthenoteratozoospermia syndrome 41
Oligomenorrhea 3, 113
Oligoovulation 117
Oligospermia 124
Omentectomy 197
Omplanon® implant 147*f*
Oncology 19
    gynecological 165
Oocyte
    cryopreservation of 130, 183, 185
    growth of 129
    maturation of 129, 129*f*
    primary 109
    retrieval 129
Oophorectomy 19, 64
Oophoropexy 185
Open surgery 80
Operative gynecology 199
Oral biguanide 117
Oral progestin pills 84
Oral progestogen 64
Orchitis, history of 113
Ormeloxifene 147
Osmotic dilators 160
    insertion of 160
Osteoporosis 11, 60, 92
    postmenopausal 46
Ovarian
    cancer 19, 27-29, 38, 41, 183, 185, 186, 197, 225
    low-grade serous 226, 226*t*
    management of 29
    staging of 185

carcinoma 225, 226
    types of 225
cycle, physiology of 115
cyst 102, 121
    complex 101
cystectomy 80
drilling 76
dysfunction 5
electrodiathermy, place of 76
failure, premature 32, 92, 115
fimbria 101*f*
follicular development 47
germ cell tumors 102
hyperstimulation syndrome 17, 89, 126, 133, 135, 136, 138
insufficiency 117
ligament 45
malignancy 28, 185
mass 175*f*
reserve 113, 135
    assessment of 116
    normal 136
    prediction of 135
    tests 116
response, prediction of 135
stimulation 128
stroma 73*f*
suppression 185
surgery 80
    conservative 185
tissue cryopreservation 183, 185
transposition 184, 185, 187
tumor 28*f*, 36, 45, 53, 174, 174*f*, 175*f*
    borderline 174
    malignant 185
volume measurement 135
Ovary 50, 112
    androgen producing tumors of 78
    carcinoma of 27
    chocolate cyst of 82, 100
    development of 41
    feminizing tumors of 51
    follicular cysts of 31
    germ cell tumor of 50
    granulosa cell tumor of 34, 50
    hormone producing tumors of 51
    neoplasms of 43
    sex cord stromal tumors of 36
    virilizing tumors of 51
Ovulation 42, 49, 109, 111, 115
    endocrine control of 109, 110
    failure of 112*fc*
    induction of 4, 16
    inhibition of 104
    physiology of 109
    process of 111
    suppression of 104
    theory 225
Ovulatory cycle 109, 111
Ovulatory disorders 16, 115, 116
    classification of 115
    management of 116
Ovulatory dysfunction 95, 115
Oxaliplatin 186
Oxygen
    dissociation curve 54
    therapy 242

P

Paclitaxel 193
Paget's disease 37
Pain 160
    causes of 83
    lower abdominal 8, 14
    management of 83, 158
    relief, surgical management of 85
    treatment of 85
Palmar plantar erythrodysesthesia 192
Papillary serous cyst adenocarcinoma 101
Para-aortic node 170, 171, 185
Paramedian incision 203
Partial mole 9, 10, 10*f*
    triploid chromosomal pattern of 10*f*
Pediatric human immunodeficiency virus, stages of 66
Pelvic 168
    adhesions 220
    angiography 236*f*
    endometriosis 5, 5*f*, 80, 87, 118, 220
    diagnosis of 5
    surgery for 6
    symptoms of 5
    therapy for 5
    treatment of 6
    endometriotic lesions, naked eye appearance of 5
    examination 12, 14
    floor muscle exercise 68
    infection 45, 118, 160
    inflammatory disease 83, 243
    lymph nodes 170
    lymphadenectomy 24, 197
    magnetic resonance imaging 187
    malignancy, staging of 31
    organ prolapse 220
    pain 5, 8, 11, 83, 84, 100, 104
    pathology 80*t*, 220
    ureter 39
Pelvis
    arterial supply of 50
    laparoscopic view of 119*f*
    ultrasonography of 4*f*
Percutaneous epididymal sperm aspiration 125
Peritoneal fluid cytology 185
Peritoneal oocyte and sperm transfer 127
Peritoneum 202
Pfannenstiel incision 201
Phimotic ostium 18*f*
Photophobia 243
Pictorial blood
    assessment chart 96*f*
    loss chart 62
Pinard's maneuvers 266
Pipelle endometrial sampling, limitations of 98
Pituitary tumor 115
Placenta
    accreta 33, 133
    previa 133
Placental site trophoblastic tumor 177, 179, 181, 182
Plasma 80

Platelet
    count 65
    dysfunction of 99
Pneumoperitoneum 40
Polycystic ovarian disease 267
    long-term consequences of 76
    surgical management of 227
Polycystic ovarian syndrome 3, 14, 37, 43, 73, 75, 76, 78, 96, 111, 113-115, 117, 126, 135, 189, 227
    diagnosis of 32, 73
    etiopathology of 73
    management of 4
    symptoms of 3
Polypoid mass, irregular 26
Polyps, endometrial 98
Pomeroy technique, modified 153
Pomeroy's method 33, 153, 153*f*
Positron emission tomography scan 29
Postcoital vaginal bleeding 21
Postmenopausal bleeding 9*f*, 11, 19, 26, 20*f*
    causes of 8, 11, 19
Postoperative surgical site infections 214
Postpartum hemorrhage 133
Post-testicular azoospermia 124
Post-tubal sterilization syndrome 154
Postvasectomy considerations 155
Pouch of Douglas 265
Pre-eclampsia 133
Pregnancy 242
    after endometrial ablation 211
    complications 211
    early diagnosis of 134
    ectopic 47, 133, 204
    loss 53
    recurrent 57
    luteal phase 154
    medical termination of 162, 179
    of unknown location 205
    persistent ectopic 205
    prevention of 104
    rates 131
    second trimester termination of 159
    test 65
Premature luteinisation 128
Presacral neurectomy 85
Preterm labor 133
Pretesticular azoospermia 124
Primordial follicles 109
Progesterone 61
    only pill 84
    use of 70
    receptors 104
    activation of 104
    supplementation 122
Progestins 84
    only pill 98
    replacement study 91
    therapy 189
Progestogen 91, 99
    only injectable contraceptive 150, 163
Prograsp forceps 233*f*
Prolactinomas 43
Prostate cancer 155
Psammoma bodies 52
Pseudohermaphroditism, male 44
Pseudomyxoma peritonei 53

Psoas hitch method 223
Pubertal ovary 186
Puberty 36, 109
    precocious 36, 44
Pubic hair distribution, male pattern of 75f
Pudendal nerve 40, 53
    supplies, sensory component of 40
Pyosalpinx 17

Q

qSOFA score 241

R

Radiation therapy 168, 195t, 196
Radiotherapy
    advantages of 21
    postoperative 194
    preoperative 194
Raloxifene 93
Rapamycin inhibitors, mammalian target of 191
Rectum 54
Rectus
    muscle 201
    sheath 201
Reinke's crystal 52
Renal dysfunction 98
Reoxygenation 196
Reproductive endocrinology 135
Reproductive organs, male 123
Retinoblastoma 22
Retroperitoneal lymph node sampling 185
Robertsonian translocation 58
Robotic surgery 170, 232
    advantages of 233
    complications of 233
    disadvantages of 233
    overall advantages of 234
Robotic system, third generation 233
Robotic technology 232
Rollerball endometrial ablation 210
Rosiglitazone 117
Round ligament 40, 50
Rubber ring pessary 20f
Rubella
    infection, maternal 52
    syndrome, congenital 52
Rutledge's classification 22

S

Sacral nerve stimulation 69
Saline infusion sonography 20, 63, 96
    contraindications of 96
    disadvantages of 96
Salpingectomy 205f
Salpingitis isthmica nodosa 118
Salpingo-oophorectomy 225
    bilateral 29, 172, 100, 168, 172, 189
Sarcoma botryoides 43
Sayana press 148
Scalpel method 155
Scanty pubic hair 13f
Scar endometriosis, treatment for 6
Scarpa's fascia 201

Schauta-Amreich operation 266
Schiller-Duval body 52
Sclerosis, multiple 92
Second-generation endometrial ablation methods 63, 210
Selective progesterone receptor modulators 70, 85, 104, 105
    contraindications of 105
    use of 104
Semen analysis 123
Semicircular fold of Douglas 265
Sentinel lymph node 173, 197
Sepsis 241, 243t
    management of 241
    organ site of 243t
    pathway 241
    recognition 241
    risk factors for 242
    screening tools 242
Septic shock 241
    multi-disciplinary team management of 242
    signs of 242
Sequential organ failure assessment score 241
Serous ovarian cancers, high-grade 225, 226, 226t
Sertoli cells 123
Serum anti-Müllerian hormone 116
Serum human chorionic gonadotropin, estimation of 204
Sex
    development, disorder of 49
    hormone binding globulin 44, 79
Sexual development, female 45
Sexual dysfunction, male 113
Sexually transmitted infections 113
Sheehan's syndrome 34
Shirodkar's operation 207
Shock 54
Sickle cell anemia 92
Signet ring cells 52
Sims' position 265
Sims' speculum 265
Sims' wire 265
Sinus, urogenital 38, 41
Skin
    bruising of 78
    changes 78
    closure 215
    Langer lines of 201
    preparation 214
    thinning of 78
Sleep disturbances 91
Somatotropic axis support 110
Sonography
    abdominal 101
    transvaginal 3, 96, 97fc
Sonohysterography, saline infusion 65
Sperm
    cryopreservation of 183
    recovery, methods of 125
Spermatogenesis 47
Spermicide 163
Stein-Leventhal syndrome 36, 267
Stereotactic body radiation therapy 195

Sterilization 118
    concurrent method of 154
    female 152, 153f, 162
    laparoscopic method of 153, 153f, 154
    male 152
    surgical 163
    voluntary 155
Stress urinary incontinence 42, 46, 68
    surgical procedures for 69
Struma ovarii 52
Subfertility, causes of 80, 80t
Submucous fibroids 71
Sunitinib 191
Superficial inguinal glands 40
Superovulation 81, 121
Suprapubic transverse incision 201
Surgery 120
    contraindications of 167
    gynecological laparoscopic 220, 221
    nonhysterectomy 63
    plan of 175
    types of 71
Surgical site infection 214
    classification of 215
    management of 216
    prevention of 216
    risk factors for 214t
Surrogacy 140, 141
    dilemmas of 140
    ethical issues of 140
    gestational 140
    procedure 140
    traditional 140
Syndactyly 10

T

Tamoxifen 71, 98
Taxanes 186
Tension-free vaginal tape 69
Teratospermia 124
Testicular feminization syndrome 13, 13f, 33
Testicular sperm
    aspiration 125
    extraction 125
Testicular tissue cryopreservation 183
Testis, function of 41
Testosterone, exogenous 124
Theca cell tumor 36
Thermal
    balloon ablation 210
    injury 223, 224
Thiazolidinediones 117
Thrombasthenia 99
Thrombocytopenia 60, 96, 99, 190
Thromboembolism, venous 92, 133
Thrombophilias 57, 59
    acquired 57
    diagnosis of 60
    inherited 57-59
Thrombophilic syndrome 117
Thyroid 12
    disease 92
    dysfunction 65, 96, 98, 115
    function 47, 54
    gland 266
    hormones 54
    stimulating hormone 65

Thyrotoxicosis 36
Tibolone 91
Tissue
    injuries 193
    inspection of 161
    sampling methods 65
Topoisomerase inhibitors 190
Topotecan 191, 193
Toxic shock syndrome 47
Trachelectomy, radical 26, 187
Tranexamic acid 64, 99
Transabdominal procedure 207
Transcervical sterilization 148
Transforming growth factor-beta 109, 135
Transobturator tape 69
Transureteroureterostomy 223f
Transvaginal scan 205
Transverse incision
    advantages of 203
    disadvantages of 203
Trichomonas vaginalis 245
Trophoblasts, persistent 205
Tubal dysfunction 5
Tubal ectopic pregnancy 204
    emergency laparotomy for 205f
    medical management of 204
Tubal endometriosis 118
Tubal intraepithelial carcinoma 225
Tubal occlusion 152, 154
    hysteroscopic method of 153
    long-term risk of 154
    methods of 153
    timing of 154
Tubal patency tests 113, 119
Tubal polyps 118
Tubal reconstructive surgery,
    contraindications of 38
Tubal sterilization
    failure of 154
    procedure 35, 153, 154
    reversal of 35, 119
Tubal surgery 118, 119
    advantages of 119
    disadvantages of 119
Tubectomy 163
Tubercular salpingitis 119f
Tuberculosis 12, 118
Tuberculous salpingitis 31, 118
Tubo-ovarian mass 97
Tuboperitoneal factors 113, 119f
Tumor 197
    endometrial 27f
    epithelioid trophoblastic 179
    invades cervical stroma 168
    low malignant potential 174
    marker 28
Turner's syndrome 49, 267
    characteristic features of 12
    features of 13f
Twin pregnancy 178, 179f, 180

U

Uchida technique 153
Ulipristal acetate 104
Ultrasonography 4f, 9f, 65, 83, 130, 207f, 209

Unruptured tubal ectopic pregnancy 205f
    expectant management for 205
    laparoscopy view of 204f
Ureter 33, 223
    accidental injury of 33
    delayed ischemic necrosis of 223
    reimplantation of 224f
    thermal injury of 224
Ureteric injury 34, 220, 222, 223, 223f
    identification of 223
    management of 223, 224
    sites of 222
    types of 222
Ureteric obstruction 224
Ureteric repair, surgical methods of 224
Ureteroneocystostomy 224f
    technique for 223f
Urethral competence, tests of 69
Urinary bladder 53
Urinary fistula, swab test for 46
Urinary incontinence 46, 68
    management of 69
    mixed 68
Urinary tract injury 220, 221
    causes of 221
    identification of 222
    management of 222, 223
    prevalence of 220
    prevention of 220
    types of 220
Urine
    analysis 68
    involuntary leakage of 68
Urodynamic stress incontinence 36
    sling procedure for 34
Urogenital system, embryology of 33
Uterine
    anomalies 60
    arteriovenous malformation 96
    causes of 97
    artery 24f, 50
    embolization 42, 63, 64, 71, 88, 90, 97, 235, 236, 236f
    ligation 88
    cavity 39, 97fc
    evaluation 95
    factors 14, 120
    fibroids 236f
    management of 71, 90
    treatment of 42
    fundus 205f
    perforation 211
    sarcoma 97
    synechiae 120, 140
Uterus 94f, 95f
    enlarged 96
    evacuation of 161
    leiomyoma of 105
    multiple fibroids of 100f
    septate 60f

V

Vagina 50
    agenesis of 33
    carcinoma of 47
    complete absence of 12f

Vaginal agenesis 12
    congenital 32
Vaginal bleeding 9
Vaginal cleansing 215
Vaginal cuff brachytherapy 171
Vaginal discharge, persistent offensive 21
Vaginal examination 83
Vaginal hysterectomy 170, 212
    limitations of 170
Vaginal ring 163
Vaginal trachelectomy, principal steps of 187
Vaginal vault brachytherapy 195
Vaginitis 43
Vaginosis, bacterial 43, 245
Varicocele repair 123, 124
Varicose veins 92
Vas
    deferens, congenital bilateral absence of 124
    dissection of 155f
    division of 155
    occlusion, methods of 155
Vascular endothelial growth factor 104, 191
Vasectomy 36, 124, 148, 149, 152, 155, 162
    complications of 155
    failure of 155
    methods of 155
    over tubectomy, advantages of 148
    prevalence rate of 149
    risks of 155
Vertical incision
    advantages of 201, 203
    disadvantages of 203
    limitations of 201
Vesicovaginal fistula repair 265
Vincristine 193
Virilization 78
Voice, change of 78
Vomiting 160, 190, 191
von Willebrand disease 96
Vulva, Paget's disease of 37
Vulvodynia 48

W

Weight
    disorders 115
    gain 78
    loss 117
Wertheim's operation 226
Wolffian duct 265
Wound
    classification of 216
    closure 203
    infection 243
    sites of 216
Wurm's operation 207

X

X-ray, chest 243

Z

Zinc, administration of 124
Zygote intrafallopian transfer 127